W9-ADW-329

NORMAN F. BOURKE
MEMORIAL LIBRARY
CAYUGA COMMUNITY
COLLEGE
AUBURN, NEW YORK 13021

Clinical
Musculoskeletal
Anatomy

J. B. Lippincott Company

Philadelphia

New York   Hagerstown   London

Neal E. Pratt
Ph.D., P.T.

Professor of Orthopedic Surgery and Rehabilitation,
and Anatomy
Director, Orthopedic Physical Therapy Program
Hahnemann University
Philadelphia, Pennsylvania

Clinical
Musculoskeletal
Anatomy

Acquisitions Editor: Andrew Allen
Assistant Production Manager: Lori J. Bainbridge
Production: P. M. Gordon Associates
Compositor: Compset
Printer/Binder: The Murray Printing Company

Copyright © 1991, by J. B. Lippincott Company. All rights reserved. No part of this book may be used or reproduced in any manner whatsoever without written permission except for brief quotations embodied in critical articles and reviews. Printed in the United States of America. For information write J. B. Lippincott Company, East Washington Square, Philadelphia, Pennsylvania 19105.

1   3   5   6   4   2

Figures 2–14, 2–17, 3–12, 3–25, 3–34, 4–6, 4–21, 4–22, 4–34, 4–35, and 4–36 are adapted with permission from Greenspan A: Orthopedic Radiology: A Practical Approach. New York, Gower, 1988.

Library of Congress Cataloging-in-Publication Data
Pratt, Neal E.
    Clinical musculoskeletal anatomy / Neal Pratt.
        p. cm.
    Includes bibliographical references and index.
    ISBN 0-397-54825-7
    1. Musculoskeletal system—Anatomy.   2. Nervous system—Anatomy.
  I. Title.
  QM100.P73 1990
  611'.7—dc20   90-24703
                                                             CIP

The authors and publisher have exerted every effort to ensure that drug selection and dosage set forth in this text are in accord with current recommendations and practice at the time of publication. However, in view of ongoing research, changes in government regulations, and the constant flow of information relating to drug therapy and drug reactions, the reader is urged to check the package insert for each drug for any change in indications and dosage and for added warnings and precautions. This is particularly important when the recommended agent is a new or infrequently employed drug.

To my darling Meredith, my dear wife and best friend.
She makes it all happen.

Preface

A detailed understanding of the nervous and musculoskeletal systems is of paramount importance for medical professionals involved in the treatment of neurologic and musculoskeletal dysfunction. This book focuses on these systems. This book is organized by anatomic region, and although each region is discussed as a unit, every effort is made to clarify continuities between regions. The discussion of each region includes sections on the bones, articulations, muscles, and neurovascular structures as well as surface anatomy. The latter subject is of particular importance because much of the clinical evaluation of the musculoskeletal system is noninvasive and based on physical examination. All structures are considered in a normal functional context; pathological considerations are included where appropriate.

The articulations of the spine, the limbs, and the temporomandibular joint are covered in detail. To facilitate the understanding of the functions of muscles, the joints are presented before the muscles that regulate their motions. The discussion of each articulation includes the shapes of the articular surfaces, the extent of the articular capsule, the supporting ligaments and their specific functions, the motions that occur at the joint, and the motors of the joint. Where appropriate, common injuries or pathologies also are considered.

The muscles of the limbs and body wall also are covered in detail. The muscle attachments are pictured and described in precise, simple terms. The major actions of each muscle, as well as the functional deficits that would result from loss of the muscle, also are included. In the chapter on the lower limb, the actions and deficits are described in the context of gait.

The courses of each peripheral nerve in the limbs and the cranial nerves are covered in detail. These descriptions include their relationships with other soft structures and bones, their locations relative to the surface, the muscles and cutaneous areas they supply, and the points where they are vulnerable to injury either from entrapment or from trauma. Also included are descriptions of the functional losses that would result from injury to each nerve and, where appropriate, both the static deformity and the dynamic losses along with various tests to evaluate the functions of each nerve. The last sections of the chapters on the upper and lower limbs are devoted to peripheral nerve injuries. Since the main function of the lower limb is gait, injuries to the peripheral nerves are considered in that context.

Hopefully, a major strength of this book is the selection of clinical information that is included. This clinical focus emphasizes the important and relevant anatomy and illustrates how a sound knowledge of anatomy facilitates the understanding of pathology. The clinical illustrations are of importance to medical professionals in the areas of orthopedics, neurology, and sports medicine. Additionally, and certainly of importance, most of these examples are commonly encountered clinical situations.

Neal E. Pratt, Ph.D., P.T.

Acknowledgments

I am particularly indebted to my teachers, friends, and colleagues in the Department of Anatomy of Temple University School of Medicine. They taught me the importance of presenting relevant anatomy and the joys of teaching so basic a subject. I wish to thank Mr. David Mascaro of the Graduate Program in Medical Illustration at the Medical College of Georgia for his masterful creation of the illustrations in this book. He was a joy to work with and was able to interpret my "mind's eye" better than I. Meredith Pratt was my daily inspiration and support. She was a kind editor; I benefited greatly from her teaching and professional skills as well as her knowledge of English. I think she learned more anatomy than I learned grammar. Mr. Colby Stong, of P. M. Gordon Associates, gently guided me through the morass of copy editing, galleys, pages, and the labeling of illustrations. This project would not have come to fruition were it not for Mr. Andrew Allen of the J. B. Lippincott Company. He answered every question and provided helpful guidance. He is a true professional. I sincerely thank you all.

Contents

Basic Anatomic Concepts

This introduction is included for the student beginning the study of gross anatomy. The chapter provides some general methods to study gross anatomy, gives an overview of the organization of this book, and presents important basic concepts pertaining to anatomic terminology, the supporting and contractile tissues, and the nervous system.

The Study of Gross Anatomy

There is no substitute for cadaver dissection in the study of gross anatomy. Gross anatomy is a visual science in that the better one can picture the anatomy in the mind's eye, the better the understanding one gains and the more useful the knowledge. One can read and memorize that the median nerve passes deep to the bicipital aponeurosis and then between the two heads of the pronator teres muscle. However, that information is more meaningful and useful, and easier to remember, when it is visualized and traced in the laboratory.

Although no single method of study is most efficient for everyone, there is a sequence that is usually helpful in learning gross anatomy. The structural framework for any region in the musculoskeletal system is the bones. Before studying the arm, between the shoulder and elbow, for example, one should master the osteology of the humerus and structure of the joints that it helps form. The muscles of the region can then be studied; their attachments and functions will have meaning, and their locations can be related to the bones. Finally, the courses of the nerves and vessels can be traced and related to various portions of the bones, the muscles, and other neurovascular structures. Also, surface anatomy is very important in the study of the musculoskeletal system. Some students believe it is best learned at the beginning of a region; others believe it is

1

easier to learn at the end; perhaps it should be learned throughout the study of a region.

Textbooks of anatomy are written by anatomists who use descriptive anatomic terminology. Before studying gross anatomy, one must learn this terminology. This language is not limited to anatomy but is a basic component of medical terminology. Thus, not only to understand anatomic textbooks, but also to be able to communicate with professional colleagues, one must understand the terminology.

Because gross anatomy is a visual science, one should continuously consult appropriate illustrations or pictures while reading. Most atlases of anatomy contain extensive illustrations that frequently are more comprehensive than those in textbooks. The use of an atlas while dissecting is imperative.

Traditionally, the study of human gross anatomy involves learning the structures of the human body. For the medical professional, however, this process should involve much more than simply learning to identify the various structures of the body. Of utmost importance is knowledge of the specific locations of the structures, their functions, their relationships to neighboring structures, their locations relative to the surface (skin), and whether they can be palpated. Accurate physical examination and evaluation depend on a sound knowledge of gross anatomy.

Anatomic Terminology

The description of all anatomic locations is based on a single position, the **anatomic position,** which is the upright position with the feet together, the upper limbs at the sides and the palms facing forward. This is the reference position for all descriptions irrespective of the position of the body—standing, lying face down (**prone**), or face up (**supine**). For descriptive purposes, the body can be sectioned in various planes. A **sagittal section** cuts the body from anterior to posterior so that there are right and left portions. There is only one **midsagittal,** or **median, section** that separates the body into equal right and left halves. There are multiple sagittal or **parasagittal sections** on either side of the midline. A horizontal cut producing upper and lower portions is a **horizontal,** or **transverse, section. Coronal,** or **frontal, sections** separate the body into anterior and posterior portions. Note that each of these sections is oriented at right angles to the other two. A section not corresponding to any of these basic planes is an **oblique section** and must be named on the basis of its orientation.

The standard images produced by high-resolution imaging techniques, such as computerized axial tomography or magnetic resonance imaging, generally correspond to the three cardinal planes of the body. Each of these images is a picture of a plane of the body that includes a cut of each structure through which the slice or plane passes. Radiographs or x-rays, conversely, are not images that correspond to the planes of the body. Each radiograph is a composite image of all structures through which the x-rays pass; that is, all structures encountered by the x-rays appear superimposed on the radiograph. In an x-ray film one structure is distinguished from another on the basis of differential absorption of the x-rays. The more dense structures (bones) absorb large numbers of x-rays and appear as light images; soft tissues (muscles, fat) are less dense and appear as darker images.

Terms of Location

The location of a specific structure is usually described on the basis of its position relative to another structure or to the entire body. For this purpose there are pairs of terms that describe relative positions. **Anterior,** or **ventral,** describes location closer to the front (anterior) of any part of the body, and **posterior,** or **dorsal,** describes location closer to the back (posterior) of any part. Structures closer to the head are **superior, cranial,** or **cephalic,** while those toward the feet are **inferior,** or **caudal.** Closer to the midline is designated by **medial,** while farther from the midline is **lateral.** The limbs are considered as lateral extensions of the body; thus the thumb is lateral to the little finger. Depth relative to the surface is indicated by **superficial,** or **external,** which is nearer the surface and **deep,** or **internal.** The terms **proximal** and **distal** are used to indicate the position relative to a specified reference point, a point that is usually centrally located. Proximal is closer to that point and distal is farther away. The reference point for an extremity is its attachment to the trunk. When referring to a nerve, the reference is the central nervous system (spinal cord and brain); for vessels, the reference is the heart.

Terms of Motion

Although there are unique terms to describe the motions that occur at certain joints, general **terms of motion** describe the movements that occur at most articulations. **Flexion** occurs as the angle formed by two bones is reduced. **Extension** is the reverse of flexion; it occurs when the flexed segment moves toward the neutral position. At certain joints extension can continue beyond the neutral position; when it does, it is called **hyperextension.** Movement of a segment toward the midline is **adduction;** movement away from the midline is **abduction.** Movement of a segment around its fixed end is **circumduction** and is really a sequence of movements: flexion, abduction, extension, and adduction. Certain bones or groups of bones can rotate around their long axes. This motion, **rotation,** can occur both **medially,** or **internally,** and **laterally,** or **externally.**

Connective Tissues

The connective tissues are the supportive tissues of the body. They provide the basic framework or base of the body and absorb most of the mechanical forces to which the body is subjected. Like all other tissues, the connective tissues are composed of both cells and intercellular material. Unlike other tissues, however, the connective tissues have large amounts of intercellular material that determine the physical properties of the tissue. The intercellular material consists of various fiber types, mostly collagen, embedded in an amorphous ground substance. The fibers resist tensile stresses, and their orientation determines the directions in which the stress is best resisted. The ground substance absorbs and resists compressive forces.

The connective tissues can be separated into *connective tissue proper, cartilage,* and *bone.* **Connective tissue proper** consists of **loose** and **dense connective tissue**; dense connective tissue is either regularly or irregularly arranged.

Loose Connective Tissue

The majority of loose connective tissue is **fascia.** Its minimal mechanical role is reflected in its composition: a small number of randomly oriented fibers are embedded within a watery ground substance. This abundant material separates and surrounds structures, serves as packing, and facilitates movement between adjacent structures. It also plays a major role in inflammation and repair because it is vascular and contains cells vital to the repair process. Fascia is present throughout the body. The single layer of **superficial fascia** (subcutaneous tissue) is just deep to the skin and continuous throughout the body. In any area, but characteristically in certain ones, like the abdominal wall, it can accumulate large numbers of fat cells (**adipose tissue**). All layers of fascia deep to the subcutaneous tissue are **deep fascia.** Adjacent layers of fascia are interconnected by varying numbers of fibers, and the amount of movement between layers is proportional to the number of fibers. The planes between adjacent layers, **fascial planes,** are natural planes of separation that can be separated by blunt dissection or an accumulation of fluid. At certain points between fascial layers, typically between tendons, ligaments, or muscles, there are no interconnecting fibers and a small space is formed. This space, a **bursa,** contains a very small amount of fluid that facilitates the movement of the two layers. A bursa is more of a potential space than an actual space because its walls are separated by only a thin layer of fluid. Only when the bursa becomes inflamed, as in **bursitis,** does the space assume its third dimension.

Dense Connective Tissue

Dense, **irregularly arranged** connective tissue contains a large number of randomly oriented fibers that permit it to resist considerable tensile stresses in multiple directions. It is found in the dermis of the skin and in the covering of bones (**periosteum**) and cartilage (**perichondrium**).

Dense, **regularly arranged** connective tissue forms ligaments and tendons. **Ligaments** typically interconnect two bones. **Tendons** connect muscles to bones. Although there are subtle differences in the arrangement of the fibers within ligaments and tendons, their composition is very similar. Both contain large numbers of collagen fibers oriented in parallel but few cells and little ground substance. As a result of this construction, both structures can withstand large amounts of unidirectional tensile force. Ligaments function to resist forces that tend to separate their points of attachment. Tendons transmit the forces generated by the muscles to which they attach. An **aponeurosis** is a flat tendon that is usually quite broad, but its construction is the same as that of other tendons.

Cartilage

There are three types of **cartilage**: *hyaline, elastic,* and *fibrocartilage.* Since the number and variety of fibers as well as the amount of ground substance differ in the three kinds of cartilage, their physical properties differ. Still, all cartilage is stiff as well as resilient. Additionally, normal cartilage is, for the most part, avascular in that no vessels enter the tissue.

Hyaline cartilage is the most prevalent cartilage in the body, covering the articular surfaces involved in the formation of most synovial joints. Therefore, the term **articular cartilage** is usually synonymous with the hyaline cartilage of joints. This type of cartilage also forms the costal cartilages, most of the fetal skeleton, the cartilages of the bronchi, and certain cartilages of the larynx. The major mechanical demands placed on this type of cartilage are compression forces across joints as well as the shear forces that accompany motion. These demands are met by both the ground substance and the fibers. The ground substance contains a large amount of proteoglycan that provides the stiffness and thus the resistance to compression. The fibers, mostly collagen, are arranged parallel to normal directions of shear, thus reinforcing the ground substance against such forces.

Fibrocartilage contains large bundles of collagen fibers and relatively little ground substance. Its major physical property is its ability to withstand large tensile forces; however, it can absorb compression as well. This type of cartilage is found in intervertebral disks, symphyses, and intra-articular disks.

Elastic cartilage has a large number of elastic fibers so it is quite flexible but resilient and thus can maintain its form after considerable deformation. It is found in cartilages of the larynx, external ear, and auditory tube.

Bone

The bones of the **skeleton** are separable into two general groups. Those of the head, vertebral column, and trunk form the **axial skeleton**; those of the limbs form the **appendicular skeleton**. On the basis of its shape, each bone can be classified as **long** (femur), **short** (carpals, tarsals), **flat** (skull), or **irregular** (vertebra, os coxae). **Sesamoid bones** are generally round or oval and located within tendons. Their presence is thought to both protect the tendon and change its angle of pull.

Parts of a long bone. The central region of a **long bone** (Fig. 1-1), the **shaft,** or **diaphysis,** is a cylinder with thick walls of compact bone. The core of this cylinder, the **marrow (medullary) cavity,** is filled with blood vessels and blood-forming and/or fatty tissue. The expanded ends, or **epiphyses,** are filled with spongy bone and covered with a thin layer

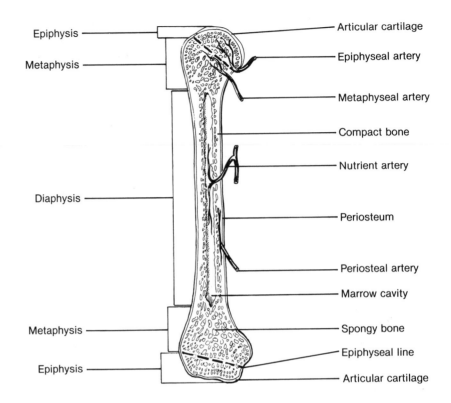

Epiphysis — Articular cartilage

Metaphysis — Epiphyseal artery

— Metaphyseal artery

— Compact bone

— Nutrient artery

Diaphysis — Periosteum

— Periosteal artery

— Marrow cavity

Metaphysis — Spongy bone

Epiphysis — Epiphyseal line

— Articular cartilage

Figure 1-1
Longitudinal section through a long bone. The regions of the bone, the major arterial supply, and the portions of the bone formed by spongy and compact bone are indicated.

of compact bone. In adult bone the thin **epiphyseal line** indicates the junction between the epiphysis and diaphysis and marks the position of the **epiphyseal disk** or **plate.** In a growing bone the epiphyseal disk is the point at which the bone grows in length. Fracture or dislocation of the epiphyseal plate (slipped epiphysis) can result in retarded longitudinal growth of the bone. The tapering region between the epiphyseal line and the main portion of the shaft is the **metaphysis.** This area is largely spongy bone and very vascular, and thus the portion of a bone in which an infection commonly settles. The **articular surfaces** (those areas participating in the formation of joints), cover either all or some portion of the epiphyses. Except for the articular surfaces, the entire bone is covered by the **periosteum,** which consists of an outer, **fibrous layer** and an inner, **osteogenic layer** (which plays an important role in fracture repair).

Composition of bone. The composition of bone is different from that of the other connective tissues because its matrix contains an inorganic component. This inorganic substance makes bone considerably more rigid than cartilage and enables it to withstand considerable compressive force. At the same time, the presence of collagen fibers renders bone flexible. The flexibility of a given bone or a portion of a bone is also dependent on the gross organization of the bone tissue. Although the basic composition of all bone is similar, it is arranged grossly into *compact* (dense, cortical) or *spongy* (cancellous, trabecular) types. **Compact bone** is tightly packed and forms the shell of all bones. **Spongy bone** is composed of trabeculae, or thin columns of bone, and is found predominantly in the ends of long bones and throughout irregularly shaped bones. Spongy bone is considerably more flexible than compact bone. In those parts of a bone that contain large amounts of spongy bone, that is, the ends of long bones or entire short bones, the compact shell covering the spongy bone is quite thin (Fig. 1-1). This combination of a thin shell and underlying spongy bone forms a resilient unit that both absorbs and cushions the force across joints. The larger sizes of the epiphyses and articular surfaces (as compared with the shafts) also serve to disperse the forces (per unit area) across joints. In addition, the resiliency of the epiphysis and the enlarged articular surface combine to protect the articular cartilage.

The orientation of the components of both spongy and compact bone reflects the stresses to which a bone is exposed. Because bone is a dynamic tissue and undergoing constant remodeling, it can adapt to either increases or decreases in force or even to changes in the directions of the forces. Such changes can occur with fracture, loss or gain of weight, or muscle paralysis and are reflected in the internal organization of the bone. However, both the overall shape and mass of a bone remain quite constant.

Blood supply of bones.   The blood supply to bones is provided by **nutrient, epiphyseal, metaphyseal,** and **periosteal arteries** (Fig. 1-1). Most of these arteries pass directly into the central portions of the bone, then branch and supply the compact bone from the inside out. Even though the periosteal vessels form anastomoses with the other vessels, they supply only the periosteum and most superficial layers of the compact bone. In long bones the nutrient arteries provide the majority of the blood supply. In bones of other shapes the amount of blood provided by each artery varies with the shape of the bone.

Nerve supply of bones.   The nerve supply to bones consists mainly of autonomic and pain fibers. The autonomic fibers enter the bone with the arteries and supply those vessels. The periosteum is richly supplied with pain fibers as evidenced by the pain that accompanies a fracture, bone bruise, or tumor that involves the periosteum. Pain fibers also enter the bone with the vessels. These fibers presumably mediate some of the pain of fracture as well as the pain associated with a bone marrow biopsy.

Articulations

The **articulations** of the body, commonly known as **joints,** can be classified in a variety of ways, and thus the terminology that describes them can be confusing and cumbersome. However, most anatomists agree that there are three basic types: *fibrous, cartilaginous,* and *synovial.* Understandably, the joints in each group have similar anatomic and functional characteristics.

Fibrous Joints

The bones forming a **fibrous joint** (synarthroses) (Fig. 1-2C) are united by dense fibrous tissue and represented predominantly by the **sutures** of

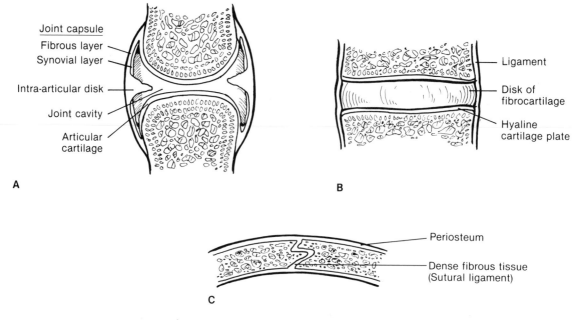

Figure 1-2
Sections through a synovial joint (*A*), a cartilaginous joint (*B*), and a fibrous joint (*C*). The basic anatomic features of each are indicated.

the skull. Although the contours of the articular surfaces that form these joints are highly irregular, the surfaces forming any specific suture match and, in fact, frequently interlock. The fibrous tissue connecting the bones is very taut and virtually fills the gap between bones. At birth the bones forming a suture are separated by several millimeters resulting in a small amount of movement between bones. As growth proceeds, the width of the space is continuously reduced. When skeletal growth is complete, the sutural spaces are very narrow; and as a result, there is virtually no motion permitted between bones. Fusion of the bones across the suture lines begins early in the third decade of life and continues thereafter. In the elderly most suture lines typically are obliterated.

Cartilaginous Joints

Cartilaginous joints (amphiarthroses) (Fig. 1-2B) are characterized by the presence of fibrocartilaginous disks between the articular surfaces and are represented by intervertebral disks and the symphysis pubis. The articular surfaces are flat and separated from the articular disks by hyaline cartilage plates. The major support of these joints is provided by strong ligaments that surround and are continuous with the disk, and interconnect the two bones. Even though these ligaments are taut, the separation of the flat bony surfaces by the disk permits a small amount of rocking or sliding motion between the bones.

Synovial Joints

Most articulations of the body are classified as **synovial joints** (diar-throses) (Fig. 1-2A). Even though they share a number of general struc-tural characteristics and permit considerable motion, there is considerable individual variation. As a result the stability and the freedom of motion varies. The motion that occurs at these joints allows the body to assume a seemingly unlimited number of positions and perform a variety of tasks. Conversely, this same motion makes these articulations vulnerable to de-generation and a myriad of mechanical dysfunctions. In addition, certain metabolic diseases, such as rheumatoid arthritis, attack these joints with gusto. Obviously, loss of motion and pain due to pathology involving these joints can affect one's ability to perform even the simplest activities of daily living.

Certain characteristics are common to all synovial joints. The **artic-ular surfaces** of the bones that form these joints are covered with **artic-ular cartilage** (hyaline cartilage). This cartilage is not covered with peri-chondrium other than at its periphery where it is continuous with the periosteum of the bone. The articular surfaces are enclosed by a **joint capsule** that forms a closed **joint (synovial) cavity** or space. The joint capsule both reinforces the joint and elaborates the synovial fluid that lubricates the articular cartilage, thereby greatly reducing the friction be-tween the surfaces. The capsule is composed of two layers: the fibrous and the synovial layers. The outer, **fibrous layer** typically attaches to the bones at the edges of the articular surfaces where it blends with the peri-osteum. This layer is formed by fibrous tissue and is the supportive layer of the capsule. Typically, it is reinforced by strong fibrous bands or liga-ments that blend with it and appear as thickenings of the fibrous layer. Other supporting ligaments of the joint do not blend with the capsule and consequently are separated from the capsule. In either case, whether the ligament blends with the capsule or is separate, it is called an **extra-capsular ligament.** The deeper, **synovial layer (synovium)** of the capsule lines the deep surface of the fibrous capsule and attaches to the bones at the edges of the articular surfaces; consequently it does not cover the articular surfaces. The synovium is very vascular and consists of an inner cellular layer that rests on an outer supporting layer of loose connective tissue. Generally, the synovial and fibrous portions of the capsule are coextensive. However, in certain instances, such as the knee, there are areas within the fibrous capsule that are not part of the synovial cavity and do not contain synovial fluid. **Synovial fluid** is a plasma dialysate containing essential lubricating agents (hyaluronic acid and glycoprotein) that are added by the surface cells of the synovium. In normal circum-stances the amount of synovial fluid is small and covers the articular sur-faces but does not interfere with motion. Injury or irritation of the syn-ovium can cause oversecretion of fluid and create an excessive amount in the joint space (effusion). This excess of synovial fluid can cause a reduc-tion of range of motion of the joint as well as considerable pain.

Certain other features of synovial joints are found in only a few joints. **Intra-articular disks,** or **menisci** (Fig. 1-2A), such as the menisci of the knee, are fibrocartilaginous structures that partially or completely separate the articular surfaces. These disks usually fill areas between poorly matching surfaces and thus improve the congruency between the surfaces. They are not covered by synovial membrane. Other joints contain **intra-articular,** or **intracapsular, ligaments**; an example is the cruciate ligaments of the knee. These ligaments are supporting ligaments but are found between the synovial and fibrous layers of the capsule, so they are not bathed by synovial fluid. A few tendons also pass through synovial joints, such as the tendon of the long head of the biceps brachii muscle. Although these tendons actually pass through the joint space, they are ensheathed by a sleeve of synovium so they also are not bathed in synovial fluid.

The directions in which motions occur and the amount of motion that occurs at synovial joints are dependent on several anatomic features. In most cases a number of structural features complement one another and thus limit or permit the same motions. The shapes of the articular surfaces and how well they fit together, as well as the locations and tautness of the ligaments and capsule, are the primary factors. For example, the ball-and-socket construction of both the shoulder and hip joints affords them virtually unlimited directions of motions. However, the congruency of the articular surfaces and the tightness of the capsule and ligaments is quite different between the two joints. The shapes of the two articular surfaces forming the shoulder joint are very different and the capsule is very loose, resulting in poor stability and very free motion. Conversely, the two articular surfaces forming the hip joint match quite well, and fit together tightly. The capsule and ligaments of the hip are taut, resulting in a stable joint, but one that permits limited motion. The muscles crossing a joint also affect motion. Obviously, the position of a muscle or its tendon determines the direction(s) in which a muscle can produce motion. The location of a muscle's attachment (near or far from the axis of motion) and the muscle's contraction range (how much it can shorten) affect the amount of motion a muscle can produce. The closer a muscle attaches to an axis of motion, the greater the range of motion it can produce. Conversely, attachment away from the axis reduces the range of motion but increases the force a muscle can generate because the longer lever arm increases the mechanical advantage. Also, the bulk of muscles and other soft tissues can affect motion; an excess can limit motion because of apposition of the segments on either side of the joint.

Muscle

There are three types of **muscle tissue** within the body: *smooth, cardiac,* and *skeletal.* **Smooth muscle** is regulated by the autonomic nervous system and found predominantly in blood vessels, the gastrointestinal tract, and in the skin, where it is associated with hair. **Cardiac muscle,** regulated by the autonomic nervous system, forms the muscular walls of the heart.

Skeletal muscle, as its name implies, forms all the skeletal muscles of the body—the muscles of the back and limbs, body wall, head, larynx and upper part of the pharynx, along with the respiratory and pelvic diaphragms. Skeletal muscle is innervated by the general somatic efferent fibers that are distributed in the spinal and several cranial nerves, and the general visceral efferent fibers in certain cranial nerves.

Function of Skeletal Muscle

The **attachments** of a skeletal muscle are its *origin* and *insertion.* Anatomically, the **origin** is the more proximal attachment, the one closer to the central portion of the body; the **insertion** is the more distal attachment. Functionally, the origin is usually the more fixed or stationary attachment and the insertion is movable. However, when a muscle contracts, it pulls equally on both attachments and the attachment that moves is simply a function of which one is the more movable. The upper limb muscles usually function to position the hand, so the origin is relatively fixed and the insertion moves. When one drinks a glass of water, the biceps brachii flexes the forearm to move the glass toward the mouth (insertion moves toward origin). However, if the hand is stationary, as in performing a pull-up, the entire body moves (origin moves toward insertion). In walking or climbing stairs, the origin usually moves and the insertion is more fixed because the foot is on the ground. In this instance, contraction of a muscle results in movement of the origin rather than the insertion.

Contraction of a muscle, by strict definition, means shortening of that muscle. The term "shortening contraction" seems redundant, but it is an important concept. A muscle can contract **isotonically,** or **concentrically** (it shortens), **isometrically** (it does not change length), or **eccentrically** (it lengthens). Motion can be produced either by muscle activity or by gravity, but it can be *controlled or regulated* only by muscle activity. As one raises a glass, the biceps brachii shortens by contracting concentrically. If the glass is held in a static position, the biceps maintains that position by contracting isometrically. When the glass is lowered toward a table, the primary force is gravity, but the biceps is regulating the motion by counteracting gravity and making the motion smooth; the biceps is contracting eccentrically.

Although muscles function synchronously as they produce motion, each plays a specific role in generating the motion. The **prime mover(s),** or **agonist(s),** performs the primary motion. Those muscles that produce the opposite motions, and are centrally inhibited when the agonists are active, are the **antagonists.** Muscles that assist the primary motion in some way are **synergists.** These muscles neutralize unwanted secondary motions of the prime movers or stabilize more proximal joints.

Construction of Skeletal Muscle

Muscle construction, the way in which the component muscle fibers (cells) are arranged within a muscle, varies considerably. The type of construction determines both the contraction range, or how far a muscle can shorten, and the relative strength of a muscle. Also, the size of a muscle is related directly to its strength. The strength of a muscle is a function of the total cross-sectional area of its fibers. The shortening length of a muscle also is a function of the individual fibers; each fiber can shorten approximately 40 to 50 percent of its length. In a **parallel, or fusiform, muscle** (Fig. 1-3A) the fibers are parallel to one another and parallel to the long axis of the muscle and its tendons; the fibers are parallel to the line of action of the muscle. This type of muscle can shorten maximally, and its strength is based on the cross-sectional area of the entire muscle (which is equal to the total cross-sectional area of its component fibers). In **pennate muscles** (Fig. 1-3B–D) the fibers are oriented obliquely to the tendons. Even though such muscles differ, having either a **unipennate** or a **multipennate** arrangement, the basic principles of contraction are the same. The individual fibers shorten the same amount as those in a parallel muscle. However, since the fibers are oriented obliquely relative to the line of action of the muscle, the distance each shortens is not reflected in equivalent shortening of the entire muscle; a pennate muscle, therefore, can shorten proportionally less than a parallel muscle. Relative to strength, the total cross-sectional area of the pennate muscle is less than the total cross-sectional area of its component fibers, thus resulting in a proportionally stronger muscle. Given muscles of exactly the same gross dimensions, the parallel muscle can shorten a greater percentage of its length and thus produce a greater range of motion; the pennate muscle produces a smaller range of motion but is capable of generating greater force.

The **sizes of muscle attachments** differ. Some muscles attach to a single point via a cordlike tendon; some attach to large areas; and some have linear attachments that may extend along a considerable portion of one or more bones. Although the motion permitted at a given joint is a factor in determining the motion a muscle can produce, so also is the size of the muscle's attachment. The force of a muscle with a small area of attachment tends to be directed toward a single motion. A muscle with a linear area of attachment may be able to generate several motions because its fibers cross several sides of an articulation; in fact, such a muscle may function as several independent muscles.

Figure 1-3
The arrangement of muscle fibers within parallel or fusiform (*A*) and pennate (*B, C, D*) muscles.

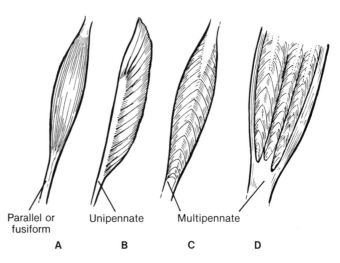

Parallel or fusiform

Unipennate

Multipennate

A   B   C   D

When one studies a muscle in the laboratory, all of the factors discussed above should be considered. The muscle attachments are important because a muscle can function only along a line or lines that connect those points. By combining the knowledge of what motions are available at a joint with the lines of muscular activity, one can determine a muscle's potential actions. The distance of an attachment from an axis of motion (length of the lever arm) provides an indication of both the range of motion and force a muscle can generate. The type of construction adds additional information regarding strength and range of motion. Finally, a muscle's peripheral nerve supply can be determined by tracing the branches of nearby nerves.

Nervous System

Anatomically, the **nervous system** is composed of two portions. The **central nervous system (CNS)** consists of the brain, which is encased within the cranial cavity, and the spinal cord, which occupies the vertebral canal. The **peripheral nervous system (PNS)** includes both the spinal and cranial nerves, which are found predominantly outside of the cranial cavity and spinal canal. Together, the spinal and cranial nerves are the means by which both the signals *from* the central nervous system are transmitted to peripheral effectors and sensory information is transmitted *to* the brain and spinal cord from peripheral receptors. The **autonomic nervous system (ANS)** is a functional division of the nervous system that regulates the visceral structures of the body.

Neuron Versus Nerve

Neuron. The basic anatomic and functional unit of the nervous system is the **neuron,** or **nerve cell.** Although there are supporting cells associated with the neurons of both the CNS and PNS, only the neurons are capable of the unique function of the nervous system: transmitting information from one point to another via conduction. Each neuron is composed of a **cell body** and **cell processes.** The cell body is the metabolic center of the cell and the cell processes, the **axons** and **dendrites,** are the conducting elements. Generally, a neuron has multiple dendrites that conduct toward the cell body and a single axon that conducts away from the cell body.

A **nerve fiber** is an axon (or axonlike dendrite) plus its supporting cells. A grouping of nerve cell bodies within the CNS is referred to as a **nucleus**; in the PNS, a similar grouping is a **ganglion.** A **synapse** is the junctional region between two neurons where impulses pass from one neuron to another. In the PNS synapses commonly occur in ganglia.

Nerve. A **nerve** consists of a large number of nerve fibers that are ensheathed in a connective tissue covering. Within a nerve the fibers are grouped into bundles, or funiculi, and both the individual fibers and the funiculi are surrounded and separated by connective tissue. These connective tissue layers are the delicate **endoneurium** around each fiber, the heavier **perineurium** around each funiculus, and the robust **epineurium** surrounding the entire nerve. This connective tissue is important because it both protects and contains the vessels that nourish the nerve and also plays a role in nerve regeneration as well as nerve entrapment.

Functional Components

Every neuron, whether in the CNS or PNS, has a single specific function. Those forming the nerves of the PNS are grouped into seven categories called the **functional components.** Four are found in all spinal nerves and certain cranial nerves; the other three are limited to the cranial nerves. Each of the functional components is named on the basis of three characteristics. First, *general* or *special* refers to the areas of the body supplied; those neurons designated as **general** supply all parts, while **special** neurons are limited to the head and neck. Second, *somatic* or *visceral* refers to the specific areas and structures innervated. **Somatic** neurons supply the body wall and limbs, specifically skeletal muscle, tendons, ligaments, joint capsules, and skin. **Visceral** neurons are associated with visceral areas (organs of the thorax, abdomen, pelvis, and perineum)—specifically, both smooth muscle and cardiac muscle and the glands. The major exceptions to this generality are the visceral structures found in the body wall and limbs (smooth muscle in blood vessels and associated with hair, and glands), which are supplied by visceral neurons. The third designation is the direction of conduction. **Efferent** (motor) fibers conduct away from the CNS; **afferent** (sensory) fibers conduct toward the CNS.

There are four functional components in spinal nerves (Fig. 1-4) and in some cranial nerves.

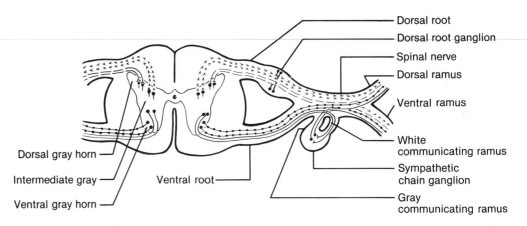

Figure 1-4

Cross section of the spinal cord showing the formation and major branches of a spinal nerve and the courses of the nerve fibers of the four basic functional components of neurons. The general somatic efferent neurons are indicated by *dotted solid lines*; the general somatic afferent neurons, by *broken* lines; the general visceral efferent neurons, by *solid lines*; and the general visceral afferent neurons by *arrowheads*.

General somatic efferent (GSE). These neurons supply the skeletal muscles that develop from somites. Their cell bodies are located within the ventral gray horn of the spinal cord, and their axons pass through the ventral root, spinal nerve, and the dorsal and ventral rami and their branches.

General somatic afferent (GSA). These neurons are associated with both the superficial (**exteroceptor**) and deep (**proprioceptor**) somatic receptors found in the body wall, limbs, head, and neck. The superficial receptors are located in the skin and are associated with sensations such as touch, temperature, and two-point discrimination. The deep receptors are in muscles, tendons, ligaments, and joint capsules; these receptors convey information regarding joint position, muscle length, and so forth. Receptors associated with somatic pain, **nociceptors,** are found both in the skin and deeper structures. The cell bodies of GSA neurons are located in the dorsal root ganglia and certain cranial nerve ganglia. At spinal levels their cell processes pass through the dorsal and ventral rami, spinal nerve, and dorsal root.

General visceral efferent (GVE). These neurons are the **sympathetic** and **parasympathetic** neurons of the ANS. They supply smooth and cardiac muscle along with glands. Their locations are described in the section on the ANS.

General visceral afferent (GVA). These neurons transmit sensory information (**interoception**) from those structures supplied by the GVE neurons. The locations of their cell bodies and proximal courses of their cell processes are similar to those of the GSA neurons. Further information on their pathways is presented in the ANS section.

There are three functional components limited to the cranial nerves:

Special visceral efferent (SVE). These neurons supply the skeletal muscles of the head and neck that develop from branchial arches (as opposed to somites). This designation is based on embryological origin rather than function, so there is no difference between the structure of these muscles and those of the back and limbs.

Special visceral afferent (SVA). These fibers transmit the sensory information associated with taste and smell.

Special somatic afferent (SSA). These fibers mediate the sensations of vision, hearing, and equilibrium (proprioceptive information from a special sense organ in the internal ear).

Spinal Nerve

A **spinal nerve** contains the nerve fibers that are associated with one-half of a single spinal cord segment and that supply a specific segment or portion of the body wall and/or limbs. Each nerve (see Fig. 1-4) is formed by the union of the **dorsal** and **ventral roots,** each of which is formed from multiple rootlets. The spinal nerve branches into the larger **ventral** and smaller **dorsal ramus.** Branches of the dorsal rami are distributed to the vertebral column, deep muscles of the back, and the skin of the medial two-thirds of the back. The distribution of the branches of the ventral rami varies with their locations. Those between the T2 and T11 spinal cord levels become the intercostal nerves that supply the body wall. Those above T2 and below T11 form the somatic plexuses (cervical, brachial, lumbosacral) that supply the limbs and neck.

A **somatic plexus** is a network of nerve bundles that undergoes multiple branchings and fusions. All plexuses are derived from the ventral rami of multiple spinal cord segments and give rise to multiple terminal or peripheral nerves. In the course of the formation of the terminal nerves, the fibers from a single spinal cord segment are distributed to multiple terminal nerves. And, each terminal nerve contains fibers from more than one spinal cord segment. These principles are important in understanding the motor and sensory symptoms that result from injuries involving the rami (or spinal nerves), the plexus itself, or the terminal nerves. Since a peripheral nerve provides the total innervation to the structures it supplies, injury of such a nerve results in complete and circumscribed paralysis and loss of sensation. This is a postplexus injury. Conversely, injury of a single spinal nerve (preplexus injury) produces more widespread symptomology, but the symptoms are less severe and segmental in distribution—muscle weakness and segmental loss of sensation. Although fibers from a single spinal nerve are found in multiple peripheral nerves, they comprise only a portion of the fibers within each nerve; loss of an entire spinal nerve causes loss of only portions of several terminal nerves. Therefore, the muscles supplied by these peripheral nerves are only partially denervated and thereby weakened, and the cutaneous loss is dermatomal. Injury of a plexus or component of a plexus (a trunk or cord) could appear as loss of two segments or two terminal nerves or a variety of other combinations.

Autonomic Nervous System

Strictly defined, the **autonomic nervous system (ANS),** or the visceral motor system, is a purely efferent system of neurons that begins in the CNS and supplies smooth and cardiac muscle and glands throughout the body. It regulates blood vessels, the gastrointestinal tract, the heart, and the lungs, along with a variety of other visceral functions. It is important to understand, however, that no part of the nervous system is autonomous and functions in a vacuum. Intimately involved in the functions of the ANS are areas in the CNS, and the GVA neurons that convey sensory information from the visceral structures to the CNS.

The ANS is composed of two portions, the **sympathetic (thoracolumbar)** and the **parasympathetic (craniosacral)** divisions, Each of these divisions is composed of two-neuron chains that extend from the CNS to the target organ or effector. The cell bodies of the **preganglionic neurons** are located in the brain stem or spinal cord, and their axons extend to ganglia outside the CNS. In these ganglia the preganglionic neurons synapse with **postganglionic neurons,** and their axons project to the target organs. The cell bodies of the preganglionic sympathetic neurons are found in the thoracic and upper lumbar levels of the spinal cord, hence, the name "thoracolumbar." The cell bodies of the preganglionic parasympathetic neurons are located both in the brain stem and spinal cord segments S2 through S4 (craniosacral).

Sympathetic versus parasympathetic divisions. Although the two divisions are similar in their general organization, they differ in several ways. The sympathetic ganglia (where the pre- and postganglionic neurons synapse) are quite near the CNS; the parasympathetic ganglia are more peripherally located, either very near or within the target organ. Anatomically, the preganglionic parasympathetic fibers are relatively long and the postganglionic fibers short, whereas the relative lengths of the sympathetic fibers are reversed. Because of this arrangement the parasympathetic fibers are more focused on specific organs while the sympathetic fibers are more widely distributed. Functionally, both divisions are important in the maintenance of the internal environment of the body. However, the parasympathetic division controls the basic visceral functions, such as peristalsis, while the sympathetic division provides overall protection in an emergency. For example, when a rapid physical response is needed, the sympathetic system effects a swift increase of the blood supply to the skeletal muscles. The chemical transmitters between the postganglionic neurons and the end organs also differ. Norepinephrine is the transmitter in the sympathetic division; adrenergic drugs can cause sympathetic responses. The parasympathetic transmitter is acetylcholine so cholinergic drugs can induce parasympathetic responses.

Also of importance in understanding the function of the two divisions of the ANS is their actions relative to each other. In some instances their actions are antagonistic. For example, sympathetic activity increases the heart rate, whereas parasympathetic activity reduces it. On the other hand, some structures are affected by only one division. A given response is regulated by more or less sympathetic or parasympathetic influence. For example, the smooth muscle in the arteries of the limbs and body wall is supplied only by sympathetic fibers. Vasoconstriction of these vessels is a sympathetic response; vasodilation occurs when there is "less" sympathetic activity.

Sympathetic system. The distribution of the sympathetic fibers (Fig. 1-5) is a bit confusing and rather circuitous. The cell bodies of the preganglionic sympathetic fibers are located in the lateral part of the intermediate gray of all thoracic and the upper two lumbar spinal cord segments. The axons of these cells pass through the ventral root into the spinal nerve and then into the **sympathetic trunk,** or **chain of ganglia,** via the **white communicating rami.** This sympathetic chain is a string of interconnected ganglia that extends from the base of the skull to the coccyx, and is positioned on the lateral aspects of the vertebral bodies. In the cervical region there are usually only three ganglia, but at other levels there is typically a ganglion associated with each spinal nerve. Once a preganglionic fiber has entered the sympathetic trunk, it traverses one of the following courses:

It synapses with a postganglionic neuron at the level it entered the trunk.

It ascends to a more superior ganglion and synapses with a postganglionic neuron.

It descends to a more inferior ganglion and synapses with a postganglionic neuron; or

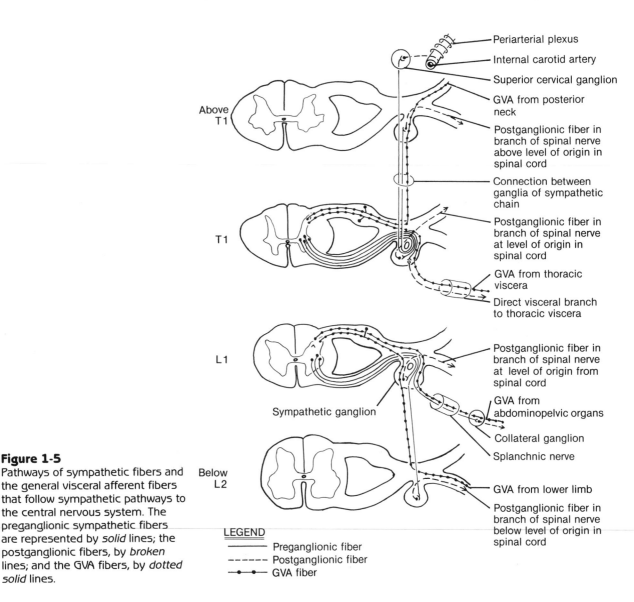

Periarterial plexus

Internal carotid artery

Superior cervical ganglion

GVA from posterior neck

Postganglionic fiber in branch of spinal nerve above level of origin in spinal cord

Connection between ganglia of sympathetic chain

Postganglionic fiber in branch of spinal nerve at level of origin in spinal cord

GVA from thoracic viscera

Direct visceral branch to thoracic viscera

Postganglionic fiber in branch of spinal nerve at level of origin from spinal cord

GVA from abdominopelvic organs

Collateral ganglion

Splanchnic nerve

GVA from lower limb

Postganglionic fiber in branch of spinal nerve below level of origin in spinal cord

Above T1

T1

L1

Sympathetic ganglion

Below L2

LEGEND
——————— Preganglionic fiber
– – – – – Postganglionic fiber
—•—•— GVA fiber

Figure 1-5
Pathways of sympathetic fibers and the general visceral afferent fibers that follow sympathetic pathways to the central nervous system. The preganglionic sympathetic fibers are represented by *solid* lines; the postganglionic fibers, by *broken* lines; and the GVA fibers, by *dotted solid* lines.

It exits from the trunk within a **splanchnic nerve.** This type of nerve contains preganglionic fibers that terminate in **collateral ganglion** located in the abdominal cavity.

Synapses between pre- and postganglionic sympathetic neurons occur in all ganglia of the chain and hence at all levels of the vertebral column. Postganglionic fibers pass from the ganglia into the nearest spinal nerve via the **gray communicating rami,** and then are distributed to all parts of the body wall and limbs through branches of the spinal nerves. The sympathetic trunk is the means by which sympathetic fibers, from the limited thoracolumbar origin, are spread to all levels of the vertebral column and thus to all spinal nerves. The ganglia associated with spinal nerves T1 through L2 are connected to the spinal nerve by both gray and white communicating rami; those above T1 and below L2 are connected by only a gray communicating ramus.

Sympathetics to the head and neck begin in the upper few segments of the thoracic spinal cord, enter the sympathetic trunk, and ascend to the cervical ganglia of the trunk. From these ganglia, principally the superior ganglion, postganglionic fibers enter periarterial plexuses around the carotid arteries and are distributed with the branches of these arteries. Postganglionic fibers also are distributed by cranial nerves and cervical spinal nerves, which acquire sympathetic fibers as they pass either branches of the carotid arteries or cervical ganglia.

Sympathetic fibers to the organs of the thoracic cavity are distributed by visceral plexuses associated with the major organs—the cardiac and pulmonary plexuses. Postganglionic fibers from the sympathetic trunk pass through **direct visceral branches** to the visceral plexuses.

Sympathetic fibers to the organs of the abdomen and pelvis are distributed through a large autonomic plexus. In the abdomen this plexus is associated with the aorta and called the aortic or preaortic plexus. The aortic plexus continues into the pelvis as the pelvic plexus. Preganglionic fibers pass from the sympathetic trunk to **collateral,** or **aortic, ganglia** via **splanchnic nerves.** These ganglia are located within the aortic plexus and named *celiac, superior mesenteric,* and so on, according to the branches of the aorta with which they are associated. The pre- and postganglionic neurons synapse in these ganglia and then the postganglionic fibers are distributed to the organs via the periarterial plexuses, which also are named for their arteries.

Parasympathetic system. The distribution of the parasympathetic fibers is rather direct and focused. The axons of the preganglionic neurons in the brain stem, the cranial portion of the parasympathetics, pass through cranial nerves III (oculomotor), VII (facial), IX (glossopharyngeal), and X (vagus). The synapses between pre- and postganglionic neurons occur in four parasympathetic ganglia in the head, and very near or within the target organs of the thorax and abdominopelvic cavities.

The sacral parasympathetic fibers are distributed to the lower portion of the gastrointestinal tract and other structures within the pelvis and perineum. The cell bodies of the preganglionic neurons are located in the lateral portion of the intermediate gray of sacral spinal cord segments 2, 3, and 4. Their axons pass through the ventral roots and spinal nerves, and then continue directly to the organs they supply where they synapse with short postganglionic neurons. Note that although the sacral parasympathetic fibers pass through the sacral spinal nerves, they are not distributed with the branches of these spinal nerves.

General visceral afferent nerves. The general visceral afferent fibers that supply the visceral structures accompany the sympathetic and parasympathetic fibers to the central nervous system. As a result, the GVA fibers are found in all spinal nerves and certain cranial nerves. The GVA fibers following the parasympathetic pathways terminate in the brain stem and the sacral portion of the spinal cord; those following sympathetic pathways terminate in the thoracic and upper lumbar portions of the spinal cord. This arrangement supplies the anatomic explanation for certain types of referred pain. For example, the pain associated with coronary artery disease is commonly felt in the medial aspect of the left arm and left pectoral region. The sympathetics that supply the heart arise in the upper thoracic spinal cord segments; the GVA fibers from the heart terminate in the same levels of the spinal cord. The pain is felt in the dermatomes supplied by the upper thoracic spinal cord segments and presumably the result of overlapping sensory neuron pools in the spinal cord.

Lesions of the autonomic nervous system.   Lesions involving components of the ANS can produce a variety of symptoms ranging from widespread trophic and constitutional disturbances to the interruption of a specific function of a single structure. In those structures that receive both sympathetic and parasympathetic innervation and their effects are opposed, loss of either results in an imbalance and the intact innervation dominates. For example, sympathetic fibers produce pupillary dilation while parasympathetics cause pupillary constriction. Loss of sympathetic innervation of the eye causes pupillary constriction; loss of parasympathetics produces pupillary dilation. Other structures receive innervation from only one component of the ANS; for example, smooth muscle in the blood vessels of the body wall and limbs is supplied only by sympathetics. Loss of this innervation results in an inability to regulate the caliber of the vessels.

Injury of a peripheral nerve includes loss of the sympathetic fibers that control the sweat glands of the skin (secretomotor fibers) and the smooth muscle of vessels (vasomotor fibers), and those supplying the hair. Loss of these fibers results in trophic changes that are apparent in the skin and nails. The skin is dry, blanched, cool, and scaly, and the nails may crack. These changes are the result of nutritional changes as well as the loss of secretion from the sweat glands. Temperature regulation is also affected, so the involved area is cool and does not adapt to changes in the external environment.

Horner's syndrome, resulting from a loss of sympathetic innervation to the eye, may involve the face as well as the eye. In addition, the interruption of the sympathetic fibers may occur at a variety of locations. The symptoms involving the eye itself are pupillary constriction (**meiosis**), a droopy eyelid (**ptosis**), and a sunken eyeball (**enophthalmus**). These symptoms occur alone if the sympathetic fibers are interrupted either within or very near the orbit. However, these same symptoms could accompany a lesion of the internal carotid artery, the superior cervical ganglion, the cervical sympathetic trunk, the upper thoracic spinal nerves, or the upper thoracic spinal cord segments. Lesions at these other locations obviously would produce additional symptoms, including trophic changes affecting the skin of the face and possibly the neck.

Loss of parasympathetic innervation usually produces changes in more specific processes or functions. Lesions involving cranial nerves III, VII, or IX affect certain glands and smooth muscles in the head. Loss of cranial nerve X affects visceral functions in the thorax and abdomen. Loss of the sacral parasympathetics affects visceral functions in the abdomen and pelvis as well as the perineum.

Back

Pathology involving the back presents a particular challenge to health professionals because the signs and symptoms resulting from dysfunction are often vague and difficult to localize, the potential causes of dysfunction are multiple and varied, and the results of intervention frequently are inconsistent. The back performs a variety of functions that require both stability and mobility, and it undergoes natural degenerative changes throughout life. Because the vertebral column is the structural base of the back, the vertebrae and their supporting tissues both absorb and resist most of the mechanical forces imparted to the back and thus are vulnerable to a variety of injuries. The vertebral column also forms the vertebral canal that houses the spinal cord and the intervertebral foramina that transmit the nerves that supply the structures of the limbs and trunk. As a result of this relationship, injury or dysfunction of the vertebral column commonly involves components of the nervous system.

Although the vertebrae of the various levels of the vertebral column are generally similar, the different levels have different mechanical functions and thus are subjected to different mechanical forces. The upper or cervical region both supports the skull and permits considerable motion so the head can be mobile. Even so, excessive motion commonly accelerates the degenerative processes, which can hasten the development of dysfunction and pain. The lower or lumbar region accommodates large mechanical stresses and allows some motion. The magnitude of these forces increases dramatically in certain postures, and, as in the cervical region, excessive use speeds degeneration. In addition, particularly in the lumbar region, the bipedal posture of man places excessive stresses on the vertebrae and their supports.

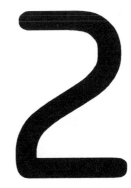

Vertebral Column

Vertebral Column as a Whole

The vertebral column, or spine, consists of a vertical stack of vertebrae that articulates with the occipital bone of the skull superiorly and the ilia of the pelvis inferiorly. The components of this column are positioned so that minimal muscular energy is needed to maintain the upright position. The column has a built-in set of spacers, the intervertebral disks, that function as shock absorbers and facilitate motion between adjacent vertebrae. The vertebral column functions to support the superincumbent weight of the head, upper limbs, and trunk; it protects the spinal cord; it provides a base of support for the head, limbs, and ribs; and it provides attachments for some of the powerful muscles of the proximal portions of the limbs.

The normal vertebral column (Fig. 2-1) has no lateral curves, but there are four anteroposterior curves. Two are present at birth and, in reality, are part of a single curve; two are acquired during growth and maturation and represent a response to man's upright posture. At birth the vertebral column exhibits a single curve, a ventral concavity, which

Figure 2-1
Anterior (*A*) and lateral (*B*) views of the entire vertebral column.

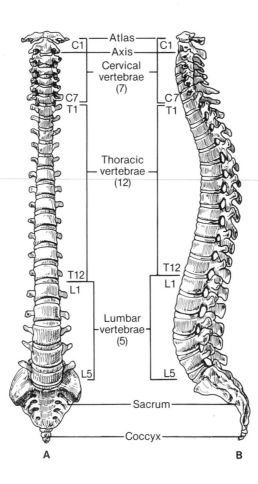

Atlas
C1
Axis
Cervical vertebrae (7)
C7
T1
Thoracic vertebrae (12)
T12
L1
Lumbar vertebrae (5)
L5
Sacrum
Coccyx

A   B

is consistent with the fetal position. Soon after birth, when the infant raises its head and looks around, the cervical portion of the curve is reversed and presents a posterior concavity. When the child sits without support, the curve in the lumbar region is reversed resulting in a posterior concavity, or **lordosis.** Each of the acquired curves—the ventral convexities in the cervical and lumbar regions—is compensatory and provides better balance of the trunk on the sacrum. Both dorsal convexities, the thoracic and sacral curves, are portions of the original single curve that was present at birth. An increased thoracic curve is known as a **kyphosis.**

Motion of the vertebral column is somewhat limited overall and represents the sum total of the motion that can occur between adjacent vertebrae. The direction of motion between any two vertebrae is determined by planes of the zygapophyseal joints; and the amount of motion is determined by the thickness of the intervertebral disk, the tightness of the ligaments and muscles interconnecting the vertebrae, and the presence of other structures, such as the rib cage. Most motion occurs in the cervical and lumbar regions, but the rib cage limits motion between thoracic vertebrae.

Typical Vertebrae

A typical vertebra (Fig. 2-2) consists of the **vertebral body** anteriorly and the **vertebral,** or **neural, arch** posteriorly. The body is cylindrical in shape, with both the side-to-side and anteroposterior diameters exceeding the height. The increasing size of the bodies from superior to inferior reflects the weight load that the vertebrae support. Each body has a collar of compact bone that surrounds a core of spongy bone, and the spongy core is separated from the intervertebral disk by a hyaline cartilage plate.

The vertebral arch consists of two **lamina** and two **pedicles,** which together with the posterior aspect of the vertebral body form the **vertebral foramen.** The contiguous vertebral foramina of all vertebrae form the vertebral canal. The pedicles project posteriorly from the posterolateral aspects of the body; the lamina extend posteromedially from the pedicles and join at the midline. The formation of this posterior arch occurs early in development, and is completed as its components meet and fuse in the midline posteriorly. Failure of this fusion produces the general group of birth anomalies referred to as **spina bifida.** Each pedicle is notched superiorly and inferiorly very close to its junction with the body; and although the depth of the notches varies, the inferior notch typically is deeper than the superior one. The superior and inferior notches of adjacent vertebrae form the respective superior and inferior boundaries of an intervertebral foramen. Typically, there are three projections from the neural arch, each of which is a lever to which muscles attach. The single **spinous process** projects posteriorly in the midline and is easily palpable at most levels of the vertebral column. The paired **transverse processes** project laterally from the junctions of the pedicles and lamina. Any of these processes, particularly the spinous processes, is subject to fracture from either violent muscle pulls or direct trauma.

Articular processes project superiorly and inferiorly from the verte-

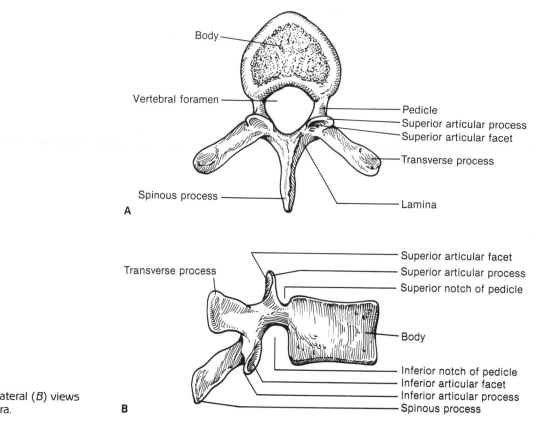

Body

Vertebral foramen

Pedicle
Superior articular process
Superior articular facet

Transverse process

Spinous process

Lamina

A

Superior articular facet
Superior articular process
Superior notch of pedicle

Transverse process

Body

Inferior notch of pedicle
Inferior articular facet
Inferior articular process
Spinous process

B

Figure 2-2
Superior (A) and lateral (B) views
of a typical vertebra.

bral arch at approximately the junction of the lamina and pedicles. There are four processes in all, two superior and two inferior. Each process bears an articular surface, or facet, and the facets of the superior and inferior processes of adjacent vertebrae articulate to form the **zygapophyseal joints.** Since the two inferior articular facets of one vertebra articulate with the superior facets of the vertebra below, there are two zygapophyseal joints between each pair of vertebrae.

Cervical Vertebrae

The bodies of the cervical vertebrae (Fig. 2-3) are the smallest of the vertebral column and are characterized by upward flares (**uncinate processes**) of their superolateral aspects. These projections are especially prominent on the lower cervical vertebrae, where those of one vertebra "articulate" with the inferolateral aspects of the body above, forming the so-called **joints of Luschka** (see page 33). The pedicles are quite short with shallow superior and inferior notches. The transverse processes of the upper six vertebrae are perforated by the **transverse foramina,** through which pass the vertebral arteries and veins, and the superior aspects of the transverse processes are indented by grooves that house the spinal nerves. The distal ends of these processes are enlarged into **anterior**

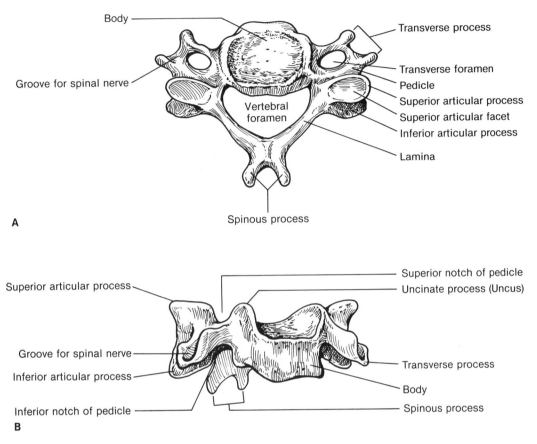

Figure 2-3
Superior (*A*) and anterolateral (*B*) views of vertebra C4.

and **posterior tubercles** with the anterior tubercle of vertebra C6 (the **carotid tubercle**) being prominent and easily palpable on the anterolateral aspect of the neck. Most spinous processes are short and bifid. Those of vertebrae C6 and C7 are considerably longer; that of C7 typically is quite long (Fig. 2-1B), and as a result, the vertebra is called the **vertebra prominens.** Although the articular surfaces of most of the cervical articular processes are oriented obliquely between the frontal and horizontal planes, the planes of the zygapophyseal joints are closer to horizontal than vertical. As a result, there is virtually no bony overlap of articular processes and dislocation without fracture is quite possible.

Vertebrae C1 (**atlas**) and C2 (**axis**) (Fig. 2-4) are constructed quite differently. The atlas has no body and consists of two **lateral masses** that are interconnected by **anterior** and **posterior arches.** The superior articular facets of the atlas are located on the lateral masses, and are concave from front to back. These facets articulate with the articular surfaces of the **occipital condyles,** which are convex from front to back. The axis is a more typical cervical vertebra except for the presence of the **dens** (odontoid process). This process represents the body of the atlas, is fused

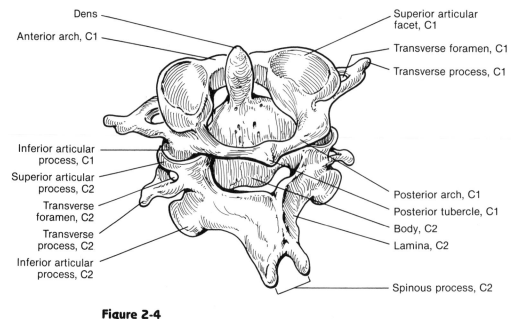

Dens

Anterior arch, C1

Superior articular facet, C1

Transverse foramen, C1

Transverse process, C1

Inferior articular process, C1

Superior articular process, C2

Transverse foramen, C2

Transverse process, C2

Inferior articular process, C2

Posterior arch, C1

Posterior tubercle, C1

Body, C2

Lamina, C2

Spinous process, C2

Figure 2-4
Posterolateral and superior view of vertebrae C1 and C2.

to the superior aspect of the body of the axis, and projects superiorly into the anterior portion of the area formed by the anterior and posterior arches of the atlas. The planes of the inferior articular facets of C1 and the superior facets of C2 are nearly horizontal and slope somewhat from medial to lateral.

Thoracic Vertebrae

Both the bodies and the transverse processes of the thoracic vertebrae (Fig. 2-5) articulate with the ribs. The heads of the ribs articulate with **costal fovea** on the posterolateral aspects of the bodies; the tubercles of the ribs articulate with costal fovea on the lateral aspects of the transverse processes. The bodies of the upper eight thoracic vertebrae usually articulate with two ribs on each side, while the lower four bodies articulate with only one. Each transverse process articulates with only one rib. Both the lamina and spinous processes overlap the next lower vertebra. As a result, the posterior boundary of the vertebral canal in the thoracic region is virtually bony. The long and obliquely oriented spinous processes extend inferiorly to the level of the next lower body; that is, the tip of the spinous process of vertebra T3 is at the level of the T4 vertebral body. The pedicles are notched unevenly, with the inferior notch considerably deeper than the superior. The articular processes overlap considerably, and the planes of the zygapophyseal joints practically parallel the frontal plane of the body.

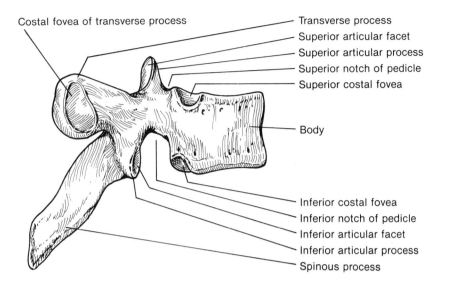

Costal fovea of transverse process

Transverse process
Superior articular facet
Superior articular process
Superior notch of pedicle
Superior costal fovea

Body

Inferior costal fovea
Inferior notch of pedicle
Inferior articular facet
Inferior articular process
Spinous process

Figure 2-5
Lateral view of vertebra T7.

Lumbar Vertebrae

The physical demands placed on the lumbar vertebrae (Fig. 2-6) are reflected in their size. The bodies are large and strong; the vertebral arch and its processes are short and heavy. The pedicles arise from the upper half of the posterolateral aspects of the bodies. The pedicles, together with the inferiorly directed lamina, create a deep inferior notch that forms a large part of the intervertebral foramen. The superior notch is quite shallow. The vertical dimensions of the laminae are less than those of the bodies, resulting in an interlaminar space between adjacent lumbar vertebrae. Because the short, posteriorly directed spinous processes do not interfere with this space, this level is ideal for spinal puncture because there is an opening between vertebrae posteriorly.

Although the surfaces of the articular facets are curved and the zygapophyseal joints therefore do not present a single plane, each presents a predominant plane. The planes in the upper lumbar levels are predominantly sagittal; at the lower levels, particularly between L5 and the sacrum, they are nearly coronal. The articular processes are large and overlap one another. This overlap provides a kind of bony strut between vertebrae so that a fracture usually accompanies a lumbar dislocation.

Sacrum and Coccyx

The sacrum (Figs. 2-7, 2-8), although composed of five vertebral segments, is a single massive bone that is tapered from superior to inferior. The bone is curved, presenting a ventral concavity, and the separation of vertebral bodies usually is marked by transverse lines on the pelvic surface. The combined spinous processes form the **median sacral crest,** and the lateral elements of the neural arches are represented by the large **lateral masses.** Laterally, the upper aspects of the sacrum present kidney-

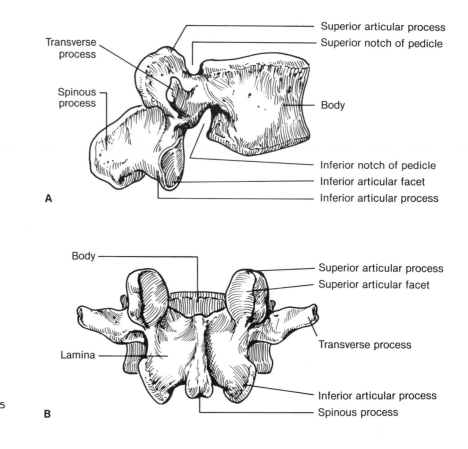

A

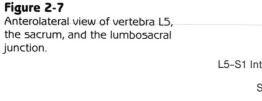

Figure 2-6
Lateral (*A*) and posterior (*B*) views
of vertebra L4.

B

Figure 2-7
Anterolateral view of vertebra L5,
the sacrum, and the lumbosacral
junction.

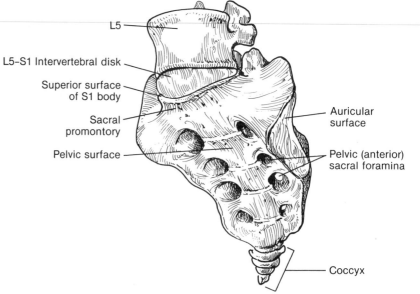

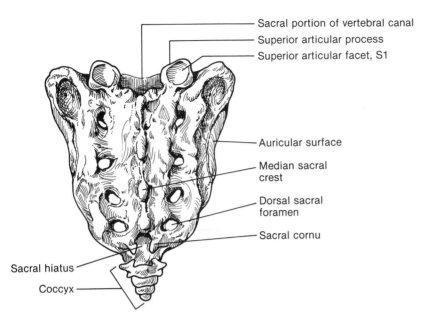

- Sacral portion of vertebral canal
- Superior articular process
- Superior articular facet, S1
- Auricular surface
- Median sacral crest
- Dorsal sacral foramen
- Sacral cornu
- Sacral hiatus
- Coccyx

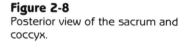

Figure 2-8
Posterior view of the sacrum and coccyx.

shaped articular surfaces, the **auricular surfaces,** that articulate with the ilia in the formation of the sacroiliac joints. The intervertebral foramina are replaced by four pairs of dorsal and ventral sacral foramina. The vertebral canal continues inferiorly into the sacrum and ends inferiorly at the **sacral hiatus,** where it opens onto the dorsal aspect of the sacrum. The location of this hiatus is marked by the palpable **sacral cornua.**

The coccyx (Figs. 2-7, 2-8) is composed of the rudiments of four vertebrae that are usually fused. It may attach to the inferior aspect of the sacrum via ligaments and, therefore, be mobile, or it may be fused with the sacrum and immovable. In either case, it is vulnerable to fracture in falls where the body weight is transferred forcibly to the buttocks.

Lumbosacral Junction

In the anatomic position the sacrum is positioned so that its longitudinal axis is considerably oblique and its superior surface is a steeply sloping anteriorly directed inclined plane. The junction between vertebra L5 and the superior aspect of the sacrum (Figs. 2-1B, 2-7) is the most angular junction between any two vertebrae, with a wedge-shaped intervertebral disk filling the interval. The natural tendency for the L5 vertebra to slide anteriorly is counteracted by the zygapophyses between vertebrae L5 and S1 as well as the ligaments of the vertebral column. **Spondylolysis** is a developmental anomaly of the lamina wherein a bony defect separates the superior and inferior articular processes, thus separating the posterior part of the neural arch from the anterior part of the arch and the vertebral body. This results in a loss of the bony support, and the potential for anterior subluxation of the body of vertebra L5 is increased. Actual anterior movement of the L5 vertebral body, **spondylolistheses,** can result in compression of the components of the cauda equina and increase the potential for other low back problems.

Although the separation between the lumbar vertebrae and the sacrum is usually definitive, vertebra L5 may assume characteristics of the sacrum or the first sacral segment may resemble a lumbar vertebra. In **sacralization,** the fifth lumbar vertebra possesses characteristics of the sacrum and may be partially or completely fused with the sacrum. In **lumbarization** of a sacral vertebra, the superior aspect of the sacrum assumes characteristics of a lumbar vertebra; in fact, six lumbar vertebrae may be present. Although the clinical implications of either situation are not fully known, fusion of vertebra L5 with the sacrum may place increased motion demands on the L4–L5 junction and consequently increase the potential for degenerative changes at that junction.

Articulations Between Vertebrae

Most vertebrae are united by a pair of synovial zygapophyseal joints and the cartilaginous intervertebral disk. None of these joints permits a large amount of motion, but all are intimately involved in the motion of the vertebral column as well as much of the pathology that frequently is difficult to diagnose and treat. The "joints of Luschka," found only between lower cervical vertebrae, are discussed later in this section.

Intervertebral disk. An **intervertebral disk** (Fig. 2-9) is found between each pair of vertebrae with the exception of the C1–C2 interval and between the segments forming the sacrum. Although the disks may vary considerably in size, their construction is similar at all levels. Each disk has a tough fibrocartilaginous cylindrical envelope that surrounds a viscous, semigelatinous core peripherally. Superiorly and inferiorly, a hyaline cartilage plate separates the semigelatinous core from the vertebral bodies.

The **annulus fibrosus,** the fibrocartilaginous envelope, is composed of concentric layers of fibrocartilage. The superficial layers attach to the peripheral compact bony collar (Fig. 2-2A) of the vertebral body, whereas the deeper layers attach to the hyaline cartilage plate. The fiber content of this cartilage is heavy, and the fibers in adjacent layers are arranged at right angles to one another and are oblique to the vertical axis of the vertebral column. This fibrous arrangement provides maximal resistance to the multidirectional stresses that are placed on the disk. These same stresses place tension on the annulus and tend to separate it from its attachments to the bodies and hyaline cartilage plates.

The central **nucleus pulposus** is mucoid in nature, contains a sparse number of irregularly arranged collagen and reticular fibers, and is composed of approximately three-quarters water. It appears to function as the fluid phase of a closed, fluid-elastic system. This means that as the disk is compressed, the resulting internal pressure is transmitted equally to all parts of the container (which in this case is composed of the annulus fibrosus and the hyaline cartilage plate). The water content of the nucleus is significant because the functional characteristics of the disk are directly related to that content. The water content, which decreases on a daily as

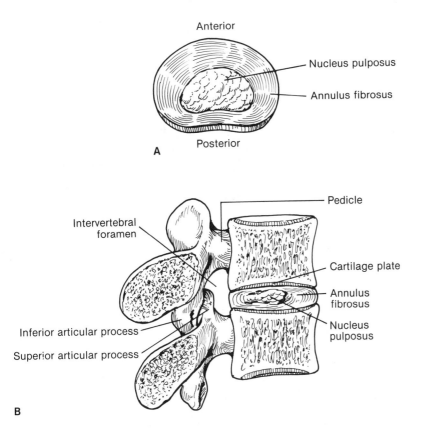

Anterior

Nucleus pulposus

Annulus fibrosus

Posterior

A

Pedicle

Intervertebral foramen

Cartilage plate

Annulus fibrosus

Nucleus pulposus

Inferior articular process

Superior articular process

B

Figure 2-9
(*A*) Transverse section through a lumbar intervertebral disk. (*B*) Sagittal section of two lumbar vertebrae and the intervening intervertebral disk.

well as a lifelong basis, affects an individual's height. The daily loss is replaced during non-weight-bearing periods (sleep), but the lifelong loss is permanent. As the water content decreases, so does the elasticity of the disk and hence the flexibility of the entire vertebral column. It is important to note that the nucleus is not centrally located but is somewhat eccentric posteriorly (see Fig. 2-9A, B), and therefore the annulus fibrosus is thicker anteriorly and laterally than posteriorly.

Functionally, the disk can absorb shock and withstand transient compression as well as permit fluid displacement within its elastic envelope. These characteristics enable each disk to undergo movement and distortion and thereby enhance motion of the vertebral column. Another characteristic of this system is that any externally applied force is distributed rather evenly over the surface of the disk and the adjoining vertebral bodies. Therefore, as the spine moves, weight is transmitted through the entire vertebral body rather than being concentrated on the side toward which the column is bending.

Zygapophyseal joints. The **zygapophyseal joints** (Fig. 2-10) are formed between the articular facets of the superior and inferior articular processes of adjacent vertebrae. Although the planes of these joints are oriented differently at various levels of the vertebral column, the joints are constructed similarly. The synovial cavity is enclosed by a loose joint capsule, and there are no reinforcing extra-articular ligaments, although

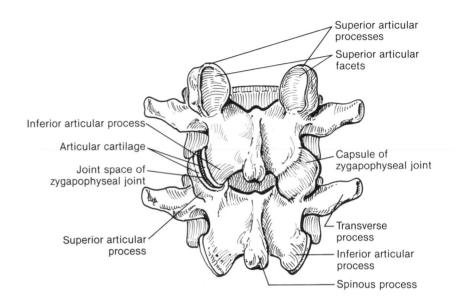

Superior articular processes

Superior articular facets

Inferior articular process

Articular cartilage

Joint space of zygapophyseal joint

Capsule of zygapophyseal joint

Superior articular process

Transverse process

Inferior articular process

Spinous process

Figure 2-10
Posterior view of two lumbar vertebrae illustrating the formation of the zygapophyseal joints.

the lateral aspect of the ligamentum flavum appears to blend with the fibrous part of the capsule (Figs. 2-11, 2-12). The major support of this joint is provided by the ligaments that bind the vertebrae together and by the deep muscles of the back. The motion that occurs at this joint is limited to a sliding motion parallel to the plane of the joint. The orientation of the articular facets dictates the direction of motion that can occur between adjacent vertebrae.

Most pathology involving these joints occurs at levels where the physical demands are greatest. Generally, the zygapophyseal joints have only a minor role in the stabilization of the vertebral column. The major exception is the lower lumbar region, particularly the lumbosacral junction, where the zygapophyses provide important support and are vulner-

Figure 2-11
Superior view of a typical vertebra illustrating the positions of the ligaments of the vertebral column.

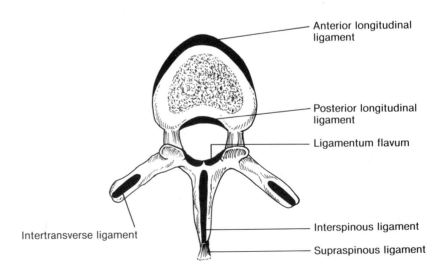

Anterior longitudinal ligament

Posterior longitudinal ligament

Ligamentum flavum

Intertransverse ligament

Interspinous ligament

Supraspinous ligament

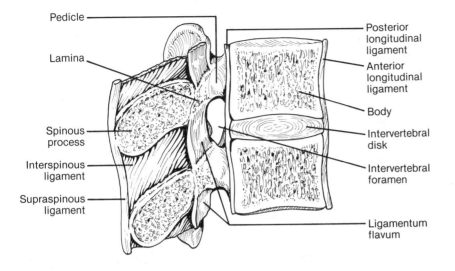

Pedicle

Lamina

Spinous process

Interspinous ligament

Supraspinous ligament

Posterior longitudinal ligament

Anterior longitudinal ligament

Body

Intervertebral disk

Intervertebral foramen

Ligamentum flavum

Figure 2-12
Sagittal section of two lumbar vertebrae illustrating the intervertebral foramen and the positions of several ligaments of the vertebral column.

able to overloading. These joints also are vulnerable to considerable trauma in areas of relatively free motion, specifically the lower cervical and lower lumbar regions. This is especially true in the lower cervical levels, where a large amount of motion occurs, and degenerative arthritis involving these joints is common.

As with all synovial joints, the joint capsule of the zygapophyseal joint contains a large number of pain endings and thus is quite sensitive. Inflammation of these joint capsules may well be the source of the local but somewhat diffuse back pain that is so common but whose cause is so difficult to pinpoint. As indicated above, these joints are vulnerable to trauma from a number of sources and injury is probably quite common.

Joints of Luschka. Not considered true articulations, the joints of Luschka are found only in the lower cervical region of the vertebral column. At these levels the intervertebral disks are rather thin, and the superolateral aspects of the vertebral bodies, the uncinate processes (Fig. 2-3B), flare superiorly. These processes may be very close to the body above and may even overlap that body. In fact, close inspection of the inferolateral aspects of the lower cervical bodies frequently reveals flattened areas that are adjacent to the uncinate processes. In prepared specimens these bony areas are very smooth and look much like the articular surfaces of other synovial joints. However, most anatomists think there is no synovial lining and that these so-called joints are in fact degenerative clefts. Motion between cervical vertebrae, particularly extreme motion, inevitably will cause contact between vertebral bodies in the regions of these clefts. Repeated contact can cause irritation and eventually the production of hypertrophic changes and exostoses. This process can be exacerbated by the natural loss of disk height that accompanies aging.

Ligaments of the Vertebral Column

The ligaments of the vertebral column (Fig. 2-11) virtually surround the column with some extending its entire length while others interconnect adjacent vertebrae. These ligaments hold the vertebrae together, add stability in the maintenance of equilibrium, and restrict or limit various motions.

The **anterior** and **posterior longitudinal ligaments** (Figs. 2-11 through 2-13) are single ligaments that extend from the atlas to the sacrum. Both attach firmly to the vertebral bodies and the intervertebral disks. The anterior longitudinal ligament covers the anterior and lateral aspect of the column and limits extension of the vertebral column. The posterior longitudinal ligament is found within the vertebral canal, where it reinforces the posterior aspects of the intervertebral disks. It is important to note that this ligament is quite narrow from side to side. In the thoracic and lumbar regions (Fig. 2-13) it flares laterally at the level of each intervertebral disk, but this lateral flare is very thin and adds very little reinforcement to the posterolateral aspects of the disks. The reinforcement provided by this ligament, then, is limited to a narrow area in the midline. The posterior longitudinal ligament restricts flexion of the vertebral column.

The transverse and spinous processes of adjacent vertebrae are interconnected by the **intertransverse** and **interspinous ligaments** respectively (see Figs. 2-11, 2-12). All of these ligaments limit flexion of the vertebral column with the intertransverse ligaments also limiting lateral bending to the contralateral side. The interspinous ligament may extend posteriorly beyond the tip of the spinous processes, thus becoming the **supraspinous ligament.** In the cervical region this ligament is the **ligamentum nuchae.**

The **ligamenta flava** (see Figs. 2-11, 2-12) are elastic ligaments that interconnect the lamina of adjacent vertebrae. These paired ligaments virtually close any interlaminar space that may exist and extend from the midline to the articular processes, where they blend with the capsules of the zygapophyseal joints. The high elastic fiber content of this ligament sets it apart from the other ligaments of the vertebral column. These ligaments are normally under tension regardless of the position of the vertebral column. Their elasticity and the continual tension preclude any

Figure 2-13
Posterior view of the posterior longitudinal ligament in the lumbar region. The pedicles have been cut and the neural arches removed.

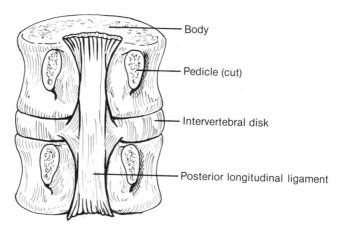

— Body

— Pedicle (cut)

— Intervertebral disk

— Posterior longitudinal ligament

bulging. As the spine is extended, the ligaments have sufficient elasticity to shorten rather than bulge anteriorly into the spinal canal. However, during extreme extension of the cervical region, the ligaments' elastic limits may be exceeded and they may bulge into the spinal canal. Although these ligaments clearly resist flexion of the vertebral column, they probably are of little importance in actually limiting flexion.

Motion and Mechanics of the Vertebral Column

The natural curves of the vertebral column are important in the maintenance of its equilibrium in the upright position. In that position the center of gravity of the entire body is slightly anterior to the second sacral vertebral segment. If a line representing the line of gravity is extended superiorly from that center of gravity, it will pass through each of the junctional regions of the vertebral column—the lumbosacral, thoracolumbar, cervicothoracic, and occipitocervical junctions. Consequently, each of the curves of the normally aligned vertebral column returns the superincumbent weight to equilibrium so virtually no muscular support is needed to maintain that posture. As soon as any movement of the vertebral column occurs, the equilibrium is lost and the muscles of the deep back, abdomen, and hips are needed to control (counteract gravitational forces) the motion.

In most instances any motion of the vertebral column is the sum total of the motion that occurs between adjacent pairs of vertebrae. Clearly, there are certain levels where considerable motion of a specific kind is available. Still, most motion is cumulative.

The direction of motion available between two vertebrae is dependent on the orientation of the articular facets that form the zygapophyseal joints. Since these joints permit only a sliding type of motion, the movement that occurs must be parallel to the plane of the joint. Virtually none of the planes of these joints corresponds exactly to any of the cardinal planes of the body; they are oblique and thus permit more than a single motion. For example, a joint that has a purely sagittally oriented plane would permit only flexion and extension. If the orientation were somewhat between the sagittal and coronal planes, rotation and side bending also would be permitted. The amount of motion between vertebrae is regulated by several structural features. These include the thickness of the intervertebral disks, the tightness of the ligaments, and the presence and characteristics of related structures. A thick intervertebral disk permits more rocking between vertebrae than a thin disk and, hence, potentially more motion. In contrast to the rest of the ligaments of the vertebral column, the capsules of the zygapophyseal joints are loose and weak and probably play little role in limiting vertebral motion. The thoracic cage clearly restricts motion in the thoracic region, and the bulk of lumbar back muscles and the abdominal contents restrict lumbar motion more than the soft tissue of the neck restricts cervical motion.

The direction and amount of motion vary from level to level in the vertebral column. With the exception of the superior two cervical levels, the cervical zygapophyseal joint planes (Figs. 2-14, 2-15) are oriented

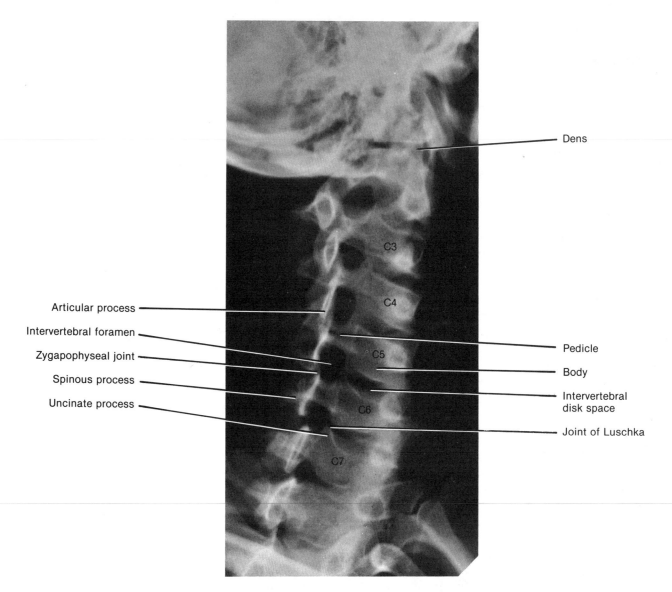

Dens

Articular process

Intervertebral foramen

Zygapophyseal joint

Spinous process

Uncinate process

C3

C4

C5

C6

C7

Pedicle

Body

Intervertebral disk space

Joint of Luschka

Figure 2-14
Anterolateral and somewhat inferior radiograph of the cervical spine.

obliquely between the horizontal and coronal planes and virtually all motions are permitted, with flexion and extension being the freest. Lateral bending is accompanied by rotation to the same side. Motion between vertebrae C5 and C6 is quite free, presumably underlying that level's excessive vulnerability to degenerative changes. The **atlantooccipital articulations** (Fig. 2-4) are between the occipital condyles and the superior articular facets of vertebra C1. These condyles are convex from front to back and thus permit the head to rock anteriorly and posteriorly on the first cervical vertebra. The **atlantoaxial junction** (Fig. 2-4) is a very dif-

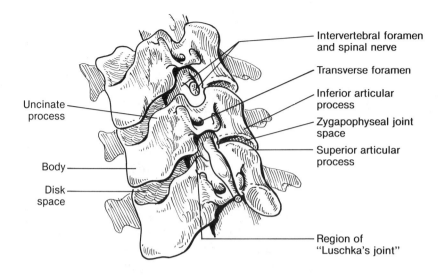

Uncinate process

Body

Disk space

Intervertebral foramen and spinal nerve

Transverse foramen

Inferior articular process

Zygapophyseal joint space

Superior articular process

Region of "Luschka's joint"

Figure 2-15
Anterolateral view of vertebrae C4–C6, illustrating the boundaries of the intervertebral foramina and the positions of the spinal nerves.

ferent arrangement because there are three synovial articulations. The planes of the zygapophyseal joints (**lateral atlantoaxial joints**) are approximately horizontal and slope somewhat inferiorly from medial to lateral. The dens articulates anteriorly with the anterior arch of the atlas, forming the **middle atlantoaxial joint.** The arrangement of these three articulations permits rotation of the atlas around the dens as well as a moderate amount of flexion and extension.

The zygapophyseal joint planes in the thoracic region (Fig. 2-5) are very nearly coronal in orientation and should permit side bending, rotation, and limited flexion and extension. All movements, however, are limited by the rib cage, which together with the vertebral column transforms that part of the trunk into a rather rigid cylinder. The thin intervertebral disks also contribute to the small amount of motion. The rigid nature of the thoracic portion of the vertebral column is significant in the etiology of compression fractures of the vertebral bodies. These fractures typically accompany a fall from a height or an automobile accident where the spine is thrown forcibly into flexion. As the flexion force is transferred inferiorly along the spine, very little of it is absorbed in the rigid thoracic region; rather, it is transferred to the next lower, more movable area. As a result, most of these fractures occur in the lower thoracic and upper lumbar areas.

In the lumbar region the planes of the upper and lower zygapophyses differ. At upper levels the planes are nearly sagittal in orientation and permit mainly flexion and extension. The lower joints, particularly those between L5 and the sacrum, are nearly coronal in orientation. In addition to flexion and extension, side bending and rotation are available. The amount of motion is enhanced by the thickness of the intervertebral disks. The motion at the lumbosacral junction is particularly free. The amount of motion, the unsteadiness of the junction, and the magnitude of the forces affecting that region undoubtedly are related to its common involvement in pathology.

Intervertebral Foramen

At all levels the intervertebral foramen is formed between vertebrae, by the pedicles superiorly and inferiorly, by the vertebral bodies and the intervening intervertebral disk anteriorly, and by the articular processes and zygapophyseal joint posteriorly. At all levels the intervertebral foramen contains the spinal nerve. Each pedicle is notched to give the superior and inferior borders of the foramen a smooth and rounded contour, although the depth of these notches varies at different levels and is significant clinically. The size of the foramen, the position of the intervertebral disk in its anterior wall, and the location of the spinal nerve within the foramen are significant relative to pathology involving the spinal nerve.

The cervical spinal nerves are vulnerable to impingement from a number of pathologic changes that involve the boundaries of the intervertebral foramina. The levels most commonly affected are in the lower half of the region, where there is considerable motion between vertebrae and the spinal nerves are large because they contribute to the formation of the brachial plexus, which innervates the upper limb. In addition, the vertebral arteries (Fig. 2-16) ascend just anterior to the spinal nerves and also are potential hazards to the nerves.

The cervical intervertebral disk is directly in the center of the anterior wall of the foramen (Figs. 2-14 through 2-16). The notches in the pedicles are similar in depth; thus roughly equal amounts of the two vertebral bodies form the anterior wall. In addition, the center of the anterior wall marks the position of the posterior aspect of the joint of Luschka. The spinal nerve occupies a large percentage of the foramen, is positioned in the center of the foramen, and is adjacent to both the intervertebral disk and Luschka's joint anteriorly and the zygapophysis posteriorly. Herniation of the intervertebral disk can impinge on the spinal nerve anteriorly. Inflammation or hypertrophic changes of either Luschka's joint or the zygapophyseal joint can impinge on the nerve anteriorly and posteriorly, respectively. These nerves also are vulnerable when cervical ver-

Figure 2-16
Anterolateral view of vertebrae C4–C6, illustrating the location of the vertebral artery relative to the spinal nerves and the vertebrae.

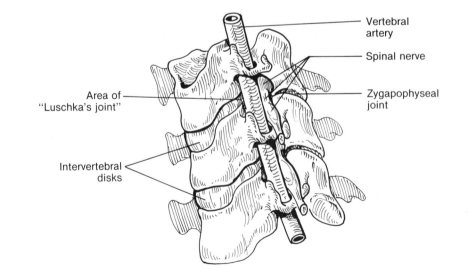

Vertebral artery

Spinal nerve

Zygapophyseal joint

Area of "Luschka's joint"

Intervertebral disks

tebrae dislocate or are fractured. Tortuous and sclerotic vertebral arteries can compress the nerves, especially when the spine is extended. The symptoms resulting from any of these situations should be segmental in distribution and consistent with those of a preplexus type of injury.

The vertebral arteries (Fig. 2-16) pass close to both the zygapophyseal and Luschka's joints and may be compressed by inflammation or hypertrophic changes involving those joints. Compression on the artery can be intensified by motion of the cervical spine. The resulting symptoms should be consistent with compromise of the blood supply to the brain stem or to the cervical portion of the spinal cord or both and would present neurological findings somewhat different from those of spinal nerve involvement.

The lumbar intervertebral foramen (Figs. 2-17 through 2-19) is large, and its anterior border is formed differently than that in the cervical re-

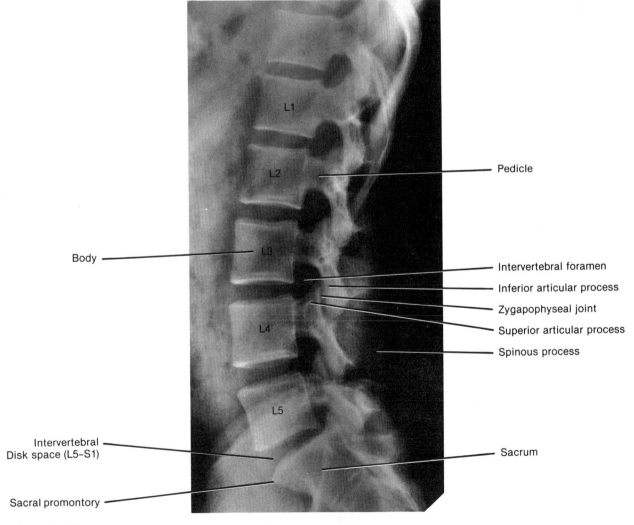

Figure 2-17
Lateral radiograph of the lumbar and lumbosacral regions of the vertebral column.

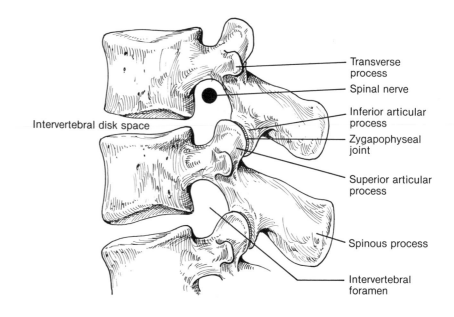

Transverse process

Spinal nerve

Inferior articular process

Zygapophyseal joint

Superior articular process

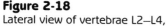
Intervertebral disk space

Spinous process

Intervertebral foramen

Figure 2-18
Lateral view of vertebrae L2–L4, illustrating the boundaries of the intervertebral foramina and the position of the spinal nerve.

gion. The notch in the inferior border of the pedicle is considerably deeper than the superior notch. As a result, the upper half of the anterior wall of the foramen is formed by the body of the upper vertebra; the lower half is formed by the intervertebral disk and only a small portion of the lower body. The spinal nerve is quite small relative to the size of the foramen and occupies only a small proportion of the foramen. All of the lumbar spinal nerves arise from the spinal cord well superior to the levels at which they pass through the intervertebral foramen; and since these nerves are somewhat taut, they pass through the most superior part of their respective foramina (Figs. 2-18, 2-19). Each nerve, then, passes through its foramen well above the level of the intervertebral disk. Herniation of a lumbar disk, assuming the herniation is small and affects a single nerve, typically does not compress the spinal nerve passing through that foramen (Fig. 2-19). As the lumbar nerves descend within the spinal canal toward their foramina, each passes inferolaterally along the anterior wall of the canal. This course places the nerve against the posterolateral aspect of the intervertebral disk; that position is maintained by the tension on the nerve. The most common point of herniation of a lumbar disk is posterolaterally where the descending nerves pass. Typically therefore, a herniated lumbar disk will involve the spinal nerve that exits through the next lower intervertebral foramen. For example, herniation of the disk between vertebrae L4 and L5 usually compresses spinal nerve L5 (Fig. 2-19). As in the cervical region, resulting symptomatology is usually consistent with the segmental pattern of innervation.

The intervertebral foramen in the thoracic region is constructed very similarly to that of the lumbar region, and the spinal nerves also pass superior to the intervertebral disks. However, the herniation of a thoracic disk is not a common occurrence, probably because of the limited motion

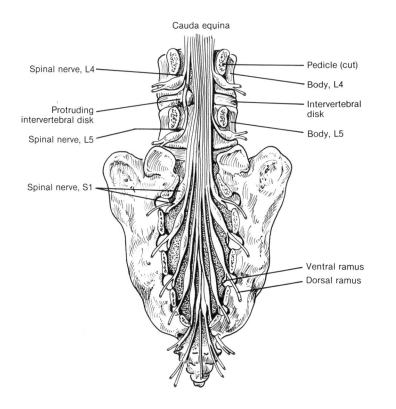

Cauda equina

Spinal nerve, L4

Pedicle (cut)

Body, L4

Protruding intervertebral disk

Intervertebral disk

Spinal nerve, L5

Body, L5

Spinal nerve, S1

Ventral ramus

Dorsal ramus

Figure 2-19
Posterior view of the vertebral canal in the lumbosacral region. The neural arches and posterior aspect of the sacrum are removed. A protruding intervertebral disk, between vertebrae L4 and L5, is indicated on the left side. (Adapted from Netter.)

of the thoracic spine as well as the thin intervertebral disks. Spinal nerve impingement does occur, but it usually is due to arthritic involvement of the zygapophyseal joints. The resulting symptomology, at least with involvement of most thoracic spinal nerves, corresponds to segmental innervation and is limited to the body wall. Involvement of a single nerve might well produce symptoms that are nearly negligible. The compression of several contiguous nerves is necessary to produce definitive sensory and motor symptoms, a circumstance that is quite possible since multiple joints are usually involved.

When an intervertebral disk compresses a single spinal nerve, the location of that disk is consistent throughout the vertebral column: The disk causing the compression is the one superior to the vertebra of the same name and number as the involved nerve. The anatomic reasons for this rule differ in the cervical and lumbar regions. The cervical spinal nerves pass through the intervertebral foramen above the vertebra bearing the same name and number; for example, spinal nerve C6 passes through the intervertebral foramen between vertebrae C5 and C6. Herniation of the disk between these two vertebrae compresses the spinal nerve (C6) passing through that foramen because the nerve virtually fills the foramen and is positioned adjacent to the disk. In the lumbar region the spinal nerves pass well above the disks and exit below their respectively named vertebrae; for example, spinal nerve L4 passes between vertebrae L4 and L5. Herniation of the disk between these two vertebrae typically does not compress spinal nerve L4, but rather nerve L5, because it crosses the posterolateral aspect of the disk (Fig. 2-19).

Reflex postural changes commonly accompany spinal nerve compression in the lumbar region. These changes, typically spinal flexion and side bending away from the side of the compression, are thought to increase the size of the intervertebral foramen and thus remove pressure from the nerve. The mechanics are logical, but the rationale is confusing as presumably the lumbar nerve is involved proximal to its passage through the foramen. A more logical explanation, perhaps, should focus on the effects of postural changes on a herniated intervertebral disk. For example, do certain postural changes reduce the degree of disk herniation?

Contents of the Vertebral Canal

Neural Elements

The **spinal cord** (Fig. 2-20) is the major structure occupying the vertebral or spinal canal, and it serves as the connecting link between higher centers of the central nervous system and most parts of the body. It is composed of multiple segments, each of which innervates a specific portion

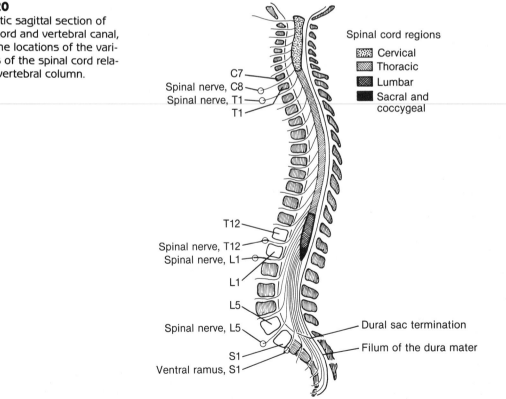

Figure 2-20
Diagrammatic sagittal section of the spinal cord and vertebral canal, indicating the locations of the various regions of the spinal cord relative to the vertebral column.

of the body wall or a limb or both. The number of spinal cord segments—8 cervical, 12 thoracic, 5 lumbar, 5 sacral, and 1 coccygeal—corresponds roughly to the number of vertebrae.

The spinal cord is composed of both white and gray matter, and its diameter at each level reflects the size of the area supplied by that segment (see Fig. 2-20). Since the amount of white matter decreases from superior to inferior, the regional changes in the diameter are due principally to the amount of gray matter. The greater diameter of those levels associated with the large somatic plexuses of the limbs, the cervical and lumbosacral enlargements, reflects the large amount of gray matter. In the thoracic region, where the muscle mass is small, the spinal cord is thin because there is less gray matter. The tapering inferior end of the spinal cord, the **conus medullaris,** is composed of decreasing amounts of both gray and white matter.

Although the vertebral canal extends nearly the entire length of the vertebral column, the spinal cord extends inferiorly only to the lower aspect of the first lumbar vertebra (Fig. 2-20). This difference in length is due to the differential growth of the vertebral column and spinal cord that occurs during development and growth. Very early in development, during the first few fetal months, the spinal cord and vertebral column are the same length, each spinal cord segment is at the same level as the vertebra for which it is named, and each spinal nerve passes horizontally toward its intervertebral foramen. Thereafter, the vertebral column grows more rapidly than the spinal cord. At birth the spinal cord extends approximately to the middle (L2–L3) of the lumbar portion of the vertebral column; and by 5 years of age, the definitive adult relationship is established. In the adult, only the upper cervical spinal cord segments are at the same level as their respectively named vertebrae. Lower cervical and upper thoracic segments are approximately one vertebral level higher; middle and lower thoracic segments are two to three vertebral levels higher; and the lumbar, sacral, and coccygeal segments are opposite vertebrae T11, T12, and L1. The courses of the spinal roots and nerves, from the spinal cord to the intervertebral foramen, become increasingly oblique from above downward. Below the spinal cord the mass of spinal nerve roots is referred to as the **cauda equina** (see Figs. 2-19, 2-20).

An understanding of the difference in the length of the spinal cord and the vertebral column is helpful in explaining the location of the symptoms that accompany a spinal cord lesion. Such lesions typically result in motor and sensory symptoms that correspond to the level of the lesion and that involve the rest of the body below that level. It is important to note that the highest level of symptoms corresponds to the level of the spinal cord lesion and not the vertebral column injury. The symptoms usually involve dermatomes and myotomes that are innervated by spinal cord segments that obviously are positioned at the same level as the vertebral injury. The name and number of the most superior spinal cord segment involved, however, typically is lower than the highest vertebra involved. For example, involvement of the spinal cord at vertebral level T11 might logically produce symptoms that correspond to spinal cord segment L1 or L2 and therefore appear to begin below the vertebral level of the lesion. This disparity is not consistent, because the differences in the levels between correspondingly named spinal cord segments and vertebrae varies; the higher the lesion, the less the disparity.

Each segment of the spinal cord communicates with the areas it innervates by means of a pair of **spinal nerves** (Fig. 2-21). The spinal nerve is formed by a pair of roots, dorsal and ventral, each of which is connected to a segment of the spinal cord by a number of rootlets. The **dorsal root** contains afferent or sensory fibers; the **ventral root** contains efferent or motor fibers. The two roots join to form the spinal nerve, which typically occupies the intervertebral foramen. The spinal nerve and its branches contain both afferent and efferent fibers and thus are called mixed nerves. Each spinal nerve branches into a **dorsal** and a **ventral** (primary) **ramus.** The dorsal rami at all levels innervate the deep muscles of the back and the skin of the medial two-thirds of the back; the ventral rami become intercostal nerves or form the somatic plexuses that innervate the limbs.

Spinal nerves T2 through T11 are considered "typical" spinal nerves because each supplies a strip of the body wall (Fig. 2-21). The ventral rami become intercostal nerves and innervate the skin, muscles, joints, and underlying parietal pleura of the intercostal spaces. The more inferior intercostal nerves continue into the abdominal wall, innervating the skin and muscles of the abdominal wall as well as the underlying parietal peritoneum. Compression of a spinal nerve at this level would produce motor and sensory symptoms limited to the body wall; the severity of the symptoms would be dependent upon the number of nerves involved.

The ventral rami of the spinal nerves above T2 and below T11 are different from those of the typical spinal nerves because they form the somatic plexuses that innervate the limbs. The lower cervical and upper thoracic ventral rami form the brachial plexus, which innervates the upper limb, and lumbar and sacral ventral rami form the lumbosacral plexus, which innervates the lower limb. The cervical plexus, formed by upper

Figure 2-21
Anterolateral view of a thoracic spinal cord segment and the formation and branches of its spinal nerves.

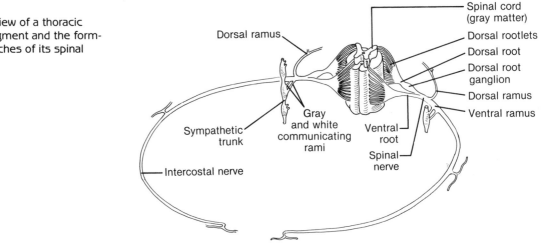

cervical ventral rami, is associated with the neck. At these levels, where the ventral rami form the somatic plexuses of the limbs, each spinal nerve also innervates a portion of the body. The dermatomes are larger than those of the thorax, and there is less overlap between adjacent ones. As a result, loss of a single spinal nerve can produce a definitive and predictable loss of cutaneous sensibility. A consequence of plexus formation is the distribution of fibers from a single cord segment into multiple terminal nerves, and hence each segment provides partial innervation to multiple muscles. Loss of a single spinal nerve that contributes to the formation of a somatic plexus produces widespread muscular weakness but typically no absolute paralysis of any single muscle.

Coverings of the Spinal Cord

The **meninges** consist of a series of coverings that surround the spinal cord and brain. The major function of these membranes is protection since they form various spaces and a fluid cushion around the central nervous system. Each of these layers has lateral sleevelike extensions that surround the spinal nerves and are continuous with the connective tissue coverings of the nerves.

The outermost covering, the **dura mater** (Fig. 2-22), is the strongest and thickest of the meninges and provides structure and shape to the entire system of spaces. It forms a closed tubular sleeve around the spinal cord that commonly is called the **dural sac** (Fig. 2-20). This sac is anchored superiorly where it passes through the foramen magnum (the opening between the vertebral canal and the cranial cavity) and is continuous with the dura mater in the cranial cavity. The dural sac extends inferiorly to the level of the second sacral vertebra (Fig. 2-20) and is anchored by an inferior extension, the **coccygeal ligament,** which passes inferiorly through the sacral hiatus and attaches to the coccyx.

The **arachnoid** (Fig. 2-22) is the intermediate layer of the meninges that virtually lines the dural sac. It is held against the dura by the cerebrospinal fluid and interconnected to the underlying pia mater by numerus trabeculae—hence, the spider-web appearance and the name arachnoid.

The deepest or innermost of the meninges is the **pia mater** (Fig. 2-22), which is closely and firmly attached to the spinal cord. The pia follows the exact contours of the cord and brain and ensheathes each of the nerve rootlets that attaches to the cord. Lateral extensions of the pia, the **denticulate ligaments,** attach laterally to the dura mater and thus provide lateral stability for the spinal cord. Each of the ligaments is attached to the dura by a series of projections or serrations that generally extend laterally between spinal nerves. These ligaments extend inferiorly through the thoracic region. The spinal cord is anchored inferiorly by an extension of the pia mater, the **filum terminale internum.** This thin cord extends inferiorly from the conus medullaris to the inferior extent of the dural sac, where it joins the coccygeal ligament.

The dura mater is separated from the periosteum of the vertebrae and the ligaments that form the vertebral canal by the **epidural space** (Fig.

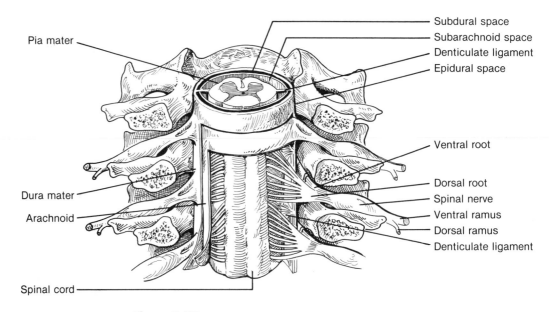

Pia mater

Dura mater

Arachnoid

Spinal cord

Subdural space

Subarachnoid space

Denticulate ligament

Epidural space

Ventral root

Dorsal root

Spinal nerve

Ventral ramus

Dorsal ramus

Denticulate ligament

Figure 2-22
Posterior view of a portion of the vertebral canal in the cervical region. The spinal cord, spinal nerves, and meninges and their related spaces are shown. (The subdural space is enlarged so it is visible.)

2-22). This space surrounds the entire dural sac and is continuous with the vertebral canal below the dural sac. The epidural space does not continue into the cranial cavity, because the cranial dura is fused with the periosteum of the bones that form the cranial cavity. This space contains fat and the internal vertebral venous plexus, a network of veins that is valveless, interconnects the body cavities and the cranial cavity, and is thought to be the pathway through which metastatic cells spread from the body cavities to the cranial cavity.

The **subdural space** (Fig. 2-22) is only a potential space because the arachnoid is pressed against the dura by the cerebrospinal fluid in the subarachnoid space. However, since there is no connection between the two layers, the space easily can be enlarged by a collection of fluid or other material.

The **subarachnoid space** (Fig. 2-22) is found between the arachnoid and the pia mater. It is filled with cerebrospinal fluid, which serves as a fluid cushion for the spinal cord as well as the brain. The subarachnoid space and the dural sac are coextensive, so the subarachnoid space extends inferiorly to the level of the second sacral vertebra. The difference in the position of the conus medullaris (lower border of vertebra L1) and the inferior extent of the subarachnoid space provides an access to cerebrospinal fluid where only the components of the cauda equina are in any jeopardy.

The anatomy of the vertebral column, spinal cord, and meningeal spaces facilitates the access to the cerebrospinal fluid in the subarachnoid space in the lumbar region of the back. **Lumbar puncture** is commonly performed inferior to vertebra L3. The interlaminar spaces between adjacent lumbar vertebrae and the short horizontally projecting spinous processes provide easy entry to the vertebral canal. Since the subarachnoid space extends inferiorly to vertebra S2 and the spinal cord ends at the inferior border of vertebra L1, only the components of the cauda equina are in jeopardy from the examiner's needle. The cerebrospinal fluid can be procured with minimal risk to the patient.

Muscles of the Back

The muscles of the back can be separated into two groups, superficial and deep, based on their location, function, and innervation. Functionally, the **superficial muscles of the back** are primary muscles of the shoulder. Most of them are innervated by branches of the brachial plexus and, for the most part, are positioned superficial to the thoracolumbar fascia. These muscles are described in Chapter 3.

The **deep,** or **intrinsic, muscles of the back** are the back muscles proper. Although this group of muscles is formed by a multitude of individual muscles, the sum total is a large mass of intertwined muscular tissue. This mass of muscle occupies the furrow formed by the transverse and spinous processes of the vertebrae (Fig. 2-23), and in the thoracic region extends about as far laterally as the angles of the ribs. These muscles are partially enclosed by the thoracolumbar fascia and innervated by the dorsal rami of the spinal nerves. The innervation is segmental, each dorsal ramus supplying a segment or section of the entire mass. These deep muscles, based on their anatomy, can be separated into four groups: spinotransversalis, erector spinae, transversospinalis, and segmental. In addition, there are the suboccipital muscles in the cervical region.

The **spinotransversalis group** consists of two muscles, the splenius

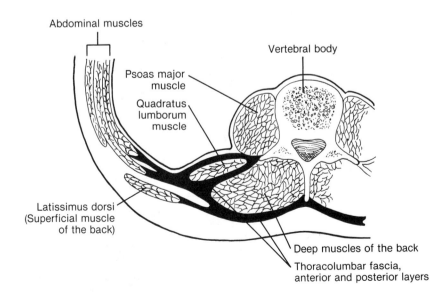

Figure 2-23
Transverse section through the lumbar portion of the back, illustrating the location of the superficial and deep back muscles.

Abdominal muscles

Vertebral body

Psoas major muscle

Quadratus lumborum muscle

Latissimus dorsi (Superficial muscle of the back)

Deep muscles of the back

Thoracolumbar fascia, anterior and posterior layers

capitis and splenius cervicis (Fig. 2-24). These muscles are the most superficial of the deep back muscles in the upper thoracic and cervical regions, and their fibers pass laterally as they ascend from their origins on the spinous processes. The **splenius capitis** extends from the spines of the lower cervical and upper thoracic vertebrae to the base of the skull; the **splenius cervicis,** from the spines of the middle thoracic vertebrae to the transverse processes of the upper cervical vertebrae.

The **erector spinae (sacrospinalis) group** is vertically or longitudinally oriented, superficially positioned, and its individual components span multiple segments. The muscles in this group constitute the true erectors of the spine and consist of three parts, each of which has subdivisions associated with various portions of the vertebral column. The **iliocostalis** (Fig. 2-24), the lateral group, consists of components that extend from ilium to rib and rib to rib. The subdivisions of the iliocostalis

Figure 2-24
Posterior view of the deep muscles of the back.

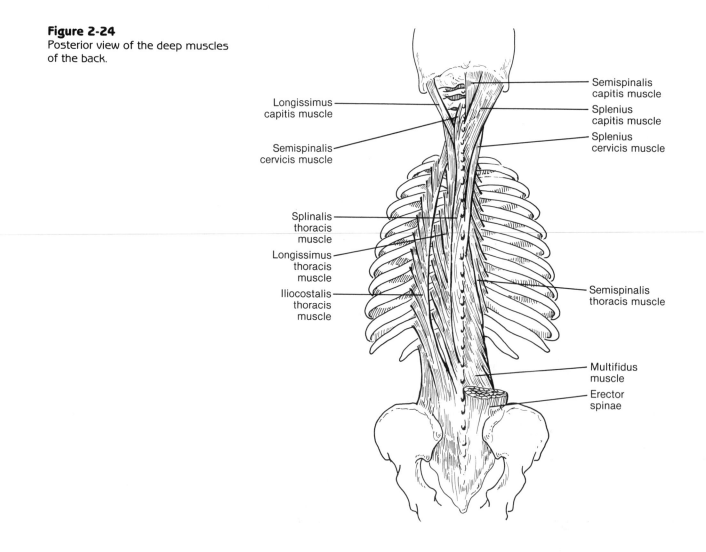

Longissimus capitis muscle

Semispinalis cervicis muscle

Splinalis thoracis muscle

Longissimus thoracis muscle

Iliocostalis thoracis muscle

Semispinalis capitis muscle

Splenius capitis muscle

Splenius cervicis muscle

Semispinalis thoracis muscle

Multifidus muscle

Erector spinae

are the iliocostalis lumborum, iliocostalis thoracis, and iliocostalis cervicis. The superior attachments of the iliocostalis cervicis are the transverse processes of the lower cervical vertebrae. The medial group, the **spinalis** (Fig. 2-24), extends from spinous process to spinous process. The components of this group usually are small and present in the thoracic (spinalis thoracis) and cervical (spinalis cervicis) regions. The intermediate group is the **longissimus** (Fig. 2-24), and its components extend from transverse process to transverse process. The longissimus is the largest and longest of the longitudinal muscles. Its components are the longissimus thoracis, longissimus cervicis, and longissimus capitis, which attaches superiorly to the mastoid process of the skull.

The **transversospinal group** is deep to the erector spinae; its component muscles span only a few segments or even one segment; and its individual muscles are oblique and extend from transverse processes to more superior spinous processes. The subdivisions of this group are the semispinalis, multifidi, and rotators. The **semispinalis** (Fig. 2-24) is not found in the lumbar region; it consists of thoracis, cervicis, and capitis portions. These muscles are the longest of the transversospinal group. The semispinalis capitis is particularly well developed and consists of fibers that are nearly vertical and ascend to the occipital bone. The **multifidi** (Fig. 2-24) extend from the sacrum to middle cervical levels. Their component muscles span only two to four segments, so they are shorter than the muscles of the semispinalis. The multifidi of the lumbar region are especially large and strong and constitute a major portion of the deep muscles in that area. The **rotators** are deep to the multifidi and extend from the sacrum to middle cervical levels. They are similar to the multifidi but span fewer vertebrae. Some rotators (short rotators) interconnect adjacent vertebrae, while others (long rotators) span two segments. Since these muscles are the shortest of the oblique muscles, they also are the most obliquely oriented.

The **segmental group** consists of the **interspinales** and the **intertransversarri muscles.** These muscles are truly segmental because they all interconnect adjacent vertebrae. Although their presence and size varies in different regions of the vertebral column, they all are vertically oriented and interconnect the parts of the vertebrae indicated by their names.

The four **suboccipital muscles** (Fig. 2-25) are associated with the most superior aspect of the cervical spine, in the interval between the skull and vertebra C2. These muscles are quite small and positioned deep to the semispinalis capitis. The **obliquus capitis superior** arises from the transverse process of the atlas and passes superiorly and medially to insert on the occipital bone of the skull. The **obliquus capitis inferior** arises from the spinous process of the axis and extends laterally and superiorly to its insertion on the transverse process of the atlas. The **rectus capitis posterior major** extends from the spinous process of the axis (origin) to the occipital bone (insertion). These three muscles form the small **suboccipital triangle.** The fourth muscle, the **rectus capitis posterior minor,** is medial to the rectus capitis posterior major which it parallels. It extends from the posterior tubercle of the atlas (origin) to the occipital bone (insertion).

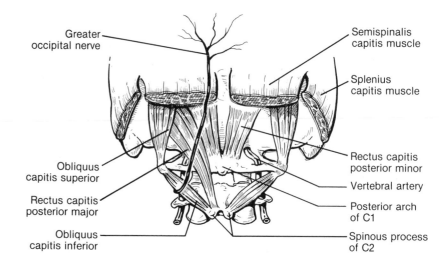

Greater occipital nerve

Semispinalis capitis muscle

Splenius capitis muscle

Obliquus capitis superior

Rectus capitis posterior major

Obliquus capitis inferior

Rectus capitis posterior minor

Vertebral artery

Posterior arch of C1

Spinous process of C2

Figure 2-25
Posterior view of the suboccipital region.

Functions of the Deep Back Muscles

The **actions** of the deep muscles of the back include extension, side bending, and rotation of the spine. This entire mass is a functional unit whose individual components work together to produce various motions. The more vertically oriented and longer muscles, primarily the erector spinae and splenius muscles, are the primary extensors when contracting bilaterally. Unilateral activity produces side bending and rotation. The deeper, shorter, and more obliquely oriented muscles, mainly the transversospinal group, are the primary rotators and side benders, although their bilateral activity can produce extension. The suboccipital muscles move the head. Contracting bilaterally, they extend the head. Contracting unilaterally, they both laterally bend and rotate the head to the same side.

Surface Anatomy of the Back

The anatomic landmarks of the back, especially the spinous processes, provide a means of assessment of both the alignment and symmetry of the back. These properties are the essence of a back examination.

The spinous processes are in a vertical line inferior to the readily palpable external occipital protuberance. The spines of the upper four or five cervical vertebrae may be somewhat difficult to palpate, but the spinous process of cervical vertebra C7 (**vertebra prominens**) is large and usually the most prominent spine at the base of the neck, although the spines of C6 and T1 also are quite long. The spinous processes of most thoracic vertebrae are easily palpable; that of T3 is at the level of the base of the spine of the scapula and that of T7 is opposite the inferior angle of the scapula. Because of the long and obliquely oriented spinous processes of the thoracic vertebrae, the tip of a thoracic spinous process is at the level of the body of the next lower vertebrae; that is, the inferior angle of the scapula is at the level of the body of vertebra T8. The spines of the lumbar vertebrae typically are somewhat difficult to palpate, although flexion of the vertebral column may help. A line interconnecting the highest levels of the iliac crests passes through the spinous process of vertebra L4; the spine of vertebra S2 is marked by a pair of dimples that indicate the positions of the posterior superior iliac spines.

Inspection and palpation of the spinous processes provides an indication of deviation from the natural anteroposterior curves as well as the presence of a lateral curve (scoliosis). A protruding or indented spine could indicate a fractured vertebra.

The large vertical muscle masses of either side of the spinous processes are the erector spinae. These muscles can be palpated from the occipital bone to the sacrum, and their symmetry and tone are important to any back examination. In the upright position and with normal alignment of the spine, there should be minimal activity in the erector spinae muscles and it should be equal from side to side. The muscles masses also should be equal in prominence. Any increase in tone or mass unilaterally may indicate the presence of a lateral curve.

The scapula and superficial muscles of the back are included as part of a back examination. The surface anatomy of those structures, however, is discussed with the upper limb.

Upper Limb

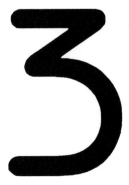

Organization of the Upper Limb

The upper limb is presented on a regional basis starting with the most proximal area and working distally. Although each region is considered as a unit and all appropriate anatomy are discussed, certain deviations from this pattern are necessary to reduce fragmentation and ensure continuity. For example, the locations of very few muscles are restricted to single regions, and muscles typically function to move segments distal to their locations. As a result, discussions of the bones and articulations typically precede discussions of the regions of which they are part. Structures that pass from region to region, the nerves and vessels, represent a challenge in a regional discussion. In this chapter the courses of these structures are described with each region, and the position from region to region is repeated. The potential injury points of nerves are indicated as the course of each nerve is described. Although the consequences of a muscle's loss are discussed with the description of each muscle, the results of nerve injuries are covered in the final section of the chapter.

Regions and Nomenclature

The **posterior cervical triangle** is included with the upper limb because it contains the major neurovascular structures that supply the limb. The general term **shoulder region** consists of the shoulder joint as well as the bones and muscles involved in its function. The bones of the **shoulder (pectoral) girdle,** the clavicle and scapula, are the foundation of the shoulder region. The shoulder region also includes the **pectoral** and **scapular regions,** which are, respectively, the anterior and posterior junctional regions between the upper limb and the trunk. The **deltoid region** is that area superficial to the deltoid muscle. The **axilla,** or **axillary re-**

gion, is also junctional; it is situated between the pectoral and scapular regions and between the lateral chest wall and the humerus. The **arm,** or **brachium** (the adjective is *brachial*), is the segment between the shoulder and elbow, and its single bone is the humerus. The **elbow** is the **cubitus,** and is generally referred to as the **cubital region.** The **forearm** is between the elbow and wrist and contains two bones, the **radius** and **ulna.** The forearm is the **antebrachium** (the adjective is *antebrachial*). The **wrist,** or **carpus,** contains the carpal bones and consists of the very small segment between the forearm and the hand. The **hand** is the **manus,** hence the term *manual.* Although the digits are numbered consecutively from the thumb to the little finger (1 through 5), the common terms **thumb, index, middle, ring,** and **little finger** will be used wherever possible. The **pollex** is the thumb, and the **digitus minimus,** the little finger.

Compartmentation of the Limb

Each limb is enclosed in a stockinglike layer of deep fascia that is found just deep to the superficial fascia (subcutaneous tissue). This **investing fascia** is connected to the deeper lying bones by **intermuscular septa;** each segment of limb is thereby partitioned into varying numbers of compartments. The muscles within a given compartment generally have similar functions and are innervated by a single peripheral nerve.

In the arm (Fig. 3-1A) the investing, or **brachial, fascia** is interconnected to the humerus by the **medial** and **lateral intermuscular septa,** and the resulting **anterior** and **posterior compartments** are easily defined. The muscles in the anterior compartment are the major flexors and supinators of the forearm, and they are innervated by the musculocutaneous nerve. The posterior compartment muscles produce forearm extension and are supplied by the radial nerve.

The forearm (Fig. 3-1B) also is divided into anterior and posterior compartments, but the arrangement is somewhat different and visualization of the separation can be quite difficult. The radius and ulna are interconnected by the interosseous membrane and are connected to the investing **antebrachial fascia** by the lateral and medial intermuscular septa, respectively. (The medial intermuscular septum is very short or nonexistent because the ulna is subcutaneous, and its periosteum blends with the antebrachial fascia.) The resulting compartments, however, are not truly anterior and posterior in location, and the position of the forearm—supination or pronation—can change the shape of the compartment. The **anterior compartment** is medial in the proximal part of the forearm and anterior at the wrist. The **posterior compartment** is lateral proximally and posterior distally. The anterior compartment muscles produce flexion of both the hand and digits along with pronation of the forearm. These muscles are supplied by the median and ulnar nerves. Contraction of the posterior muscles causes extension of the hand and digits and supination of the forearm. The radial nerve supplies all posterior muscles.

Although the hand contains a myriad of compartments and spaces, only those areas that contain muscles are considered compartments and are described here. The other spaces are described with the discussion of

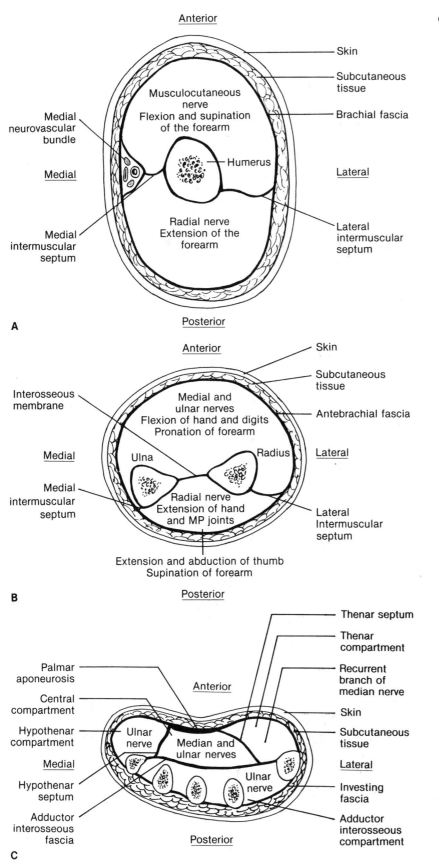

Figure 3-1
Cross sections of the arm (*A*), forearm (*B*), and hand (*C*), illustrating the formation of the compartments of each.

the hand. The compartments of the hand (Fig. 3-1C) are located in the palm and between the metacarpals. The **thenar** and **hypothenar compartments** are associated with the thumb and little finger, respectively. Each is formed by the investing fascia and a septum, the **thenar** and **hypothenar septum,** that extends from the investing fascia to the appropriate metacarpal. The thenar compartment muscles are innervated by the recurrent branch of the median nerve and produce motions of the thumb, particularly opposition. The hypothenar muscles are supplied by the ulnar nerve and produce movements of the little finger. A deep layer of fascia, the **adductor-interosseous fascia,** separates the central portion of the hand into **central** and **adductor-interosseous compartments.** The more superficial central compartment contains the lumbrical muscles, which function in flexion and extension of the digits and are innervated by branches of the median and ulnar nerves. The muscles in the adductor-interosseous compartment, which are located primarily between the metacarpals, are innervated by a branch of the ulnar nerve and function in producing adduction, abduction, flexion, and extension of the digits.

Superficial Structures

The superficial structures of the limb are found superficial to the investing fascia and include the superficial veins (Fig. 3-2) and the cutaneous

Figure 3-2
Anterior view of the superficial veins of the upper limb.

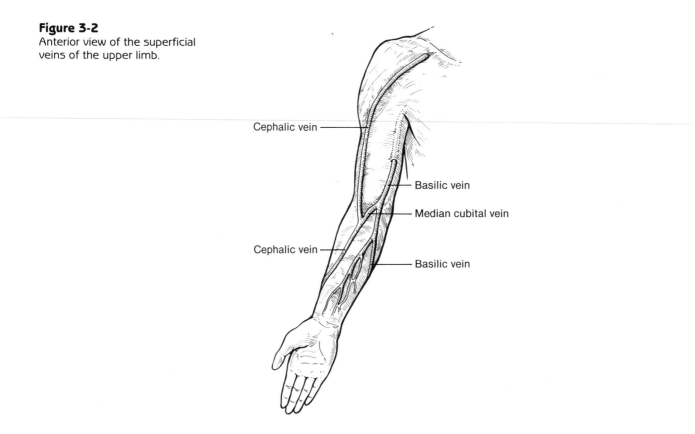

Cephalic vein

Basilic vein

Median cubital vein

Cephalic vein

Basilic vein

nerves (Fig. 3-55). A venous network on the dorsum of the hand gives rise to two venous networks, each of which is usually represented by a single prominent vein. The **basilic vein** ascends along the medial aspect of the forearm and typically passes through the investing fascia in the proximal part of the arm to join the brachial vein. The **cephalic vein** ascends along the lateral aspect of the forearm and arm and passes across the shoulder region in the groove that separates the pectoralis major and deltoid muscles. It joins the axillary vein just distal to the clavicle. These two veins are interconnected by the **median cubital vein,** which passes obliquely across the ventral aspect of the elbow, where it is commonly used for venipuncture. Although definitive veins are described, there occasionally are multiple veins representing each system.

Most cutaneous nerves are branches of the major peripheral nerves that innervate the upper limb. The locations of these cutaneous nerves are indicated in Figure 3-55. The **medial brachial** and **medial antebrachial cutaneous nerves,** which respectively innervate the skin of the medial arm and forearm, are direct branches of the brachial plexus. The lateral aspect of the proximal arm is innervated by the **superior lateral brachial cutaneous nerve,** a branch of the axillary nerve. The lateral forearm is supplied by the terminal portion of the musculocutaneous nerve, the **lateral antebrachial cutaneous nerve.** The remainder of the arm and forearm, mostly the posterior aspect, is innervated by the **posterior brachial** and **antebrachial cutaneous nerves,** respectively. These two nerves, along with the **inferior lateral brachial cutaneous nerve,** which supplies the lower lateral arm, are branches of the radial nerve. Both dorsally and ventrally the medial aspect of the hand is innervated by the ulnar nerve; the dorsolateral aspect, by the radial nerve; and the ventrolateral aspect, by the median nerve. A superficial injury that includes one of these cutaneous nerves results in a circumscribed loss of cutaneous sensibility but no involvement of muscles. Injury of a major peripheral nerve typically results in paralysis of a defined group of muscles as well as loss of sensation in the cutaneous areas supplied by the nerve's cutaneous branches.

Posterior Cervical Triangle

The posterior cervical triangle (posterior triangle of the neck) is included in this section because it contains the major neurovascular structures, the brachial plexus and subclavian artery, that supply the upper limb. These structures are vulnerable to mechanical interference as they pass through this region, and thus the area of the posterior triangle can be the source of considerable upper limb pathology.

Boundaries of the Posterior Cervical Triangle

The posterior cervical triangle (Fig. 3-3) is bounded anteriorly by the posterior border of the sternocleidomastoid muscle, posteriorly by the superior border of the trapezius muscle, and inferiorly by the middle third of the clavicle, which is the segment of bone between the attachments of the sternocleidomastoid and trapezius muscles. These boundaries can

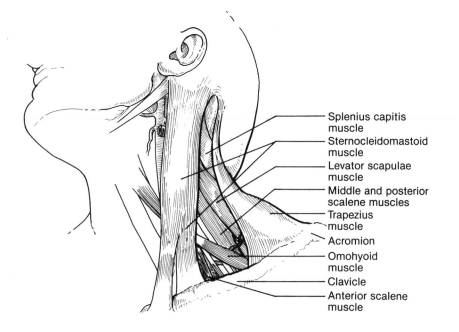

Figure 3-3
Posterior cervical triangle.

be identified easily by inspection and palpation; they are more obvious if the head is rotated to the contralateral side and the shoulder moved superiorly and anteriorly.

The floor of the posterior cervical triangle (Fig. 3-3) is muscular. The muscles extend from the cervical vertebrae to the upper ribs and scapula. From anterior to posterior these muscles are the anterior, middle, and posterior scalenes, and the levator scapulae. This floor is not complete because there is a gap, the **scalene groove,** between the anterior and middle scalene muscles. The floor typically is quite deep, and the structures that occupy this triangle are embedded in a loose connective tissue packing.

Contents of the Posterior Cervical Triangle

The proximal part of the **brachial plexus** (Fig. 3-4), the ventral rami (roots) and/or trunks, enters the triangle through the scalene groove and passes through the inferomedial aspect of the triangle before passing deep to the clavicle. The few branches that arise from this part of the plexus are described with the brachial plexus on page 64. The nerve trunks of the plexus are large and firm, and thus usually palpable in the inferomedial portion of the posterior triangle.

The **subclavian artery** enters the posterior triangle by arching over the first rib and passing through the scalene groove (Fig. 3-5). Its course through this triangle is very short as it follows the most inferior portion of the brachial plexus. This artery is usually palpable, and the subclavian pulse can be felt in the inferomedial aspect of the triangle in the angle formed by the first rib and sternocleidomastoid muscle. A branch may or may not arise from the artery in the triangle; if one does, it typically winds

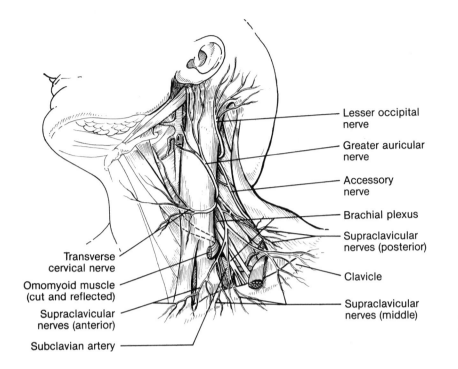

Lesser occipital nerve

Greater auricular nerve

Accessory nerve

Brachial plexus

Supraclavicular nerves (posterior)

Clavicle

Supraclavicular nerves (middle)

Transverse cervical nerve

Omomyoid muscle (cut and reflected)

Supraclavicular nerves (anterior)

Subclavian artery

Figure 3-4
Contents of the posterior cervical triangle.

Figure 3-5
Anterolateral view of the scalene triangle.

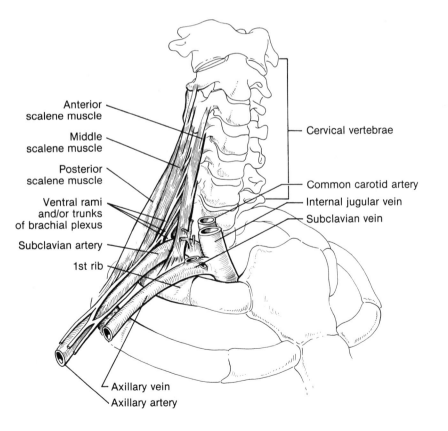

Anterior scalene muscle

Middle scalene muscle

Posterior scalene muscle

Ventral rami and/or trunks of brachial plexus

Subclavian artery

1st rib

Cervical vertebrae

Common carotid artery

Internal jugular vein

Subclavian vein

Axillary vein

Axillary artery

through the brachial plexus as it passes posterolaterally toward the shoulder.

The **accessory nerve** (Fig. 3-4) passes superficially across the posterior triangle of the neck. After passing through or deep to the sternocleidomastoid muscle, which it innervates, the accessory nerve emerges from the middle third of the muscle's posterior border. Its course through the triangle parallels a line connecting the ear lobe and the point of the shoulder. It disappears under the superior border of the trapezius muscle two to three centimeters from its clavicular attachment. The nerve's relatively superficial course makes it vulnerable to lacerations and blunt trauma. It is especially vulnerable to surgical approaches through the posterior triangle. It is also vulnerable to either compression or stretch by excessive use of heavy backpacks.

From their origins from the ventral rami of the upper cervical spinal nerves, the **cutaneous branches of the cervical plexus** (Fig. 3-4) enter the subcutaneous tissue just posterior to the middle third of the sterno-cleidomastoid muscle. From that point each of the four nerves travels a different course, supplying the skin of the anterolateral neck, and the occipital, supraclavicular, and shoulder regions. The **lesser occipital nerve** ascends along the posterior border of the sternocleidomastoid muscle; the **greater auricular nerve** ascends obliquely across the same muscle toward the ear; the **transverse cervical nerve** passes horizontally across the muscle toward the anterior neck; the **anterior, middle,** and **posterior supraclavicular nerves** descend across the posterior triangle toward the clavicular and shoulder regions.

Multiple lymph nodes, all of which are along the tributaries to the lower deep cervical lymph nodes, are found within the posterior triangle. The inferior belly of the **omohyoid muscle,** an infrahyoid muscle, passes across the inferolateral aspect of the triangle.

Scalene Triangle

The scalene triangle (Fig. 3-5) is the interval in the floor of the posterior triangle that is formed anteriorly by the anterior scalene muscle, posteriorly by the middle scalene muscle, and inferiorly by a small portion of the first rib. The base of this triangle is quite small, so the term **scalene groove** may be more descriptive. The significance of the scalene triangle is related to the vulnerability of the structures that pass through it; both the roots or trunks of the brachial plexus and the subclavian artery are vulnerable to potential mechanical pressure from the borders of the triangle or from other structures.

The more inferior structures in the triangle, the inferior trunk of the brachial plexus and the subclavian artery, appear to be more susceptible to pressure than the middle or superior trunks. Their vulnerability may be related to their locations adjacent to the bone, or perhaps their arching courses across the first rib make them particularly susceptible to tension exerted by the dependent limb. Hypertrophy of the scalene muscles, sharp fibrous bands associated with the scalene attachments to the first rib, and developmental variations have all been implicated as potential hazards. The presence of a cervical rib, whether partial or complete, usually reduces the vertical dimension of the triangle and clearly has been identified as the cause of symptomology. The presence of an additional muscle, the scalene minimus, is quite frequent, and, although its position is variable, it usually reduces the size of the triangle.

Although all of the above are thought to be potential causes of the anterior scalene syndrome (thoracic outlet, scalenus anticus), the cause-and-effect relationship between a cervical rib and the symptoms has been documented most consistently. Posture clearly is an important consideration; in fact, much conservative management addresses that issue first.

The size of the scalene triangle can be reduced by utilizing Adson's maneuver. This maneuver includes rotation of the head to the ipsilateral side and extension of the cervical spine, followed by a deep breath. The rotation and extension reduce the width (anteroposteriorly) of the triangle; and the deep breath elevates the first rib, which further narrows the width of the triangle as the scalene muscles contract. During this maneuver, inferior traction is placed on the upper limb and the radial pulse is palpated to provide a means of monitoring constriction of the subclavian artery. The efficacy of this maneuver as a diagnostic tool should be questioned, however, because loss of the radial pulse commonly accompanies this maneuver in people who are asymptomatic.

Axilla

Boundaries of the Axilla

The **axilla** (Fig. 3-6), or axillary region, is the junctional region between the thorax and upper limb that transmits the large nerve trunks and vessels that supply the limb. Although quite irregular in shape, the axilla can be compared to a pyramid. It does have four sides, but they are very unequal in size and shape. As this area is visualized it is important to remember that the floor is convex superiorly, its sides are tall and tapering, and it is directed superomedially toward its apex, which is not closed but open to the inferior aspect of the posterior triangle.

The anterior wall of the axilla is entirely muscular and consists of the pectoralis major and minor muscles. The posterior wall is formed by the subscapularis muscle, which covers the ventral aspect of the scapula and portions of both the latissimus dorsi and teres major muscles. The humeral attachments of these three muscles are separated from that of the pectoralis major by a narrow strip of humerus, the intertubercular groove. This thin strip of bone is commonly considered the lateral wall of the axilla. The medial wall is the muscular covering of the lateral thoracic wall, the serratus anterior. The dome-shaped floor is a strong fascial layer, the axillary fascia, that is continuous with the fascial layers of the axillary walls—that is, the latissimus dorsi and pectoral muscles, the lateral chest wall, and the investing fascia of the arm. The anterior, medial, and posterior walls converge superomedially to form the apex, which in reality is a narrow channel between the clavicle, first rib, and superior border of the scapula.

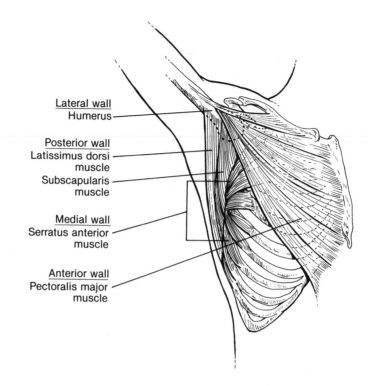

Lateral wall
Humerus

Posterior wall
Latissimus dorsi
muscle
Subscapularis
muscle

Medial wall
Serratus anterior
muscle

Anterior wall
Pectoralis major
muscle

Figure 3-6
Anterolateral and inferior view of
the structures forming the axilla.
The humerus is abducted.

Contents of the Axilla

The brachial plexus and subclavian artery (the latter becomes the axillary artery as it crosses the first rib) enter the axilla from the posterior triangle where they are joined by the axillary vein. These structures are enclosed in a sleeve of fascia, the **axillary sheath,** which is continuous with the prevertebral layer of cervical fascia. The axilla also contains multiple lymph nodes that filter lymphatic fluid from the entire upper limb as well as the scapular and pectoral regions, including the breast. All lymphatic fluid from the upper limb drains through the most superior or apical nodes before passing proximally. All structures in the axilla are embedded in fatty connective tissue.

The **axillary artery** (Figs. 3-5, 3-7) is the direct continuation of the subclavian artery, extending from the first rib to the inferior border of the teres major muscle where it becomes the brachial artery. The artery passes posterior to the pectoralis minor muscle and is separated into three parts relative to that muscle: The first part is proximal; the second, posterior; and the third, distal. The vessel is ensheathed in the same connective tissue bundle as the axillary vein and brachial plexus, and it is surrounded by the plexus throughout most of its length. Its branches supply the pectoral, scapular, and shoulder regions. Although variable in number, the typical branches are the supreme thoracic, thoracoacromial, lateral thoracic, subscapular, and humeral circumflex arteries. The **supreme thoracic artery** is a small branch that descends a short distance along the thoracic wall. The **thoracoacromial artery** has branches that supply the

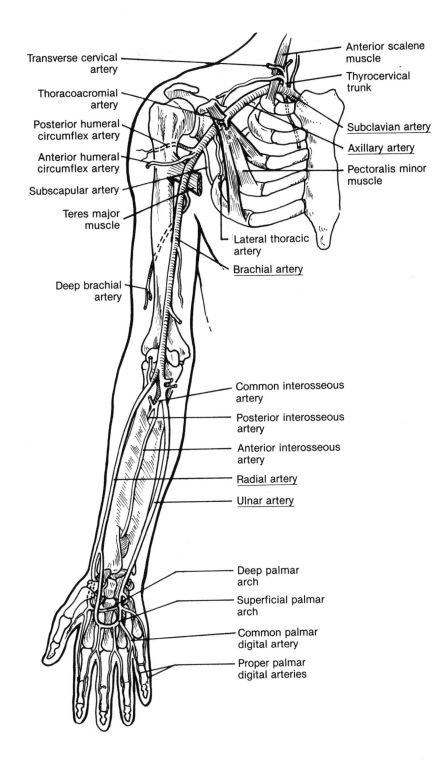

Transverse cervical artery

Thoracoacromial artery

Posterior humeral circumflex artery

Anterior humeral circumflex artery

Subscapular artery

Teres major muscle

Deep brachial artery

Anterior scalene muscle

Thyrocervical trunk

Subclavian artery

Axillary artery

Pectoralis minor muscle

Lateral thoracic artery

Brachial artery

Common interosseous artery

Posterior interosseous artery

Anterior interosseous artery

Radial artery

Ulnar artery

Deep palmar arch

Superficial palmar arch

Common palmar digital artery

Proper palmar digital arteries

Figure 3-7
Summary of the arterial supply of the upper limb.

clavicular, pectoral, deltoid, and acromial regions. The **lateral thoracic artery** descends along the anterolateral aspect of the thoracic wall somewhat lateral to the pectoralis minor muscle. The large **subscapular artery** branches into the **circumflex scapular artery,** which passes around the axillary border of the scapula, and the **thoracodorsal artery,** which descends on the deep surface of the latissimus dorsi muscle with the thoracodorsal nerve. The **anterior** and **posterior humeral circumflex arteries** are typically the most distal branches and arise at the level of the surgical neck of the humerus. Each branch passes around the surgical neck, with the larger posterior vessel accompanying the axillary nerve. The suprascapular and transverse cervical branches of the subclavian artery and the subscapular branch of the axillary artery form potential anastomoses around the scapula within the substance of its muscles. This area of anastomosis is a potential alternate route around the distal portion of the subclavian artery and the proximal portion of the axillary artery, an area that is vulnerable to thrombosis that can result from stretching trauma of the vessel, as might occur when the upper limb is forcibly and excessively abducted.

Brachial Plexus

Formation of the brachial plexus.   The brachial plexus (Fig. 3-8) is the somatic plexus that gives rise to the peripheral nerves that innervate the upper limb. Its component nerve fibers are derived from spinal cord segments C5 through T1. On occasion there is a large contribution from spinal cord segment C4 and very little from T1, a prefixed brachial plexus. The reverse, a plexus arising from segments C6 through T2, is a postfixed brachial plexus. From proximal to distal, the plexus consists of the **ventral rami,** which contribute to the plexus, the **trunks,** the **divisions,** the **cords,** and the **terminal peripheral nerves. Smaller branches** arise from the plexus proper and supply muscles in the shoulder region. The formation of the plexus extends from the posterior cervical triangle well into the axillary region; small branches arise from the plexus in both the posterior triangle and the axilla, but the terminal nerves begin only in the axilla.

After branching from the spinal nerves, the ventral rami pass laterally through the scalene triangle. The ventral rami of C5 and C6 join to form the **superior trunk,** the ventral ramus of C7 continues as the **middle trunk,** and the C8 and T1 rami join to form the **inferior trunk.** Each of the trunks then branches into **anterior** and **posterior divisions.** This branching is significant because terminal nerves derived from cords formed by anterior divisions innervate the muscles in anterior compartments of the limb, and posterior division nerves innervate posterior compartment muscles. The posterior divisions from all three trunks converge to form the **posterior cord.** The anterior divisions of the superior and middle trunks form the **lateral cord,** while that of the inferior trunk becomes the **medial cord.** The cords surround the second part of the axillary artery and are named on the basis of their relationships with that vessel.

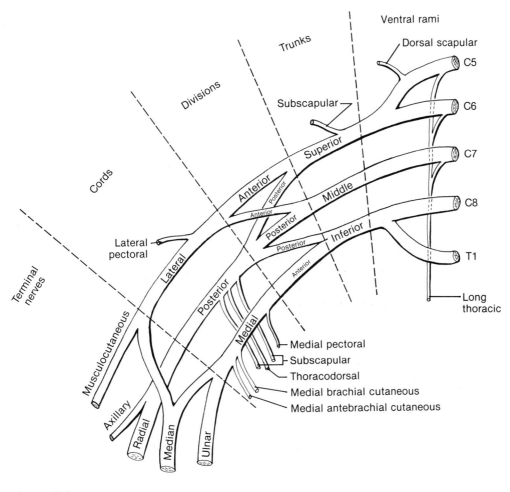

Figure 3-8
Organization of the brachial plexus.

The posterior cord typically branches most proximally so that the **radial** and **axillary nerves** are formed high in the axilla. The medial and lateral cords branch in a pattern that resembles the letter **M**, giving rise to the **median, ulnar,** and **musculocutaneous nerves.** The median nerve is formed on the anterior aspect of the axillary artery by contributions from both the medial and lateral cords. The ulnar and musculocutaneous nerves are the continuations of the medial and lateral cords, respectively.

It is important to note that the segmental content of the peripheral nerves is rather constant, as is the branching pattern that forms the nerves. However, the branchings and fusions may occur more proximally or distally than indicated in illustrations, or a single interconnection may be multiple. The end result of the plexus, however, is quite predictable.

On the other hand, even though the specific segmental content of a given peripheral nerve is predictable, it is not necessarily logical on the basis of the branching pattern of the brachial plexus. The axillary nerve is a good example. This nerve is a branch of the posterior cord that is formed by the posterior divisions of all three trunks, which in turn are composed of the ventral rami of spinal nerves C5 through T1. The posterior cord thus contains nerve fibers from all five spinal cord segments and, although it would be logical to assume that the axillary nerve contains fibers from the same number of segments, it does not. It contains fibers from spinal cord segments C5 and C6 only. As will be evident in the section covering lesions of the brachial plexus, an understanding of both the formation of the brachial plexus and the segmental content of its terminal nerves is essential to the understanding of the symptoms and locations of various lesions.

Smaller branches of the brachial plexus. The majority of the smaller branches of the brachial plexus innervate both the intrinsic and extrinsic muscles of the shoulder, others innervate cutaneous areas. The **dorsal scapular** and **long thoracic** nerves branch from the ventral rami. The dorsal scapular nerve arises from the C5 ventral ramus proximal to the scalene triangle. It passes posteriorly and inferiorly, typically piercing the middle scalene muscle and then passing deep to the levator scapulae and rhomboid muscles, which it innervates. Its innervation of the levator scapulae is variable. The long thoracic nerve is formed by branches of the C5, C6, and C7 ventral rami. These branches join posterior to the trunks of the plexus and form a single nerve that descends along the lateral aspect of the thoracic wall on the surface of the serratus anterior muscle, which it innervates. Its course is long and, since it sends a branch to each serration of the muscle, it is anchored firmly to the lateral chest wall. Since this nerve is fixed throughout its course, it is vulnerable to stretching injuries during extreme motion (abduction) of the shoulder; it also is vulnerable to the surgeon's knife during radical dissection procedures in the axillary region.

The **suprascapular nerve** is the only branch of any of the trunks of the brachial plexus. It branches from the superior trunk and passes inferiorly, laterally, and somewhat posteriorly before going deep to the trapezius muscle. It is joined by the suprascapular vessels as it passes toward the scapular notch on the superolateral aspect of the scapula. The nerve passes through the **scapular foramen,** the supraspinous fossa, and around the neck of the spine of the scapula. It innervates both the supraspinatus and infraspinatus muscles, and provides a sensory branch to the posterior and lateral aspects of the shoulder joint capsule. This nerve may well be a major source of pain that accompanies shoulder joint pathology, or in fact the cause of certain problems such as adhesive capsulitis. It is vulnerable to entrapment as it passes through the scapular foramen. The course of the nerve is short and the nerve is taut. As the scapula moves, particularly during extreme motions, the nerve pistons back and forth through the scapular foramen. The foramen is small relative to the size of the nerve, and its edges are sharp. If the nerve becomes inflamed, it is more sensitive and more vulnerable to impingement. Movement thus produces pain, which in turn is apt to limit motion.

Multiple branches arise from the cords of the brachial plexus. The **medial** and **lateral pectoral nerves** branch from the proximal portions, respectively, of the medial and lateral cords. These two nerves, usually interconnected, pass anteriorly directly into the deep aspects of the pectoral muscles. Both nerves innervate the pectoralis major muscle, but only the medial pectoral supplies the pectoralis minor. A number of **subscapular nerves** arise from the posterior cord, which is situated on the ventral aspect of the subscapularis muscle. Although three such nerves are described, more may be present. The **upper subscapular** nerve passes directly into the subscapularis muscle; the **lower subscapular** nerve supplies the teres major as well as the subscapularis. The **middle subscapular** nerve, which is almost always a single nerve, is called the **thoracodorsal nerve.** It descends along the lateral border of the scapula in company with the thoracodorsal artery and enters the deep aspect of the latissimus dorsi muscle, which it innervates. The **medial brachial** and **antebrachial cutaneous nerves** arise from the distal portion of the medial cord. Each descends through the medial aspect of the limb to supply the skin of the medial arm and forearm, respectively.

Thoracic outlet syndrome. The brachial plexus is thought to be vulnerable to entrapment (either compression or stretch) at various points (Fig. 3-9). Its relationship to the scalene triangle and the first rib was discussed previously. As the plexus exits from the posterior triangle, it passes between the clavicle and the first rib. This bony interval is a potential hazard because the nerve trunks or axillary vessels can be compressed by the viselike action of the bones. The interval between the two bones is smaller medially than laterally, and as the clavicle is depressed, or the rib cage elevated, the space becomes even smaller. Since the axillary vein is medial to the axillary artery and the brachial plexus, it passes

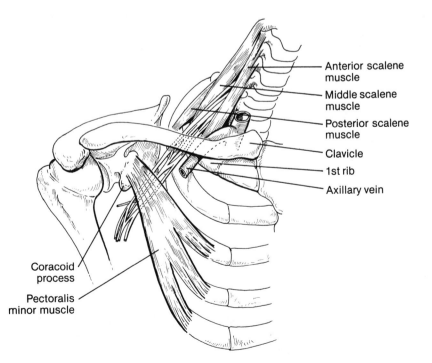

Anterior scalene muscle

Middle scalene muscle

Posterior scalene muscle

Clavicle

1st rib

Axillary vein

Coracoid process

Pectoralis minor muscle

Figure 3-9
Anterior view of the brachial plexus indicating its location and relationships in both the posterior cervical triangle and the axilla.

through the narrowest portion of the interval. As a result, it presumably is more vulnerable to compression at that point than either the plexus or the artery. More laterally, the neurovascular bundle passes inferior to the coracoid process and posterior to the pectoralis minor muscle, which attaches to the coracoid. During extreme excursions of the upper limb, especially abduction and external rotation at the shoulder, the brachial plexus is stretched around the coracoid where it is thought to be vulnerable to stretching injuries. The types of lesions described here (as well as those described with the scalene triangle) commonly fall under the general diagnosis of **thoracic outlet syndrome.** Although the anatomic rationale for entrapment at these various points might seem quite plausible, a clear cause frequently is difficult to substantiate because of the multiple potential points of involvement.

Symptoms of brachial plexus injury.   The symptoms involving lesions of the brachial plexus obviously differ depending on the location of the lesion. However, it is helpful to compare a lesion of a ventral ramus (preplexus injury) and one of a terminal nerve (postplexus injury). Ventral ramus C6 and the axillary nerve are convenient examples. As discussed in the introduction to somatic plexuses, the nerve fibers from spinal cord segment C6 (or any other segment involved in the formation of a somatic plexus) are distributed to multiple peripheral nerves, and the axillary nerve contains fibers from more than one spinal cord segment. Specifically, nerve fibers from spinal cord segment C6 are found in the axillary, radial, musculocutaneous, and median nerves. The axillary nerve contains fibers from segments C5 and C6. The axillary nerve supplies the teres minor and deltoid muscles and a small patch of skin in the region of the insertion of the deltoid muscle. Loss of the axillary nerve causes an absolute paralysis of the two muscles and anesthesia of the indicated area of skin. The loss is complete and restricted to a limited area. The nerve fibers in the ventral ramus of spinal nerve C6 partially supply many muscles, including the teres minor and deltoid, and some skin of the lateral forearm. Loss of the C6 ventral ramus causes weakness in the teres minor and deltoid muscles (as well as in many others) and a potential anesthesia of the skin of the lateral forearm. (The area of anesthesia is somewhat variable because of dermatomal overlap.) This loss is partial but widespread. Knowledge and understanding of the brachial plexus is necessary to localize the site of a lesion given the symptoms; it also permits anticipation of symptoms given the site of the lesion.

Shoulder Region

Bones of the Shoulder Region

Scapula.   The **scapula** (Fig. 3-10) is an irregularly shaped flat bone that is basically triangular in shape. Its slightly concave **costal (ventral) surface** fits against the posterosuperior aspect of the thoracic wall, and, except for certain of its prominences, it is covered by the muscles that use it for attachment. It is positioned so that its base, the **superior border,**

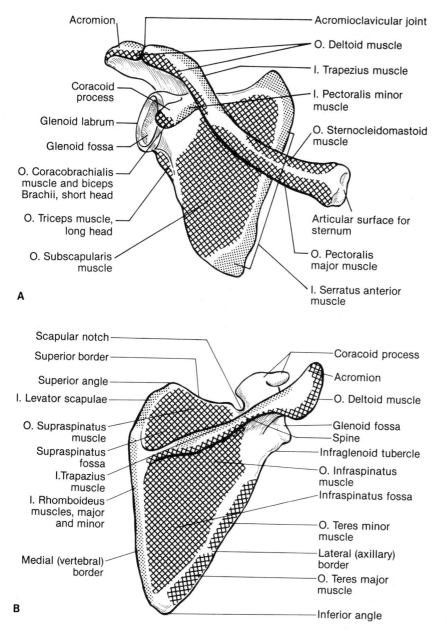

Acromion

Acromioclavicular joint

O. Deltoid muscle

I. Trapezius muscle

Coracoid process

I. Pectoralis minor muscle

Glenoid labrum

O. Sternocleidomastoid muscle

Glenoid fossa

O. Coracobrachialis muscle and biceps Brachii, short head

O. Triceps muscle, long head

Articular surface for sternum

O. Subscapularis muscle

O. Pectoralis major muscle

I. Serratus anterior muscle

A

Scapular notch

Superior border

Superior angle

I. Levator scapulae

Coracoid process

Acromion

O. Deltoid muscle

O. Supraspinatus muscle

Supraspinatus fossa

Glenoid fossa

Spine

Infraglenoid tubercle

I. Trapazius muscle

O. Infraspinatus muscle

I. Rhomboideus muscles, major and minor

Infraspinatus fossa

O. Teres minor muscle

Medial (vertebral) border

Lateral (axillary) border

O. Teres major muscle

B

Inferior angle

Figure 3-10
Anterior view of the right scapula and clavicle (*A*); posterior view of the right scapula (*B*). The areas of muscle origin are indicated by crosshatch, and insertions by stipple.

is superior and its apex, its **inferior angle,** is directed inferiorly. The **medial (vertebral) border** joins the superior border at the **superior angle;** the **lateral (axillary) border** joins the superior border at the **lateral angle,** which is the **glenoid cavity.**

The **spine** of the scapula projects posteriorly from the dorsal surface, separating the **supraspinatus** and **infraspinatus fossae.** The spine is obliquely oriented so that from its base at the medial border it extends

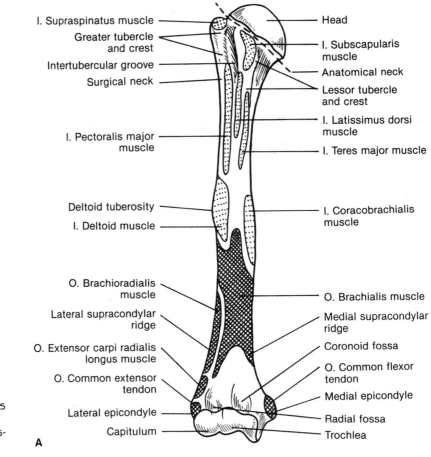

I. Supraspinatus muscle

Greater tubercle and crest

Intertubercular groove

Surgical neck

I. Pectoralis major muscle

Deltoid tuberosity

I. Deltoid muscle

O. Brachioradialis muscle

Lateral supracondylar ridge

O. Extensor carpi radialis longus muscle

O. Common extensor tendon

Lateral epicondyle

Capitulum

Head

I. Subscapularis muscle

Anatomical neck

Lessor tubercle and crest

I. Latissimus dorsi muscle

I. Teres major muscle

I. Coracobrachialis muscle

O. Brachialis muscle

Medial supracondylar ridge

Coronoid fossa

O. Common flexor tendon

Medial epicondyle

Radial fossa

Trochlea

A

Figure 3-11
Anterior (*A*) and posterior (*B*) views of the right humerus. Areas of muscle origin are indicated by cross-hatch, and insertions by stipple.

superolaterally toward the lateral angle and ends as the expanded **acromion process,** the bony point of the shoulder. The **coracoid process** projects anteriorly and then laterally from the lateral aspect of the superior border of the scapula. The **scapular notch** indents the superior border just medial to the coracoid process.

The glenoid cavity is the articular surface that forms the shoulder joint. It is important to note that this surface is directed somewhat anterolaterally, a factor that presumably contributes to anterior dislocation of the shoulder. The roughened areas just superior and inferior to the glenoid cavity are the **supraglenoid** and **infraglenoid tubercles,** respectively.

Clavicle. The **clavicle** (Fig. 3-10) represents the only bony link, through the sternoclavicular and acromioclavicular joints, between the upper limb and the axial skeleton. The medial half of this bone is convex anteriorly, the lateral half concave. Since this is the only bony link between the limb and axial skeleton, all force transmitted proximally through the limb must pass through this bone. The junction between the lateral and middle thirds of the bone is its most acute bend and hence

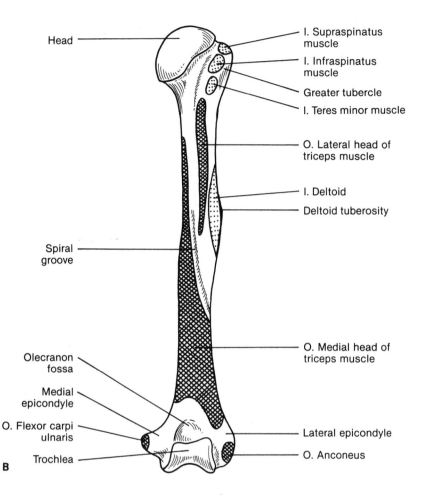

Head

I. Supraspinatus muscle

I. Infraspinatus muscle

Greater tubercle

I. Teres minor muscle

O. Lateral head of triceps muscle

I. Deltoid

Deltoid tuberosity

Spiral groove

O. Medial head of triceps muscle

Olecranon fossa

Medial epicondyle

O. Flexor carpi ulnaris

Trochlea

Lateral epicondyle

O. Anconeus

B

the area where proximally directed force must change direction most dramatically. That point is the most common fracture site in the body.

The medial end of the clavicle is expanded and covered with articular surface, and it articulates with the manubrium of the sternum. The lateral third of the bone is flattened and has a small articular surface that articulates with the acromion. The two prominences that project from the inferior surface of the bone's lateral aspect, the **conoid tubercle** and **trapezoid line,** provide the attachments for the two portions of the coracoclavicular ligament.

Humerus. The **humerus** (Fig. 3-11) is the only bone in the arm and thus participates in the formation of both the shoulder and elbow joints. Its proximal end consists of the rounded **head** and the **greater** and **lesser tubercles.** The lesser tubercle is smaller and projects anteriorly. The larger, greater tubercle is situated superiorly and laterally. The tubercles are separated by the **intertubercular groove,** which is bordered inferior to the tubercles by the **crests of the greater and lesser tubercles.** The head and tubercles are separated by the **anatomic neck;** the proximal part of the humerus joins the shaft at the **surgical neck.** The surgical neck is not an anatomic structure but rather the location of most of the proximal shaft fractures of the humerus.

At about the midshaft level of the humerus the **deltoid tuberosity** projects laterally. The **sulcus for the radial nerve** (spiral groove), a rather subtle indentation, descends posteriorly and then laterally around the midshaft region and the deltoid tuberosity. Midshaft fractures tend to follow the spiral of this groove.

The distal portion of the shaft of the humerus, the **supracondylar** area, flattens anteroposteriorly and widens medially and laterally into the **medial** and **lateral supracondylar ridges.** This distal portion of the humerus is inclined anteriorly, and in supracondylar fractures this inclination is typically reversed. The ridges end inferiorly in the **medial** and **lateral epicondyles.** The medial epicondyle is the more prominent and is notched posteriorly and inferiorly by an **ulnar nerve sulcus.** The distal aspect of the humerus has two articular surfaces: the medial **trochlea** and the lateral **capitulum.** The central portion of the supracondylar part of the humerus is thinned by depressions both anteriorly and posteriorly, the **coronoid** and **olecranon fossae,** respectively, which accommodate the coronoid and olecranon processes of the ulna in full motion.

Articulations of the Shoulder Region

Shoulder (glenohumeral) joint. The **shoulder (glenohumeral) joint** (Figs. 3-12 through 3-14) is formed by the articulation of the head of the humerus and the glenoid cavity of the scapula. Both the shapes and the

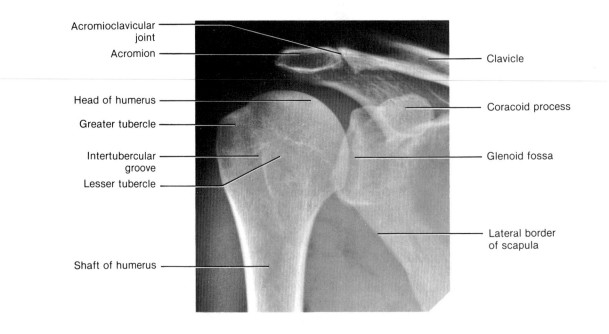

Figure 3-12
Anteroposterior radiograph of the shoulder joint.

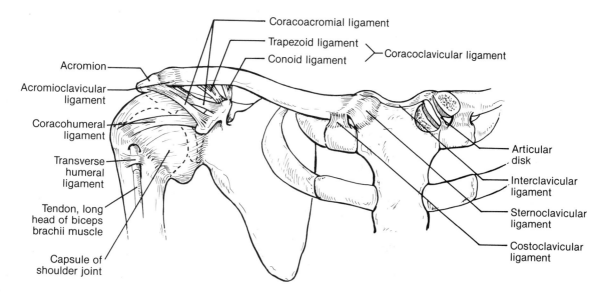

Figure 3-13
Anterior view of the glenohumeral, acromioclavicular, and sternoclavicular
joints and certain of their supporting ligaments.

sizes of the two articular surfaces are considerably different. The glenoid
cavity is small and quite shallow, while the humeral head is much more
curved and larger in surface area. In any position of the arm, the area of
contact between the two bones is small and of virtually no consequence
relative to support or stabilization of the joint. Any motion between the
two bones involves the gliding of the humeral head on the relatively small
glenoid surface. Since the surface area of the humeral head is relatively
extensive, a large amount of motion is available; and since the humeral

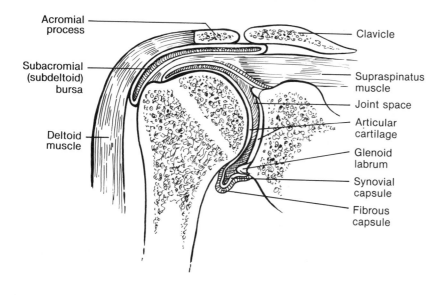

Figure 3-14
Coronal section through the glenohumeral joint and the suprahumeral
space.

head is a portion of a sphere, motion is available in all directions. The shapes of the bony surfaces that form this joint ensure maximal mobility at the expense of stability.

The glenoid cavity is deepened and enlarged by the **glenoid labrum,** a fibrocartilaginous lip that attaches to the periphery of the cavity. This labrum increases the congruency between the two surfaces but adds little support to the joint.

The **capsule of the glenohumeral joint** (Figs. 3-13, 3-14) extends from the edge of the glenoid cavity and the labrum to the anatomic neck of the humerus. This capsule in and of itself provides very little support to the joint. In fact, if all muscles that cross the shoulder joint were removed, the two bones literally would fall apart. The capsule not only is thin, it is also loose. In most positions of the arm a part of the capsule is loose and even redundant. For example, in the anatomic position the superior part of the capsule is taut, but the inferior part is very loose and hangs in folds. As the arm is elevated or abducted, the situation reverses: The inferior aspect of the capsule tightens, while the superior aspect loosens and is thrown into folds. This looseness of the capsule is essential for full motion. Inactivity or a reduction of motion at the shoulder joint can lead to a reduction in the motion available because of shortening of the capsule. It is essential that the joint capsule be stretched on a regular basis, particularly the redundant inferior portion.

Several ligaments are associated with the joint capsule. The **coracohumeral ligament** (Fig. 3-13) is an anterior thickening of the capsule that interconnects the base of the coracoid process and the anterosuperior aspect of the anatomic neck of the humerus. This ligament is somewhat obliquely oriented and may assist in maintaining the position of the humerus when the arm is at the side. A "shelf mechanism" has been proposed to explain the support of the shoulder joint when the limb is unloaded and at the side. In the anatomic position the inferior aspect of the glenoid cavity, most likely the inferior portion of the glenoid labrum, is lateral to the superior aspect. In this position the superior portion of the articular capsule and the coracohumeral ligament are taut; the proposal is that these ligaments hold the humeral head on the inferior lip of the glenoid cavity. This theory is supported by electromyographic studies that show a lack of activity in the intrinsic muscles of the shoulder, particularly the supraspinatus. As soon as motion occurs or the limb is loaded, the mechanism is destroyed and the intrinsic muscles become active. The **glenohumeral ligaments** are variably developed ligaments associated with the anterior aspect of the capsule and typically are visible from the joint cavity. However, they are of questionable functional value.

The synovial cavity of the glenohumeral joint generally is limited to the area within the joint capsule. A common but variable extension of the joint capsule is a communication with the **subscapular bursa,** which is deep to the tendon of the subscapularis muscle. This bursa is anterior and medial to the joint; and if the communication between bursa and joint is large, the humeral head may be more prone to anterior dislocation. A superior communication between the synovial cavity and the **subacromial (subdeltoid) bursa** is not normally present.

The tendon of the long head of the biceps brachii muscle occupies the intertubercular groove and passes across the joint space to attach to the supraglenoid tubercle. The synovial layer of the capsule forms a sheath around this tendon that extends from the tendon's attachment distally into the intertubercular groove, where both tendon and sheath are held in place by the **transverse humeral ligament** (Fig. 3-13). Since the tendon is ensheathed by the synovial layer of the capsule, it is not in contact with the synovial fluid.

The shoulder joint is a very loosely constructed ball-and-socket arrangement that permits motion in an infinite number of planes around an infinite number of axes. The motions described, however, are those that occur in the cardinal planes of the body. **Flexion** and **extension** occur in the sagittal plane, flexion occurring as the arm moves anteriorly to the overhead position and extension occurring with the reverse motion. Extension beyond the plane of the body is sometimes referred to as **hyperextension. Abduction** and **adduction** take place in the coronal plane, abduction occurring as the entire limb moves laterally to the vertical position and adduction occurring when the limb is returned to the side. **Circumduction** of the humerus is rotation around its fixed proximal end, and **rotation** is rotation around its long axis. Rotation is termed **medial,** or **internal,** and **lateral,** or **external.** Motion anteriorly across the chest is sometimes referred to as **horizontal adduction,** while the reverse would be **horizontal abduction.** In reality, motion at the shoulder joint seldom is limited to these specific planes but is a complex combination of several motions.

Dislocation of the shoulder joint is quite common; most commonly the head of the humerus passes anteroinferiorly and lodges in the infraclavicular fossa, which is inferior to the lateral aspect of the clavicle. This is an anterior dislocation of the shoulder. Several anatomic factors predispose this injury. The looseness of the joint capsule and the common communication between the joint space and the subscapularis bursa were mentioned previously. Muscular support of the shoulder joint essentially is absent inferiorly, and the glenoid labrum provides only a minimal barrier against a sliding humeral head. The etiological motions that produce the initial dislocation usually are predictable: A patient frequently recalls falling forward and trying to break the fall with outstretched upper limbs. At the time of impact the humerus is forcibly externally rotated and extended; the humeral head slides anteriorly and inferiorly across the glenoid cavity and is forced against the anteroinferior aspect of the joint capsule. The region of the surgical neck may contact the acromion process, which then becomes a fulcrum, and the humeral head is thus propelled across the glenoid cavity with greater force. The joint capsule is usually torn or stretched, also, the labrum may be torn.

Sternoclavicular joint. The **sternoclavicular joint** (Fig. 3-13) is a synovial joint formed between the cylindrical and flattened medial end of the clavicle and the superolateral aspect of the manubrium of the sternum. The joint contains an **articular disk,** which is usually complete so that two separate joint spaces exist. This disk has an important functional value in that it strongly reinforces the joint. The disk attaches superomedially to the upper aspect of the sternal end of the clavicle and inferolaterally to the first costal cartilage. The disk thus resists any force that tends to dislocate the clavicle medially. The presence of the disk also increases the distance between the two articular surfaces; the result is an increase in the amount of motion available between the clavicle and the sternum. The joint is reinforced by the **anterior** and **posterior sternoclavicular ligaments,** an **interclavicular ligament,** and the **costoclavicular ligament.** The motion available is that of a restricted ball and socket joint. The lateral end of the clavicle can move anteriorly (protraction) and posteriorly (retraction), superiorly (elevation) and inferiorly (depression); the bone also can rotate around its long axis. Because of the curved shape of the clavicle, posterior rotation results in elevation of its lateral aspect. This is known as the "crank-handle" mechanism.

Acromioclavicular joint. The **acromioclavicular joint** (Figs. 3-12, 3-13) is a junction between the lateral end of the clavicle and the anteromedial aspect of the acromion process. This joint usually contains an articular disk, frequently incomplete. Although a synovial articulation, very little motion occurs between the two bones. The joint capsule is thin and somewhat loose so that a small amount of sliding is permitted between the articular surfaces. The main stabilization is provided by the **coracoclavicular ligament,** which consists of two separate ligaments, the **conoid** and **trapezoid ligaments,** that interconnect the clavicle and the coracoid process. These ligaments are strong and ensure that the relationship between the scapula and clavicle is maintained statically and during motion. Since the fibers of the conoid ligament are oriented vertically, it prevents vertical separation of the clavicle and scapula. The trapezoid ligament, consisting of oblique fibers that pass laterally from coracoid to clavicle, resists medial displacement of the scapula relative to the clavicle. The acromioclavicular joint is marked on the surface by a slight elevation or a small "step"; the acromion is somewhat inferior to the lateral end of the clavicle. A marked step-off usually indicates a **shoulder separation** (dislocated acromioclavicular joint), which usually results from a forceful downward blow on the point of the shoulder that separates (depresses) the scapula from the clavicle.

Thoracoscapular articulation. The **thoracoscapular articulation** is a misnomer because there is no true anatomic articulation between the scapula and the posterolateral thoracic wall. However, the scapula must move on the thoracic wall if full motion of the shoulder region is to occur. The only bony connection between the scapula and the axial skeleton is through the clavicle via the sternoclavicular and acromioclavicular articulations. Otherwise, the **extrinsic muscles of the shoulder** both maintain the position of the scapula and produce its movement. The major control of the scapula is provided by the trapezius and serratus anterior muscles. Although the movement of the scapula is seldom of a single kind, specific motions are generally defined. The scapula can slide laterally (**abduction** or **protraction**) and medially (**adduction** or **retraction**); also it can be **elevated** or **depressed.** Rotation of the scapula occurs around an anteroposterior axis just below the middle of the spine, and the direction the lateral angle moves determines whether it is **superior (upward)** or **infe-**

rior (downward) rotation. It is important to note that the orientation of the glenoid cavity changes when the scapula either is abducted or rotated superiorly. With abduction, the scapula slides anteriorly as well as laterally and the glenoid cavity faces more and more anteriorly. With superior rotation, the glenoid faces superiorly.

Extrinsic Muscles of the Shoulder

The extrinsic muscles of the shoulder include the superficial muscles of the back and the pectoralis major and minor muscles. All of these muscles arise from the axial skeleton and insert on the scapula, clavicle, or humerus. This group of muscles functions to stabilize and move the shoulder girdle; two of these muscles cross the shoulder joint and thus move the humerus. Overall, these muscles move and stabilize the scapula and thus provide maximal mobility of the hand while providing a firm base on which the arm, forearm, and hand function. With one exception, the trapezius, they are innervated by the small branches of the brachial plexus.

The **trapezius muscle** (Figs. 3-10, 3-15) arises from the external occipital protuberance of the occipital bone and the spinous processes (or supraspinous ligament) of the cervical and thoracic vertebrae. From this rather extensive origin the fibers converge as they pass toward the shoulder. The upper fibers insert on the posterolateral aspect of the clavicle, the middle on the acromion and lateral aspect of the scapular spine, and the lower fibers, on the medial aspect of the scapular spine. The fibers are arranged so that there are three distinct potential lines of action of the muscle: the upper, middle, and lower portions. The three acting in concert are strong adductors of the scapula. Simultaneous action of both the upper and lower parts produces upward rotation of the scapula. The superior part is important in maintaining the static position of the scapula, which is the base of the entire shoulder. It also elevates the scapula as in shrugging the shoulder. The middle part is the strongest adductor of the scapula and resists any force that tends to cause scapular protraction. The lower part depresses the scapula.

Loss of the trapezius produces postural changes as well as clear functional deficits. The contour between the head and point of the shoulder changes and the shoulder sags; the lateral angle (point of the shoulder) drops, and the scapula may be somewhat protracted. Shoulder shrugging and humeral flexion and abduction are greatly weakened. The trapezius muscle is innervated by the accessory (11th cranial) nerve and by branches of the third and fourth cervical nerves.

The **latissimus dorsi muscle** (Figs. 3-11A, 3-15) occupies a large portion of the lower back. It has a large origin via the thoracolumbar fascia to the lumbar and lower thoracic vertebrae, the sacrum, and the posterior part of the iliac crest. Its fibers converge as they pass superolaterally toward the axilla where a flat tendon is formed. This tendon spirals around the teres major muscle and tendon and inserts into the floor of the intertubercular groove of the humerus. The latissimus dorsi is a strong extensor and medial rotator of the humerus. Loss of this muscle produces no easily

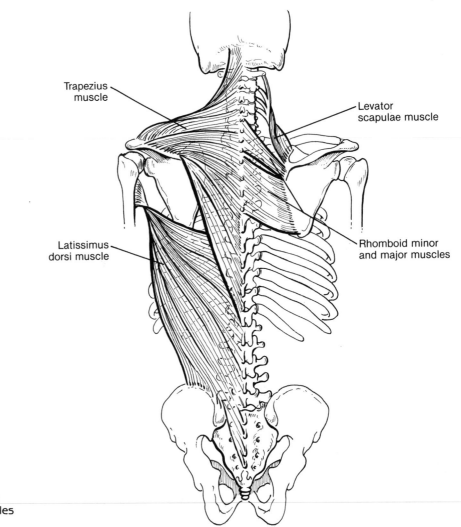

Trapezius
muscle

Levator
scapulae muscle

Latissimus
dorsi muscle

Rhomboid minor
and major muscles

Figure 3-15
Posterior view of the extrinsic
muscles of the shoulder that are
located in the back. (These same
muscles are the superficial muscles
of the back.)

discernible postural change; but the ability to perform activities such as
rowing a boat or crutch walking is greatly reduced. This muscle's innervation is provided by the thoracodorsal nerve.

The **levator scapulae** and **rhomboid major** and **minor muscles** (Figs.
3-10B, 3-15) are deep to the trapezius and interconnect the vertebral
column and the medial border of the scapula. The levator scapulae arises
from the transverse processes of the upper three or four cervical vertebrae;
its fibers descend and insert on the superior portion of the medial border
of the scapula. The rhomboid muscles arise from the spinous processes of
the lower cervical and upper thoracic vertebrae and insert on the rest of
the medial border of the scapula below the levator scapulae. All three
muscles are downward rotators of the scapula. The levator scapulae contracting alone elevates the superior angle of the scapula; the rhomboids
retract the scapula. Although these muscles participate in the overall

control of the scapula, their loss produces neither a noticeable postural change nor a significant functional loss. The static position of the scapula may be changed somewhat in that it may be rotated somewhat superiorly. The rhomboid muscles are innervated by the dorsal scapular nerve and the levator scapulae by branches of cervical nerves three and four. On occasion, the dorsal scapular nerve also innervates the levator scapulae.

The **serratus anterior muscle** (Figs. 3-10A, 3-16) covers a large portion of the lateral aspect of the thoracic wall. The muscle arises by individual attachments from the anterolateral aspects of the upper eight or nine ribs. From this rather extensive origin the fibers converge somewhat as they pass posteriorly between the scapula and thoracic wall and insert onto the ventral aspect of the medial border of the scapula. It is important to note that the fibers that comprise the origin from the lower four or five ribs ascend considerably toward their insertion, which is concentrated on the inferior angle. The position of the medial border of the scapula, against the ribs, is maintained by the serratus anterior. Contraction of this muscle produces upward rotation and protraction of the scapula. This upward rotation is essential for full abduction and/or flexion of the arm. Loss of the serratus anterior produces both a static and a dynamic loss. The static or postural loss is apparent from inspection of the position of the scapula; its medial border protrudes away from the thoracic wall producing a "winging" of the scapula. The functional loss is manifest in an inability to fully abduct or flex the arm, which is due to a loss of full upward rotation of the scapula. Both the trapezius and the serratus anterior muscles are necessary for complete upward rotation of the scapula with full power. The serratus anterior is innervated by the long thoracic nerve.

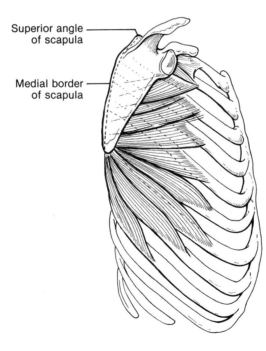

Superior angle of scapula

Medial border of scapula

Figure 3-16
Lateral view of the serratus anterior muscle.

The **pectoralis major muscle** (Figs. 3-11A, 3-17) essentially defines the pectoral region since it virtually forms that region. This muscle has an extensive origin that includes the anteromedial aspect of the clavicle, the manubrium and body of the sternum and adjacent portions of the ribs and/or costal cartilages, and usually the deep fascia of the abdominal wall. From this wide origin the muscle fibers converge as they pass laterally, the upper fibers descending and the lower fibers ascending, and form a flat tendon that inserts on the crest of the greater tubercle of the humerus. The insertion of the fibers is somewhat reversed in that the clavicular fibers insert inferiorly and the abdominal and lower sternal fibers insert superiorly. The entire muscle is a strong adductor and medial rotator of the humerus. The sternocostal and abdominal portions, together with the latissimus dorsi muscle, depress the entire shoulder region in activities such as crutch walking. The upper and lower portions of the muscle are antagonistic in certain movements, the clavicular part assisting in the initial segment of humeral flexion and the sternocostal part extending the humerus, especially from full extension. Paralysis of this muscle produces no apparent static deformity, but atrophy leads to a flattening of the contour of the pectoral region. Adduction, medial rotation, flexion, and extension of the humerus all are weakened with loss of the pectoralis major. Both the medial and lateral pectoral nerves innervate this muscle.

The **pectoralis minor muscle** (Figs. 3-10A, 3-17) is deep to the pectoralis major and is much smaller. From an origin on three or four ribs, usually ribs 2–5, its fibers pass superolaterally to insert on the coracoid process. It functions to stabilize and depress the scapula; its loss produces

Figure 3-17
Anterior view of the pectoralis major and minor muscles.

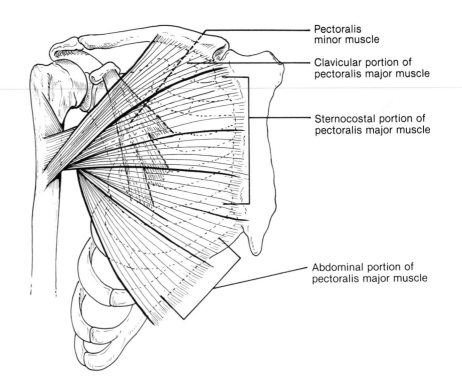

Pectoralis minor muscle

Clavicular portion of pectoralis major muscle

Sternocostal portion of pectoralis major muscle

Abdominal portion of pectoralis major muscle

neither a discernible postural change nor a functional loss. Only the medial pectoral nerve innervates this muscle.

Intrinsic Muscles of the Shoulder

The intrinsic muscles of the shoulder include the deltoid, teres major, and muscles of the **rotator (musculotendinous) cuff**: the subscapularis, supraspinatus, infraspinatus, and teres minor. All of these muscles arise from the scapula or clavicle and insert on the humerus, functioning to move the humerus and stabilize the shoulder joint. The specific motions of abduction and lateral rotation at the glenohumeral joint are produced only by certain of these muscles. Innervation is provided by spinal cord segments C5 and C6 through the axillary nerve and several of the small branches of the brachial plexus.

Deltoid. The **deltoid muscle** (Figs. 3-10, 3-11, 3-18) produces the rounded contour of the shoulder. This muscle has three rather distinct parts. The anterior part arises from the anterolateral aspect of the clavicle, the middle arises from the acromion, and the posterior arises from the posterolateral aspect of the spine of the scapula. The fibers of the three parts pass across the head of the humerus and converge toward the lateral midshaft region of the humerus, the deltoid tuberosity, on which

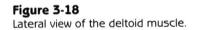

Figure 3-18
Lateral view of the deltoid muscle.

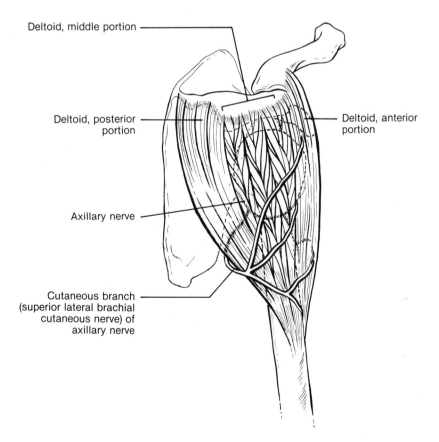

Deltoid, middle portion

Deltoid, posterior portion

Deltoid, anterior portion

Axillary nerve

Cutaneous branch (superior lateral brachial cutaneous nerve) of axillary nerve they insert. These three components can function either independently or as a unit. The fibers of the anterior and posterior parts are arranged in parallel. The anterior part is a major flexor of the humerus as well as a medial rotator; the posterior part extends and laterally rotates. Both parts assist in humeral abduction. The fibers of the middle portion are arranged in a multipennate pattern, a construction that provides maximal strength per unit volume of muscle. Even though this middle part is at great mechanical disadvantage, it is ideally constructed and situated to be the primary abductor at the glenohumeral joint. It is important to note that this part of the muscle is not ideally situated to initiate abduction because in the anatomic position its line of pull parallels the long axis of the humerus; without any help with the initial few degrees of abduction, the middle deltoid would pull the head of the humerus vertically into the acromion. This help is provided by the supraspinatus muscle. Loss of deltoid function produces a profound loss of mobility at the shoulder joint. Theoretically, the humerus would not sublux if the scapular position were maintained and the supraspinatus intact. Still, there may be some degree of subluxation. The rounded contour of the shoulder definitely would be flattened and the point of the shoulder more angular. Both the range of motion and the strength of humeral abduction would be greatly reduced; in fact, any remaining motion would be of little functional value. The deltoid muscle is innervated by the axillary nerve.

Teres major.   The **teres major muscle** (Figs. 3-10B, 3-11B, 3-19), together with the latissimus dorsi muscle and tendon, forms the posterior

Figure 3-19
Posterior view of the intrinsic muscles of the shoulder and the triceps brachii muscle.

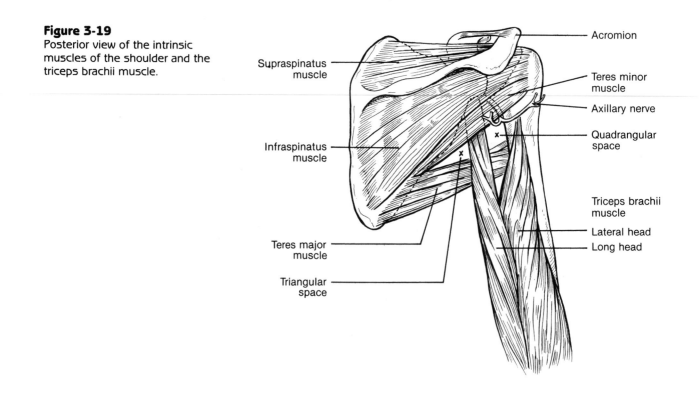

axillary fold. It arises from the inferolateral aspect of the posterior surface of the scapula and inserts on the crest of the lesser tubercle of the humerus. This muscle is a medial rotator, extensor, and adductor of the humerus. Loss of the teres major causes neither postural changes nor significant functional loss. The muscles that adduct, medially rotate, and extend the humerus are numerous and powerful; loss of the teres major weakens those movements, but not significantly. This muscle is innervated by the lower subscapular nerve.

Rotator cuff. The **muscles of the rotator cuff** provide the major stabilization of the shoulder joint. The tendons of each of these muscles blend with the fibrous portion of the shoulder joint capsule and thus hold the humeral head against the glenoid cavity. Loss of these muscles removes that support and the joint subluxes—the head of the humerus literally falls away from the glenoid cavity. These muscles reinforce the joint anteriorly, superiorly, and posteriorly but not inferiorly, a factor that predisposes dislocation of the humeral head.

The **subscapularis muscle** (Figs. 3-10A, 3-11A, 3-20) supports the anterior aspect of the shoulder joint. It arises from the majority of the anterior surface of the scapula, the subscapular fossa, and inserts on the lesser tubercle of the humerus. Its tendon blends with the anterior aspect of the fibrous portion of the joint capsule; and the subscapular bursa separates the lateral aspect of the muscle and the scapula. In addition to reinforcing the shoulder joint, this muscle is a medial rotator of the humerus. The strength and length of this muscle are factors in anterior shoulder dislocation because a strong subscapularis muscle can be a deterrent to anterior dislocation. Shoulder joint stabilization is more of a problem than loss of motion when this muscle is paralyzed, since other

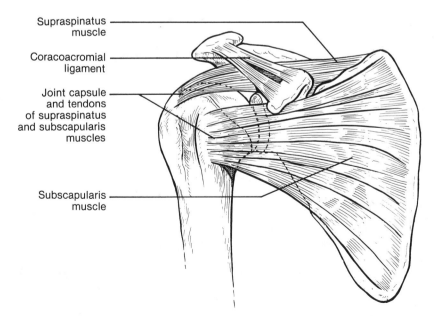

Supraspinatus muscle

Coracoacromial ligament

Joint capsule and tendons of supraspinatus and subscapularis muscles

Subscapularis muscle

Figure 3-20
Anterior view of the subscapularis and supraspinatus muscles, both intrinsic muscles of the shoulder.

strong medial rotators are still intact. It is supplied by the upper and lower subscapular nerves.

The **supraspinatus muscle** (Figs. 3-10B, 3-11, 3-20) is the most superior of the rotator cuff muscles and is perhaps subject to more trauma on a daily basis than any other muscle. After arising from the supraspinatus fossa, the fibers of this muscle pass across the superior aspect of the head of the humerus and insert on the most superior aspect of the greater tubercle of the humerus. Its tendon blends with the superior aspect of the fibrous portion of the articular capsule. Although this muscle is a weak abductor of the humerus, its role is essential in the natural smooth rhythm of abduction at the glenohumeral joint. It is positioned ideally to initiate abduction, augment the action of the deltoid, and hold the head of the humerus "down" (in the glenoid cavity) throughout the abduction range of motion. However, its mechanical advantage is poor, it is small, and great stress is placed on this muscle and its tendon during virtually any upper limb activity. By and large, the purpose of any motion of the entire limb is to position the hand so it can function most effectively. The initial phase of any motion is a small amount of glenohumeral abduction to get the hand and elbow away from the body, a task that falls largely to the supraspinatus muscle. Loss of this muscle produces no postural change, but a definite "hitch" in humeral abduction is usually present. The initial few degrees of abduction, normally produced primarily by the supraspinatus, may be provided by dropping the shoulder so that gravity pulls the humerus laterally. This muscle is innervated by the suprascapular nerve.

The **infraspinatus** and **teres minor muscles** (Figs. 3-10B, 3-11B, 3-19) support the shoulder joint posteriorly. The infraspinatus muscle arises from the majority of the infraspinatus fossa, and the teres minor arises from a portion of the posterior aspect of the lateral border of the scapula. Both muscles cross the posterior aspect of the humeral head and insert on the middle and inferior aspects of the greater tubercle, respectively. Both muscles externally rotate the humerus. Their loss leaves the posterior part of the deltoid as the only external rotator so that motion is weakened. There is no static deformity. The infraspinatus is innervated by the suprascapular nerve; the teres minor, by the axillary nerve.

Unified Motion of the Shoulder Region

Full motion of the humerus, particularly abduction and flexion, requires movement of the scapula and motion at both the sternoclavicular and acromioclavicular joints in addition to that which occurs at the glenohumeral articulation. Loss of motion at any of these joints, be it from joint pathology or muscle weakness, can limit the range, force, and smoothness of the overall motion. Motion in the shoulder region is a symphony of movement of all components.

For the most part abduction of the arm is a combination of abduction at the glenohumeral joint and upward rotation of the scapula. However, appropriate movement of the clavicle also is essential. The motion between the humerus and the glenoid cavity is produced by the deltoid and rotator cuff muscles; it is a coordinated combination of external rotation as well as abduction. Abduction is initiated predominantly by the supraspinatus muscle. Simultaneously, all rotator cuff muscles contract to maintain contact between the articular surfaces. Soon after a few degrees of abduction have occurred, the deltoid provides the force necessary to overcome gravity and complete the motion. Although the middle portion of the deltoid is the prime mover, the anterior and posterior parts assist during the end of the range of motion. As the motion proceeds the rotator cuff muscles continue to contract, maintaining the integrity of the joint; they "hold down" the head of the humerus and thus maintain contact between the humeral head and the glenoid. The subscapularis, infraspinatus, and teres minor are particularly important because their downward pull counteracts the tendency of the humeral head to move superiorly. Before the humerus is abducted to 60 degrees, the differential contraction force between the subscapularis (internal rotator) and infraspinatus and teres minor (external rotators) muscles changes to favor the external rotators, and the humerus rotates externally. This rotation moves the greater tubercle of the humerus posteriorly and allows it to pass under the highest portion of the coracoacromial arch, the acromion process. Otherwise, abduction would be limited to about 60 degrees, because the greater tubercle cannot pass under the more anterior portion of the coracoacromial arch. Upward rotation of the scapula begins soon after the glenohumeral motion has been initiated. This motion is produced by the trapezius and serratus anterior muscles and occurs in concert with the glenohumeral motion throughout the entire range of motion. Scapular rotation is essential to a full range of motion of abduction of the arm and comprises approximately 60 degrees of that motion. Overall, the humerus is abducted approximately 2 degrees for each degree of scapular rotation. At the completion of full humeral abduction, the face of the glenoid cavity has changed to a superolateral orientation.

Since the relationship between the scapula and clavicle is maintained by the coracoclavicular ligament, upward rotation of the scapula requires elevation of the lateral end of the clavicle. This elevation is approximately 60 degrees and is accomplished by elevation of the lateral end of the clavicle and rotation around its longitudinal axis. Elevation of the lateral end of the clavicle is limited by the costoclavicular ligament. Even though the elevation stops, the scapula continues to rotate superiorly and the coracoclavicular ligament tightens. Tightness of this ligament, particularly the more posterior conoid portion, produces posterior rotation of the clavicle, which produces further elevation of the acromioclavicular joint. This final elevation via the "crank-handle" mechanism permits sufficient upward rotation of the scapula for full abduction of the humerus.

Suprahumeral Space

The **suprahumeral space** (Figs. 3-14, 3-21) is the narrow interval between the head of the humerus and the **coracoacromial arch.** This arch provides a protective roof above the anterior and superior aspects of the shoulder joint and is formed by the coracoid process, the acromion, and

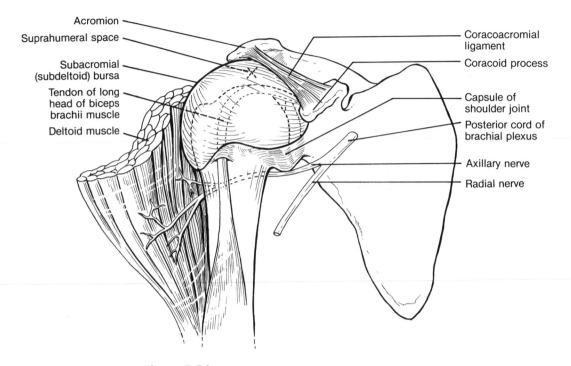

Acromion
Suprahumeral space
Subacromial (subdeltoid) bursa
Tendon of long head of biceps brachii muscle
Deltoid muscle

Coracoacromial ligament
Coracoid process
Capsule of shoulder joint
Posterior cord of brachial plexus
Axillary nerve
Radial nerve

Figure 3-21
Anterior view of the shoulder region illustrating the suprahumeral space and the course of the axillary nerve.

the intervening **coracoacromial ligament.** The health of the structures occupying this space is critical to the normal functioning of the entire shoulder region. However, these structures are vulnerable to a variety of pathologic problems that inevitably lead to a reduction in shoulder mobility.

From superior to inferior, this space is occupied by the subacromial (subdeltoid) bursa, the supraspinatus muscle and tendon, the superior part of the shoulder joint capsule, a portion of the synovial cavity of the shoulder joint, and the tendon of the long head of the biceps brachii muscle (Fig. 3-14). These structures are packed closely together and move synchronously during shoulder motion. Since the supraspinatus is active during any shoulder motion, there is movement in this space with virtually any activity of the upper limb. During extreme motions, particularly flexion and abduction of the arm, the structures in this space are compressed. Inflammation of any of these structures, **subacromial bursitis** and **supraspinatus tendonitis** are common, causes pain that usually increases with motion. As described previously, even relatively short-term inactivity of the glenohumeral joint can lead to a debilitating and long-standing loss of shoulder motion.

Axillary Nerve

The **axillary nerve** (see Figs. 3-8, 3-18, 3-19, 3-21) is the smaller of the two terminal branches of the posterior cord. Arising in the axilla ventral to the subscapularis muscle, it passes horizontally and laterally toward the shoulder. This course takes it anterior to the inferiormost part of the shoulder joint. As this nerve approaches the proximal aspect of the humerus, it is joined by the posterior humeral circumflex vessels, which, together with the nerve, pass posteriorly around the surgical neck of the humerus and through the **quadrangular space** (Fig. 3-19). This space is formed laterally by the surgical neck of the humerus, medially by the long head of the triceps brachii muscle, superiorly by the teres minor and subscapularis muscles, and inferiorly by the teres major muscle. The axillary nerve innervates both the deltoid and teres minor muscles and a small area of skin in the region of the insertion of the deltoid muscle.

This nerve is vulnerable to injury at various points along its course, but most injuries occur at one of two points. The first is where the nerve passes the inferior aspect of the shoulder joint. During an anterior dislocation of the shoulder, the nerve may be stretched by the head of the humerus. The course of the axillary nerve is relatively short, it is fixed at either end, and it is under some tension. As a result it moves very little. The course of the humeral head during anterior dislocation is usually anterior, inferior, and medial into the infraclavicular fossa, a course that takes the head through the position of the axillary nerve. In most cases the nerve apparently slips around the bone, but occasionally it is caught by the bone and stretched anteriorly with resulting potential nerve damage. The second common point of injury is where the nerve passes around the surgical neck of the humerus. Both the nerve and posterior humeral circumflex vessels are adjacent to the bone and are vulnerable to sharp edges when the bone is fractured. Most fractures of the proximal part of the humerus occur in the region of the surgical neck, and therefore accompanying injuries of the nerve or vessels are common. This nerve potentially is vulnerable to entrapment as it passes through the quadrangular space. Fibrous bands associated with the muscles forming this space are thought to be the culprits.

Surface Anatomy of the Shoulder Region

The sternoclavicular joint is palpable just superolateral to the **suprasternal,** or **jugular, notch**; its location can be verified by asking the patient to circumduct his or her arm. From that point laterally the examiner can follow the entire length of the clavicle, palpating its medial anterior convexity and lateral anterior concavity. Tenderness at any point along the bone is readily detectable. The **infraclavicular fossa** is inferior to the lateral half of the clavicle, and the coracoid process is palpable in the depths of that fossa. This fossa typically disappears when the humerus dislocates anteriorly because of the presence of the humeral head. The lateral end of the clavicle typically is marked by a small elevation or step off that indicates the location of the acromioclavicular joint and possible shoulder separation, which would be marked by a pronounced step off.

The acromion process, the bony point of the shoulder, is lateral to the acromioclavicular joint. Inferolaterally from the acromion, the greater tubercle of the humerus is palpable through the deltoid muscle. Directly inferior to the greater tubercle, at about the midarm level, the deltoid tuberosity is easily palpable. Anteromedially from the greater tubercle, both the lesser tubercle and the intertubercular groove of the humerus also are palpable through the deltoid muscle.

The majority of the scapula, with the exception of the superior border and lateral angle, can be palpated. The entire length of the spine of the scapula can be palpated as it passes inferomedially from the acromion to its base on the medial border. The medial border also is easily followed. The lateral border is palpable from the inferior angle to a variable point inferior to the glenoid cavity.

The pectoralis major muscle is readily palpable at any point in the pectoral region, and it can be followed laterally as it forms the anterior axillary fold. The three parts of the deltoid can be evaluated separately, especially if each is palpated close to its origin. The infraspinatus and teres minor muscles are, for the most part, deep to the posterior part of the deltoid and difficult to palpate. The teres major can be followed laterally as, together with the latissimus dorsi, it forms the posterior axillary fold. The supraspinatus, levator scapulae, and rhomboid muscles are deep to the trapezius and thus not readily palpable.

Arm and Elbow

Radius and Ulna

The proximal epiphysis, or **head,** of the **radius** (Figs. 3-22, 3-23) is cylindrical in cross section and concave on its end; the entire surface is covered by articular cartilage. The **neck** of the radius unites the head and shaft; and just distal to the neck, the large **radial tuberosity** projects anteromedially. The majority of the shaft is marked by a sharp medial ridge to which the interosseous membrane attaches. Distally, the shaft enlarges smoothly into the distal epiphysis, which is somewhat rectangular in cross section with the greater dimension oriented transversely. The medial aspect is indented by the **ulnar notch,** an articular surface, and dorsally the prominent **dorsal radial tubercle (of Lister)** is present. The **radial styloid** projects distally from the lateral aspect of the bone and represents the most distal part of the radius. The distal surface of the radius, an entirely articular surface, is biconcave and obliquely oriented so that both its dorsal and lateral aspects extend more distally than its anterior and medial aspects.

The proximal aspect of the **ulna** (Figs. 3-22, 3-23) is much larger than the distal portion. The deep **trochlear notch** is lined by articular surface and directed anterosuperiorly. The **olecranon process** is the most proximal part of the ulna, bordering the trochlear notch proximally. Distally, the notch is bordered by the **coronoid process.** The **ulnar tuberosity** is the roughened area just distal to the coronoid process, and the **radial notch,** an articular surface, indents the lateral aspect of the coronoid process. The shaft of the ulna has two ridges. The more prominent is the lateral ridge, which provides attachment for the interosseous membrane; the posterior ridge is the palpable subcutaneous portion of the bone that extends from the olecranon to the **styloid process.** This styloid process is

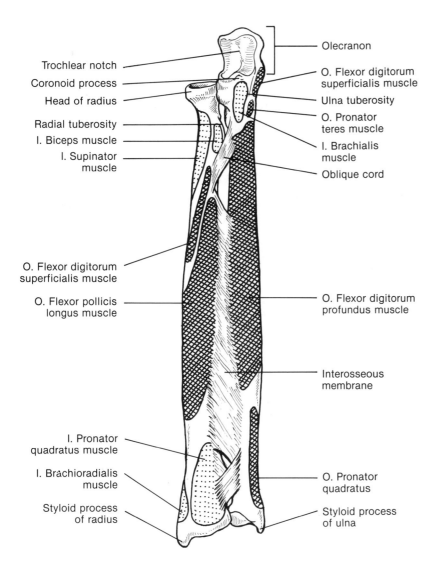

Trochlear notch

Coronoid process

Head of radius

Radial tuberosity

I. Biceps muscle

I. Supinator muscle

O. Flexor digitorum superficialis muscle

O. Flexor pollicis longus muscle

I. Pronator quadratus muscle

I. Brachioradialis muscle

Styloid process of radius

Olecranon

O. Flexor digitorum superficialis muscle

Ulna tuberosity

O. Pronator teres muscle

I. Brachialis muscle

Oblique cord

O. Flexor digitorum profundus muscle

Interosseous membrane

O. Pronator quadratus

Styloid process of ulna

Figure 3-22
Anterior view of the radius and ulna. The areas of muscle origin are indicated by crosshatch, the insertions by stipple.

an extension of the small, cylindrically shaped **head** of the ulna, which is covered by articular surface distally and peripherally.

Elbow Joint

The elbow joint (Figs. 3-24, 3-25) is formed between the trochlea of the humerus and trochlear notch of the ulna medially, and the radial head and capitulum of the humerus laterally. The direction of motion that occurs between the arm and forearm is determined by the humeroulnar articulation. That union acts like a hinge, with the trochlear notch sliding around the trochlea, resulting in flexion and extension of the forearm. Extension is limited by contact between the olecranon process and the olecranon fossa. Flexion generally is limited by contrast between the cor-

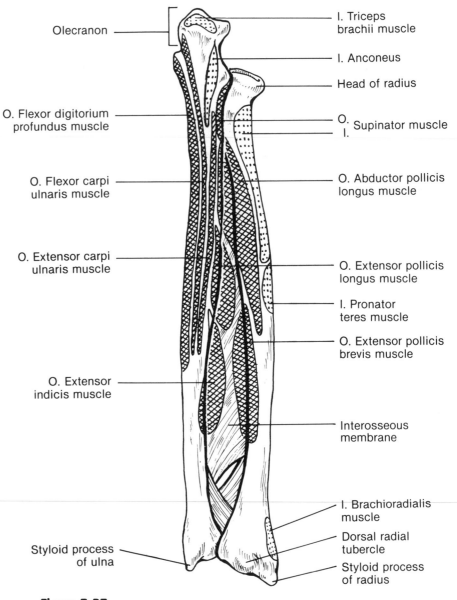

Olecranon

I. Triceps brachii muscle

I. Anconeus

Head of radius

O. Flexor digitorium profundus muscle

O. Supinator muscle
I.

O. Flexor carpi ulnaris muscle

O. Abductor pollicis longus muscle

O. Extensor carpi ulnaris muscle

O. Extensor pollicis longus muscle

I. Pronator teres muscle

O. Extensor pollicis brevis muscle

O. Extensor indicis muscle

Interosseous membrane

I. Brachioradialis muscle

Dorsal radial tubercle

Styloid process of ulna

Styloid process of radius

Figure 3-23
Posterior view of the radius and ulna. The areas of origin are indicated by crosshatch, the insertions by stipple.

onoid process and coronoid fossa, but in some very muscular individuals it may be limited by soft tissue bulk.

A single joint capsule encloses both parts of the elbow joint and the proximal radioulnar joint. This capsule is large, attaching proximally to the borders of the olecranon and coronoid fossae and distally to the edges of the olecranon and coronoid processes and the radial neck. It is loose anteriorly and posteriorly, it is reinforced on either side by the collateral

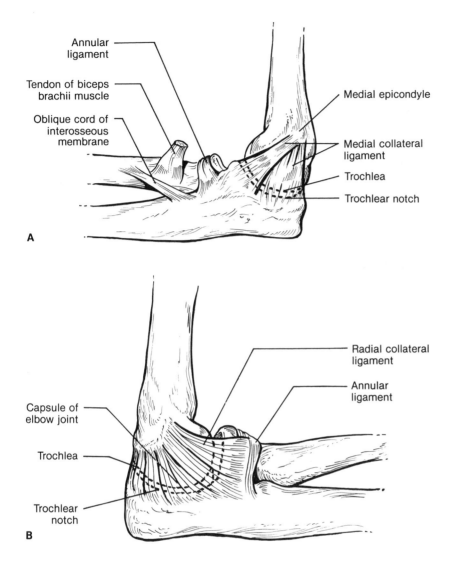

Annular ligament

Tendon of biceps brachii muscle

Oblique cord of interosseous membrane

Medial epicondyle

Medial collateral ligament

Trochlea

Trochlear notch

A

Radial collateral ligament

Annular ligament

Capsule of elbow joint

Trochlea

Trochlear notch

B

Figure 3-24
Medial (A) and lateral (B) views of the elbow and proximal radioulnar joints.

ligaments. The **radial (lateral) collateral ligament** extends from the lateral humeral epicondyle to the annular ligament and lateral aspect of the ulna adjacent to the attachment of the annular ligament. The **ulnar (medial) collateral ligament** is triangular in shape. From an attachment to the medial humeral epicondyle, its fibers diverge and attach to the ulna along a line from the medial aspect of the coronoid process to the olecranon process. These ligaments protect the joint against medial and lateral forces and are taut throughout flexion and extension. They are most taut in full extension.

The major flexors of the forearm are the biceps brachii and the brachialis muscles. The brachioradialis also flexes the forearm, especially when the forearm is midway between pronation and supination. The superficial muscles in the anterior compartment of the forearm are weak

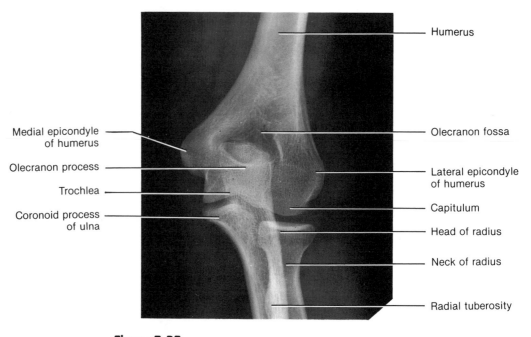

Humerus

Medial epicondyle of humerus

Olecranon process

Trochlea

Coronoid process of ulna

Olecranon fossa

Lateral epicondyle of humerus

Capitulum

Head of radius

Neck of radius

Radial tuberosity

Figure 3-25
Anteroposterior radiograph of the elbow.

flexors at the elbow. The triceps brachii is the single major extensor of the forearm.

Articulations Between the Radius and Ulna

The radius and ulna are united by two radioulnar joints and the **interosseous membrane.** This membrane (Figs. 3-22, 3-23) is a strong, fibrous sheet that binds the bones together and interconnects them through most of their lengths. The majority of the fibers forming this membrane are obliquely oriented and pass distally from radius to ulna. This membrane appears to facilitate the transfer of proximally directed force from the radius to the ulna because such a force tightens the majority of the fibers. A smaller proximal portion of the membrane, the **oblique cord** (Fig. 3-22), is oriented at about 90 degrees to the rest of the membrane and resists distal traction on the radius.

The articular surfaces forming the **proximal** and **distal radioulnar joints** are similar: Each consists of the cylindrically shaped head of one bone that fits into a shallow notch in the other. Specifically, the proximal radioulnar joint is formed by the head of the radius and the radial notch of the ulna, and the distal by the head of the ulna and the ulnar notch of the radius.

The proximal radioulnar joint (Figs. 3-24 through 3-26) is enclosed by the articular capsule of the elbow joint and reinforced primarily by the **annular ligament.** This ligament attaches to the edges of the radial notch, surrounding the head of the radius and extending distally along the neck

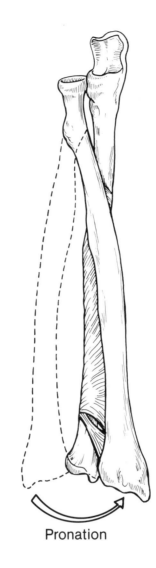

Pronation

Figure 3-26
Anterior view of the radius and ulna in the pronated position. The broken line indicates the position of the radius in the supinated position.

of the radius so it is somewhat funnel-shaped. The smaller diameter distally helps this ligament resist traction on the radius. In children, prior to calcification of the radial head, the annular ligament provides only minimal resistance to traction because the head is small and malleable.

The distal radioulnar joint (Fig. 3-35) is reinforced by both the interosseous membrane and the strong articular disk that extends from the distal medial aspect of the radius to the styloid process of the ulna. The joint space is between the ulnar head and both the ulnar notch and articular disk, and is separated completely from the radiocarpal joint space by the articular disk.

During supination and pronation, motion occurs at the two joints simultaneously. Proximally, the radial head spins within the radial notch and annular ligament; distally, the ulnar notch slides around the head of the ulna. Since the ulna is fixed at the elbow, only the radius and hence the hand, moves. During pronation, the radius crosses the ulna in such a way that its distal end passes ventral and then medial to the ulnar head (Fig. 3-26). During supination, the radius returns to the anatomic position where it is parallel to the ulna.

The biceps brachii and supinator muscles are the major supinators of the forearm. The supinator muscle is a strong supinator irrespective of the forearm position (flexion or extension), but the biceps is most efficient in the midrange of forearm flexion. Pronation is produced by both the pronator teres and pronator quadratus muscles. The brachioradialis muscle is both a pronator and a supinator; from full supination it can pronate to about the midposition and vice versa.

Anterior Compartment of the Arm

The anterior compartment of the arm (Figs. 3-1A, 3-27, 3-29) contains the biceps brachii, brachialis, and coracobrachialis muscles. The **biceps brachii muscle** (Figs. 3-10A, 3-22, 3-27, 3-29) occupies a major portion of the anterior compartment and is largely responsible for its contour. Its two heads arise from the scapula. The tendon of the long head occupies the intertubercular groove of the humerus and passes across the head of the humerus to attach to the supraglenoid tubercle. This tendon is ensheathed by a layer of synovium as it passes through the joint space and is subject to degeneration and rupture in the later years of life. The short head is muscular almost to its attachment on the coracoid process. From their origins the two heads converge and join in the proximal part of the arm. The tendon of insertion crosses the ventral aspect of the elbow and inserts into the radial (bicipital) tuberosity. A strong, flat extension of the tendon, the **bicipital aponeurosis,** extends medially and distally and blends with the investing fascia of the forearm. The biceps is a flexor and supinator of the forearm. It is a weak flexor when the forearm is pronated, because in that position the biceps is an antagonist and thus is centrally inhibited. Performing pull-ups with the forearm supinated and pronated illustrates this point quite well. The biceps also is a weak abductor and flexor of the arm. Its ability to abduct is enhanced somewhat if the arm is laterally rotated so the tendon of the long head passes directly across the superior aspect of the humeral head. If this lateral rotation accompanies an attempt to abduct the arm, the major abductors of the arm are usually greatly weakened or paralyzed. Loss of this muscle produces a significant weakness in both forearm flexion and supination, but there is virtually no change in function at the shoulder. The static position of the upper limb may change so that the forearm would tend to be somewhat pronated. More noticeable would be the change in contour of the anterior compartment. The biceps is innervated by fibers from spinal cord segments C5 and C6 through the musculocutaneous nerve.

The **brachialis muscle** (Figs. 3-11A, 3-22, 3-27) is deeply situated in the distal half of the anterior compartment. It arises from the distal half of the anterior aspect of the humerus and inserts on the ulnar tuberosity. This muscle is wide and covers most of the anterior aspect of the elbow joint. It is a pure flexor of the forearm, flexing equally well regardless of the position (supination or pronation) of the forearm. Loss of the bra-

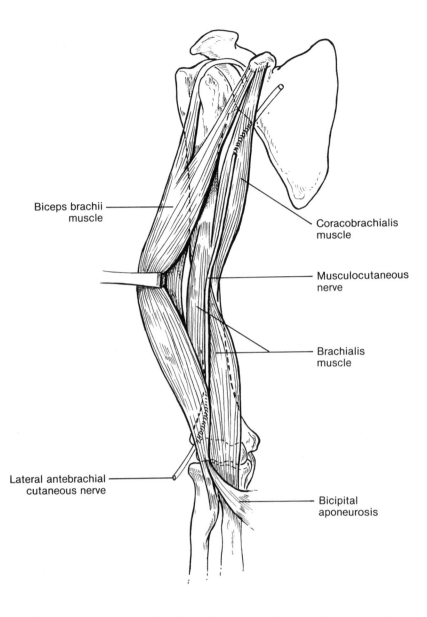

Biceps brachii
muscle

Coracobrachialis
muscle

Musculocutaneous
nerve

Brachialis
muscle

Lateral antebrachial
cutaneous nerve

Bicipital
aponeurosis

Figure 3-27
Muscles of the anterior compartment of the arm. The biceps brachii
muscle is retracted laterally.

chialis muscle causes a marked loss of power in forearm flexion, yet there
is no discernible change in the static position of the forearm. This muscle
is supplied by the musculocutaneous nerve.

The **coracobrachialis muscle** (Figs. 3-10A, 3-11A, 3-27, 3-29) is a
small muscle in the medial aspect of the proximal arm that blends with
the short head of the biceps brachii muscle. It extends from the coracoid
process (origin) to the medial aspect of the midshaft region of the humerus. A weak flexor and adductor of the arm, its loss produces neither
a functional loss nor a positional change. Along with the rest of the muscles in this compartment, it is innervated by the musculocutaneous
nerve.

The **musculocutaneous nerve** (Figs. 3-8, 3-27, 3-29) supplies the muscles in the anterior compartment of the arm and the skin of the lateral forearm. From its origin as the direct continuation of the lateral cord of the brachial plexus, this nerve passes inferiorly and laterally, first piercing the coracobrachialis muscle and then passing between the biceps and brachialis muscles. In the distal arm it passes through the investing fascia just lateral to the biceps and descends in the subcutaneous tissue of the lateral forearm as the **lateral antebrachial cutaneous nerve.** There are two points along this nerve's course where entrapment has been implicated. The first is where it passes through the coracobrachialis muscle. The second involves the lateral antebrachial cutaneous nerve as it pierces the investing fascia and assumes its superficial position. The cause of entrapment at this point is probably an external force, such as the strap of a heavy handbag compressing the nerve against the edge of the investing fascia or other underlying structures.

Posterior Compartment of the Arm

The **triceps brachii muscle** (Figs. 3-10A, 3-11B, 3-19, 3-28) fills the posterior compartment of the arm and is responsible for its surface contours. This muscle has three heads of origin, two from the humerus and one from the scapula. The long head crosses the shoulder joint and arises from the infraglenoid tubercle. The medial and lateral heads arise from the posterior aspect of the humerus and are separated by the spiral groove. The lateral head arises from a vertical line superior to the spiral groove; the medial head arises from most of the remaining surface medial and inferior to the spiral groove. The three heads attach to a strong flat tendon that inserts on the olecranon process of the ulna. The triceps muscle is the major extensor of the forearm, and its long head can assist in extension and adduction of the arm. Loss of the triceps muscle results in a virtual absence of active forearm extension. In the upright position gravity would keep the forearm extended so any static positional change would depend on the position of the limb. Also, the contour of the posterior compartment would become flattened. This muscle is supplied by the radial nerve.

The **anconeus muscle** (Fig. 3-28) is a small muscle in the distal posterior arm that extends from the lateral epicondyle of the humerus to the lateral aspect of the olecranon process of the ulna. Although it extends the forearm, it is very weak and of little practical value. The anconeus is innervated by the radial nerve.

The course of the **radial nerve** (Figs. 3-8, 3-28) through the arm for the most part is in the posterior compartment. From its beginning as the continuation of the posterior cord of the brachial plexus, this nerve inclines laterally as it passes across the subscapularis, teres major, and latissimus dorsi muscles. It crosses the inferior border of the latissimus dorsi in an angle formed by that muscle and the long head of the triceps. In reality, both muscles are tendons at that point and usually connected by fibrous material. The radial nerve is vulnerable to those tendinous edges; it can be traumatized as it rubs against them, or it can be compressed against them by external force such as an axillary crutch. The nerve con-

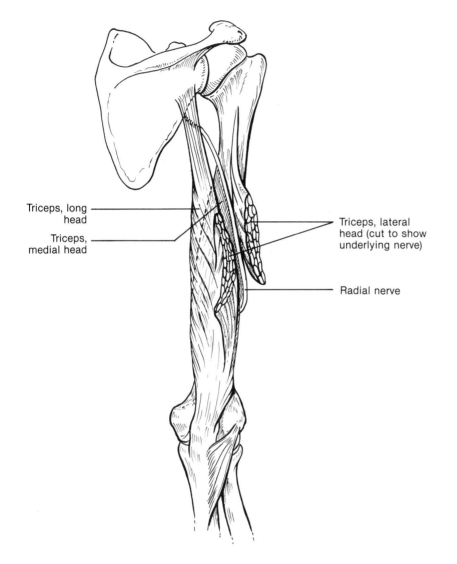

Triceps, long head

Triceps, medial head

Triceps, lateral head (cut to show underlying nerve)

Radial nerve

Figure 3-28
Muscles of the posterior compartment of the arm and the radial nerve.

tinues into the posterior compartment and spirals around the posterior aspect of the midshaft of the humerus in the spiral groove, passing between the medial and lateral heads of origin of the triceps. It is accompanied by the deep brachial vessels. This nerve is vulnerable to injury as it passes along the spiral groove immediately adjacent to the bone. Midshaft fractures of the humerus frequently spiral around the spiral groove, and the nerve and vessels are vulnerable to laceration by sharp bony edges. Since several branches to the triceps arise high in the axilla and thus are not vulnerable to this type of injury, the triceps muscle may be at least partially intact even though the nerve is severed at the midshaft level. If an injury of this type is suspected, it is important to test radial nerve functions in the forearm and hand to ensure that the nerve is functioning. The radial nerve passes posterior and then inferior to the deltoid tuberosity, then pierces the lateral intermuscular septum to enter the anterior compartment in the distal lateral arm where it is in a deep position between the brachialis and brachioradialis muscles. It enters the forearm by crossing the anterolateral aspect of the elbow deep to the brachioradialis muscle. Again, this nerve is vulnerable as it passes inferior to the deltoid tuberosity: It is superficial, it is positioned on the humerus, and it is fixed as it passes through a small fibrous opening in the lateral intermuscular septum into the anterior compartment. Any blunt trauma or constricting band can compress it against the bone, and entrapment can occur as it passes through the intermuscular septum.

Medial Neurovascular Bundle

Several nerves and the brachial vessels form a neurovascular bundle (Fig. 3-29) that passes through the arm at the junction of the investing fascia and the medial intermuscular septum. The **brachial artery** (Figs. 3-7, 3-29) descends through the arm in this bundle and, proximal to the elbow, inclines laterally to enter the cubital fossa, where it passes deep to the bicipital aponeurosis. Its largest branch in the arm is the **deep brachial artery,** which usually arises in the proximal half of the arm, even in the axilla, and accompanies the radial nerve into the posterior compartment. **Collateral** branches of both the brachial and deep brachial arteries, together with **recurrent** branches of the radial, ulnar, and interosseous arteries distal to the elbow, form potential anastomoses around the elbow region.

The **median** and **ulnar nerves** supply no structures in the arm but descend in the neurovascular bundle (Fig. 3-29). After its formation on the ventral aspect of the axillary artery in the axilla, the median nerve accompanies the artery through the arm and into the cubital fossa. Especially at this origin, this nerve is vulnerable to compression by aneurysm within the neurovascular bundle. The connective tissue forming the axillary sheath is strong, and the structures are packed tightly so there is little room for additional material. The presence of an anomalous muscle associated with the latissimus dorsi and pectoralis major, Langer's muscle, also may entrap the median nerve near its origin. The nerve's superficial course through most of the arm makes it somewhat vulnerable to superficial lacerations but well protected from injury that might accompany a fracture of the humerus.

The ulnar nerve is the direct continuation of the medial cord. It descends in the neurovascular bundle (Fig. 3-29) to approximately the midarm level, where it enters the posterior compartment and follows the medial intermuscular septum to the medial epicondyle of the humerus. It enters the forearm by passing posterior to that epicondyle and deep to the flexor carpi ulnaris muscle. This nerve occupies the same connective sleeve in the proximal part of the arm as the median nerve and is, therefore, also vulnerable to aneurysm. As the nerve enters the posterior compartment, it passes through a fibrous opening where it is subject to entrapment. In the posterior compartment the nerve occupies a groove in the medial head of the triceps brachii muscle where it is quite firmly anchored and has little padding between it and the bone. At this point

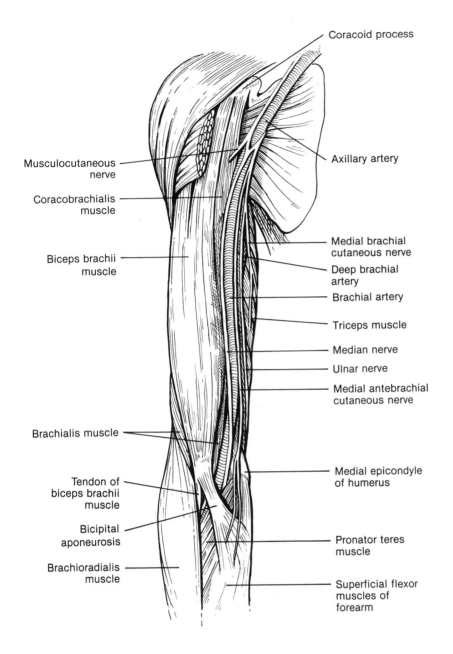

Coracoid process

Musculocutaneous
nerve

Coracobrachialis
muscle

Biceps brachii
muscle

Axillary artery

Medial brachial
cutaneous nerve

Deep brachial
artery

Brachial artery

Triceps muscle

Median nerve

Ulnar nerve

Medial antebrachial
cutaneous nerve

Brachialis muscle

Tendon of
biceps brachii
muscle

Bicipital
aponeurosis

Brachioradialis
muscle

Medial epicondyle
of humerus

Pronator teres
muscle

Superficial flexor
muscles of
forearm

Figure 3-29
Anterior view of the shoulder, arm,
and cubital fossa.

it is vulnerable to external pressure such as a tourniquet or a hard surface
such as the edge of an operating table. Needless to say, the ulnar nerve
is vulnerable to both major and minor trauma as it passes posterior to the
medial humeral epicondyle.

Surface Anatomy of the Arm

The surface anatomy of the proximal humerus is described with the discussion of the shoulder. Distally both the medial and lateral epicondyles
and portions of their supracondylar ridges are easily palpable. The medial

epicondyle should be palpated carefully due to the presence of the ulnar nerve. The deltoid tuberosity is palpable laterally at the level of the mid-arm, and the radial nerve can be felt just distal to that same prominence. The contours of the two compartments of the arm, the anterior formed primarily by the biceps and the posterior by the triceps, are easily defined and clearly demarcated medially and laterally by a vertical depression. The deltoid is easily defined superolaterally, as are the anterior and posterior muscle groups of the forearm, where they extend superior to the medial and lateral aspects of the elbow, respectively. Medially, the position of the neurovascular bundle is marked by a vertical indentation between the anterior and posterior compartments, and the components of the bundle can be palpated throughout the arm. The brachial artery not only is easily palpated, but its pulsation frequently can be visualized.

Figure 3-30
Anterior view of the bones of the wrist and hand.

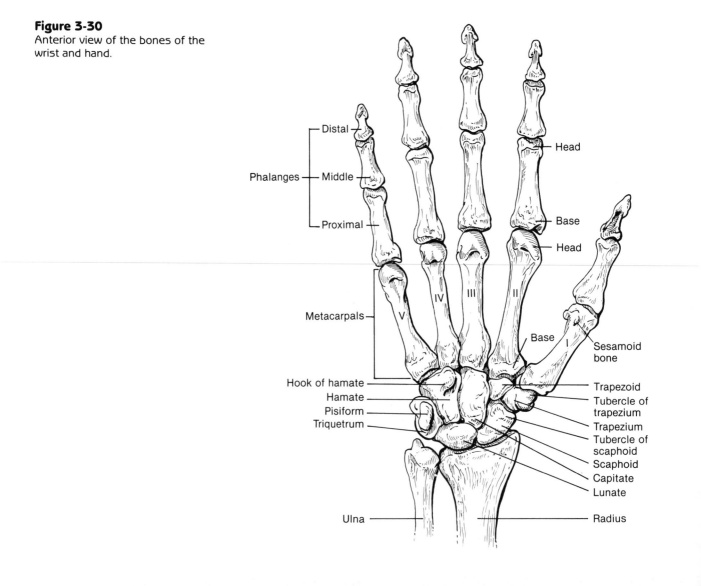

Forearm and Wrist

Bones of the Wrist and Hand

The irregularly shaped **carpal bones** (Figs. 3-30 through 3-34) fill the small interval between the forearm and hand. Their arrangement forms a ventral groove that connects the forearm and hand; the wedge-shaped configuration of certain of these bones contributes to this arch. These bones are arranged in two rows with four bones in each row. From lateral to medial the proximal row consists of the **scaphoid, lunate, triquetrum, and pisiform;** the distal row consists of the **trapezium, trapezoid, capitate, and hamate bones.**

The four most ventral points of these carpal bones are palpable, and are the attachments for the **deep part of the flexor retinaculum** (transverse carpal ligament). These points (Fig. 3-30) are the pisiform, which is positioned on the ventral aspect of the triquetral, the **hamulus (hook)**

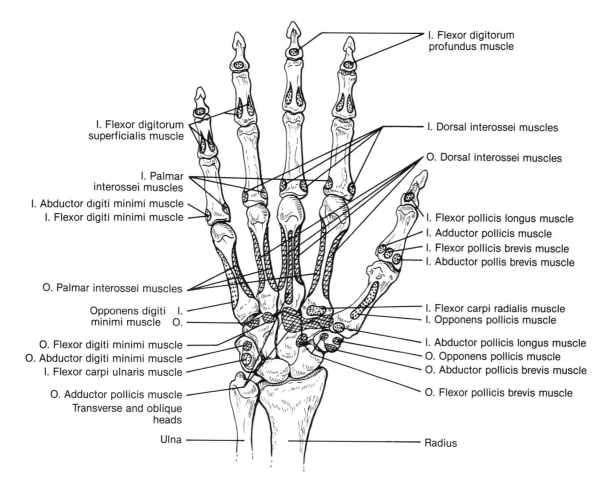

Figure 3-31
Anterior view of the bones of the wrist and hand. The areas of muscle origin are indicated by crosshatch, the insertions by stipple.

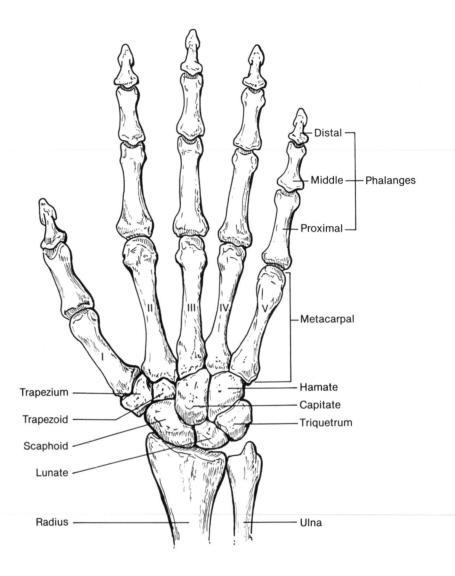

Figure 3-32
Posterior view of the bones of the wrist and hand.

of the hamate, the **tubercle** of the trapezium, and the **tubercle** of the scaphoid. Note that no muscles attach to the dorsal aspect of these bones (Fig. 3-33) and that ventrally (Fig. 3-31), with the exception of the pisiform, only intrinsic muscles of the hand attach.

The **metacarpals** and **phalanges** (Figs. 3-30 through 3-34) are the bones of the hand. The five metacarpal bones are similar, each having a proximal **base,** a distal **head,** and a **body** that is somewhat ventrally concave longitudinally. This shape facilitates the basic function of grasping and allows efficient packing of the soft structures so the bulk of the palmar aspect of the hand is kept to a minimum. The third metacarpal is the longest, the first the shortest. The proximal aspect of each base is flattened and covered by articular surface proximally and on the sides. These surfaces form articulations with the carpal bones and adjacent metacarpals. The proximal articular surface of the first metacarpal is saddle-

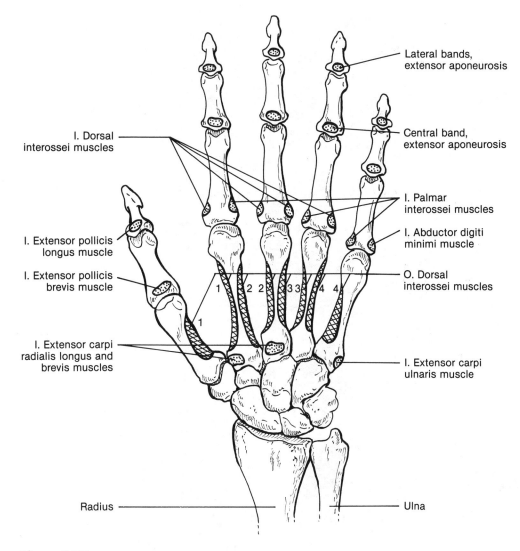

Lateral bands, extensor aponeurosis

Central band, extensor aponeurosis

I. Dorsal interossei muscles

I. Palmar interossei muscles

I. Abductor digiti minimi muscle

I. Extensor pollicis longus muscle

I. Extensor pollicis brevis muscle

O. Dorsal interossei muscles

I. Extensor carpi radialis longus and brevis muscles

I. Extensor carpi ulnaris muscle

Radius

Ulna

Figure 3-33
Posterior view of the bones of the wrist and hand. The areas of muscle origin are indicated by crosshatch, the insertions by stipple.

shaped—concave in one direction and convex in the opposite direction—and forms a specialized articulation with the trapezium. The metacarpal heads are rounded but basically cylindrically shaped and present articular surface distally and ventrally. **Tubercles** project from either side of the dorsal aspects of the heads.

The fourteen phalanges (Figs. 3-30 through 3-34) are designated as **proximal, middle,** and **distal** for each digit other than the thumb, which has only proximal and distal phalanges. The bones decrease in size from proximal to distal. Each, however, has a base, a head, and a body that is somewhat ventrally concave longitudinally. The articular surfaces of the bases of proximal phalanges are biconcave. The articular surfaces of the

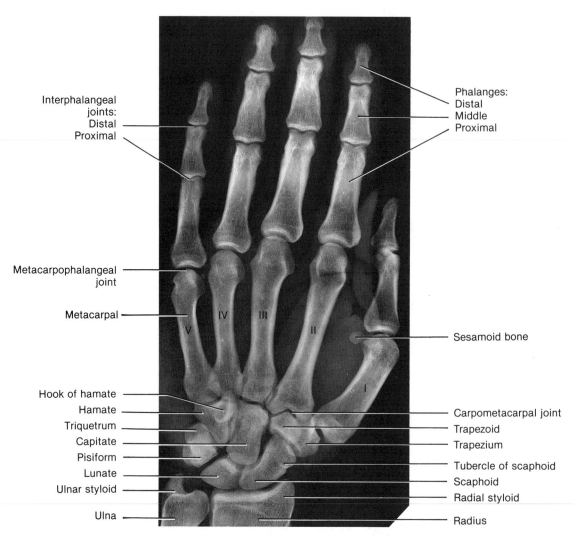

Figure 3-34
Anteroposterior radiograph of the wrist and hand.

bases of the middle and distal phalanges are similarly shaped but have ridges that cross the surfaces from anterior to posterior. The articular surfaces of the heads of the proximal and middle phalanges are cylindrical in shape and grooved to accommodate the ridges of the adjacent phalangeal bases. The heads of the distal phalanges have roughened tubercles that are directed ventrally.

Articulations of the Wrist and Hand

Radiocarpal and midcarpal joints.   The area of the wrist has two major articulations (Figs. 3-34, 3-35), the **radiocarpal joint (wrist joint**

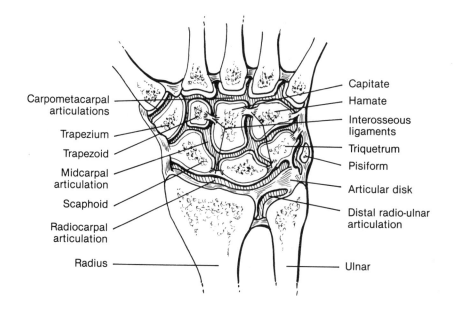

Figure 3-35
Coronal section through the distal portions of the radius and ulna, the carpal bones, and the proximal portions of the metacarpals.

proper) and the **midcarpal joints.** The radiocarpal joint is formed between the distal end of the radius and the adjacent articular disk and the proximal row of carpal bones. The major contact is between the distal surface of the radius and the scaphoid and lunate. The midcarpal joint is formed between the proximal and distal rows of carpal bones. The articular surfaces forming the radiocarpal joint present single overall contours; the radius and articular disk are biconcave—concave from medial to lateral and from anterior to posterior—and the proximal row of carpal bones forms a biconvex surface. The articular surfaces forming the midcarpal joint present two contours. The medial portion of the joint, between the capitate and hamate distally and the scaphoid, lunate, and triquetrum proximally, is biconcave proximally and biconvex distally. The lateral portion of midcarpal joint, between the trapezoid and trapezium distally and the scaphoid proximally, is more of a single plane.

The joint cavities of the radiocarpal and midcarpal joints are separate, and the joint capsules attach to the edges of the articular surfaces of the involved bones. In the case of the radiocarpal joint, the capsule also attaches to the edge of the articular disk that is distal to the ulna. Because the spaces between adjacent carpal bones in each row are closed by interosseous ligaments (Fig. 3-35), typically there is no communication between the two cavities. The radiocarpal and midcarpal articulations are reinforced by **radial** and **ulnar collateral ligaments,** along with a complex system of **dorsal** and **palmar intercarpal, radiocarpal,** and **ulnocarpal ligaments.** The palmar ligaments are more extensive and stronger. Both the dorsal and ventral radiocarpal ligaments are oriented obliquely; that is, they pass medially as they pass distally, and thus strengthen the relationship between the forearm and hand during pronation and supination. As the forearm is pronated or supinated, the dorsal or palmar radiocarpal ligament, respectively, is tightened. The hand not only follows the fore-arm but does so with minimal lag.

The motion at the wrist is the sum of motion that occurs at the radiocarpal and midcarpal joints. In the resting position the hand tends to be deviated toward the ulnar, or little finger, side and somewhat flexed. This is because the radius extends more distally than the ulna, and the lateral and posterior aspects of the radius extend more distally than its medial and anterior portions, respectively. For these same reasons the hand can be moved farther medially and anteriorly than it can laterally and posteriorly. Movement of the hand medially is termed **adduction** or **ulnar deviation,** movement laterally is **abduction** or **radial deviation.** The hand also can be **flexed** (anterior motion) and **extended** (posterior mo-tion). And, as a result of the combination of these four motions, it can be **circumducted**—rotated so the fingers circumscribe a circle. Any ap-parent rotation of the hand is actually the supination and pronation that occurs at the proximal and distal radioulnar joints.

Certain muscles, the flexors and extensors of the carpus, act only on the wrist joint. Others, the long flexors and extensors of the digits, act primarily on the digits and only affect the wrist secondarily. None of the primary muscles of the wrist is positioned so that it can produce a single pure motion such as flexion, extension, adduction, or abduction. Rather, the tendons of these muscles cross the wrist at its four corners and thus produce two motions simultaneously. For example, the flexor carpi ulnaris muscle produces flexion and adduction of the hand, and the extensor carpi ulnaris muscle causes extension and adduction. Pure adduction can occur only if these two muscles function simultaneously. On the radial side of the wrist there are three primary tendons whose muscles control wrist motion. The flexor carpi radialis is a flexor and abductor; both the extensor carpi radialis longus and brevis muscles are extensors and abduc-tors.

Because the lunate and scaphoid are the major carpal bones forming the radiocarpal joint, force transmitted proximally from the hand to the wrist is concentrated on these two bones. As a result, they are the most commonly injured of the carpal bones. The upper limbs commonly are used reflexly to break a fall, and, at the time of impact, the hands are forced into extension and some radial deviation. The lunate is somewhat wedge-shaped with its narrow portion directed posteriorly. During forced extension it is compressed between the scaphoid and radius and can be forced (dislocated) anteriorly into the carpal tunnel. The scaphoid is vul-nerable to fracture. This bone is somewhat kidney-shaped (Fig. 3-34), having two expanded ends that are connected by a narrower "waist" area. As the hand is extended and radially deviated, the waist area is forced against the radial styloid. Most commonly, the scaphoid is fractured through this waist area. This fracture is often complicated by retarded healing or the absence of healing. Most scaphoids receive a dual blood supply, one artery going to each of its ends. One of these vessels is absent approximately one-third of the time, which corresponds to the incidence of poor fracture repair involving this bone.

Carpometacarpal joints.   The **carpometacarpal (CM) joints** (Fig. 3-35) are commonly confused with the joints forming the "knuckles," but they are not as they are found proximally in the hand where it joins the wrist. The CM joints of the four medial digits can be discussed together. The four medial metacarpals articulate with the trapezoid, capitate, and hamate bones, and with the bases of each other. A common joint cavity separates the metacarpals and the carpals, and extends distally between the bases of the metacarpals. The joint capsule is reinforced by **dorsal** and **palmar carpometacarpal** and **metacarpal ligaments.** The bases of these metacarpals also are held together by **interosseous metacarpal ligaments.** Virtually no definitive motion occurs at this set of articulations.

Unlike those of the digits, the **carpometacarpal joint of the thumb** (Fig. 3-35), is quite mobile. It is formed between the saddle-shaped articular surfaces of the base of the first metacarpal and the trapezium. The relative looseness of the joint capsule and reinforcing ligaments permits considerable motion but also makes the joint vulnerable to dislocation. At this joint the first metacarpal can be both flexed and extended, and adducted and abducted. Most importantly, it can be rotated around its longitudinal axis, the motion that is necessary for opposition of the thumb.

It is important to note that the motion of the thumb, although described similarly to the movements of the other digits, occurs in different planes. The resting position of the thumb is different; that is, it is rotated approximately 90 degrees relative to the other digits. As a result, flexion and extension occur in a plane that is parallel to the palm. The thumb moves across the palm as it is flexed. Abduction and adduction occur in a plane (the sagittal plane) that forms a right angle with the palm. The thumb moves ventrally away from the palm when it is abducted, and it moves dorsally toward the pad of the index finger when it is adducted.

Metacarpophalangeal joints. The **metacarpophalangeal (MP) joints** (Figs. 3-30 through 3-34) are formed between the rounded heads of the metacarpals and the concave bases of the proximal phalanges. These joints form the knuckles, and each has its own synovial cavity and joint capsule. Ventrally, the capsules are reinforced by strong **palmar ligaments** (volar plates). These ligaments are interconnected with the **deep transverse metacarpal ligament,** which in turn binds the heads of metacarpals 2–5 together. Dorsally, the capsules blend with the extensor tendon sheaths. The **collateral ligaments** are obliquely oriented and pass from the dorsal aspects of the metacarpal heads to the palmar aspects of the bases of the proximal phalanges. As a result of this placement, these ligaments tighten as the proximal phalanx is flexed. The proximal phalanx can be flexed and extended, and while extended, abducted and adducted. When the proximal phalanx is flexed, the tightness of the collateral ligament precludes adduction and abduction.

Interphalangeal joints. The **interphalangeal (IP) joints** (Figs. 3-30–3-34) are all simple hinge joints. Those between the proximal and middle phalanges are the **proximal interphalangeal (PIP) joints**; those between the middle and distal phalanges are the **distal interphalangeal (DIP) joints.** The thumb has a single IP joint. At each joint a pulley-shaped head articulates with a rounded base that has a ridge that tracks in the pulley's groove. The joint capsule is reinforced by **collateral** and **palmar ligaments**; dorsally it blends with the extensor tendon sheath. The muscles controlling the digits are described on page 146.

Cubital Fossa

The **cubital fossa** (Fig. 3-29) is the depression anterior to the elbow and the proximal part of the forearm. Its presence reduces the soft tissue bulk in that area and thus permits the final degrees of forearm flexion that are important in performing many everyday tasks. This fossa is bounded laterally by the brachioradialis muscle, medially by the pronator teres muscle, and proximally by a line interconnecting the medial and lateral epicondyles of the humerus. Its floor is the brachialis muscle. The tendon of the biceps brachii muscle disappears into this fossa as it passes toward the radial tuberosity; the bicipital aponeurosis extends medially from the biceps tendon to the investing fascia on the forearm. This aponeurosis separates structures passing through the fossa from those passing superficially. The median nerve and brachial artery enter the fossa from the medial aspect of the arm. In the fossa the artery is medial to the biceps tendon and the nerve is medial to the artery, and both are deep to the bicipital aponeurosis. Importantly, the median cubital vein is in the superficial fascia and separated from the brachial artery by the bicipital aponeurosis. Since this vein is commonly used for venipuncture, its differentiation from the artery is important.

Anterior Compartment of the Forearm

The complexity of the compartmentation of the forearm is described in the beginning of this chapter (Fig. 3-1B). The anterior compartment is associated with the medial epicondyle of the humerus so it is positioned medially in the proximal aspect of the forearm. The tendons of the muscles in this compartment cross the anterior aspect of the wrist, so distally this compartment is located truly anteriorly. The major actions of its muscles are flexion of the hand and digits and pronation of the forearm. Its nerves are the median and ulnar; its vessels, the ulnar and radial. With the exception of the radial artery, these nerves and vessels pass distally into the anterior aspect of the hand.

Understanding forearm muscles.   A student's first contact with the muscles of the forearm, whether in the laboratory or textbook, can be a bit overwhelming. The first point to remember is that the muscles are grouped, both anteriorly and posteriorly, into superficial and deep groups. Second, the names of the muscles describe function, or location, or both. For example, the flexor carpi radialis muscle is a flexor of the carpus on the radial side. Since it is a flexor, it is in the anterior compartment; since it produces flexion at the wrist, its tendon crosses the wrist but does not pass into the digits; and since it is called "radialis," its tendon is on the radial side. The pronator quadratus is a square muscle that pronates the forearm. From a practical standpoint it is important to note that the majority of the muscle bellies of these muscles, both in the anterior and posterior compartments, cannot be palpated definitively. These muscle bellies blend together in their groups or are positioned deeply. For the most part, the muscle-tendon junctions are in the distal aspect of the forearm, and therefore only tendons cross the wrist. A number of individual tendons are palpable, and thus a muscle can be evaluated definitively. The deeper tendons cannot be palpated at the wrist, but their insertions are all on the digits. As a result, specific resistance can be applied to the digits, and thus these muscles also can be evaluated definitively. Obviously, relationships around the wrist and the specific insertions of the forearm muscles are important.

Muscles of the anterior compartment of the forearm.   The muscles in the anterior compartment of the forearm are separated into the **superficial** and **deep groups.** The muscles in the superficial group, the **pronator teres, palmaris longus, flexor carpi radialis, flexor carpi ulnaris,** and **flexor digitorum superficialis,** for the most part arise from the medial epicondyle of the humerus via the common flexor tendon. These muscles include the primary wrist flexors, a pronator, and the shorter of the long digital flexors. There are three deep muscles, the **pronator quadratus, flexor pollicis longus,** and **flexor digitorum profundus.** These muscles arise from the ventral aspects of the radius, ulna, and interosseous membrane and include a pronator and the longer of the long digital flexor muscles.

The **pronator teres muscle** (Figs. 3-11A, 3-23, 3-29, 3-36) is the shortest of these superficial muscles. From two separate origins, the medial humeral epicondyle and the medial side of the coronoid process of the ulna, the fibers of the two heads converge as they pass inferiorly and laterally toward an insertion on the lateral midshaft region of the radius. This muscle is wrapped around the anterolateral aspect of the radius when the forearm is supinated; and when it contracts, it unwraps and pronates the forearm. Loss of this muscle results in a marked loss of pronation power but no apparent static deformity. It is innervated by the median nerve as it passes between the muscle's two heads of origin.

The **flexor carpi radialis muscle** (Figs. 3-11A, 3-31, 3-36) is the only one of the principal muscles of the wrist that is not positioned exactly at one of the wrist's four corners. From its common humeral origin its fibers pass inferiorly and slightly laterally to join its strong tendon in the distal half of the forearm. This large tendon inserts on the ventral base of the second metacarpal and is prominent at the wrist where it is positioned just lateral to the midpoint. The flexor carpi radialis is the strongest flexor at the wrist; it also is an abductor of the hand. Loss of this muscle greatly reduces the strength of flexion at the wrist, but grasp is not greatly affected. The posture of the relaxed hand changes somewhat in that the hand is statically extended, resulting in an increase in the passive stretch of the long digital flexor tendons around the extended wrist and thus more digital flexion. The flexor carpi radialis is innervated by the median nerve.

The **palmaris longus muscle** (Fig. 3-36) is a small muscle that is absent approximately 15 percent of the time. It has a small belly and a long tendon; and although its belly is usually positioned in the proximal

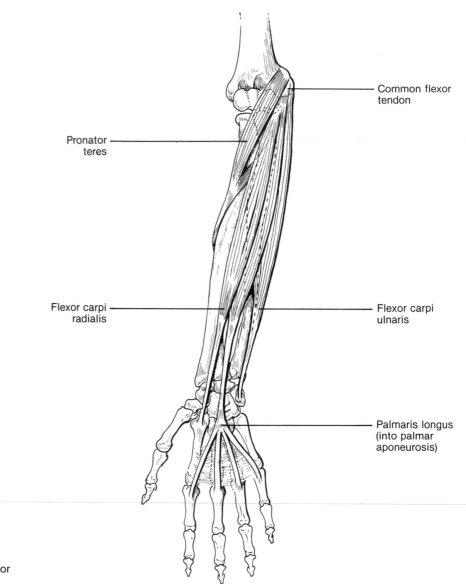

Figure 3-36
Superficial muscles of the anterior compartment of the forearm.

Common flexor tendon

Pronator teres

Flexor carpi radialis

Flexor carpi ulnaris

Palmaris longus (into palmar aponeurosis)

part of the forearm, it may be found in the middle of the forearm or just proximal to the wrist. Its small tendon is prominent at the wrist, and just distal to the wrist, it blends with the palmar aponeurosis. Contraction of this muscle tenses the palmar aponeurosis and flexes the hand; however, its functional usefulness is questionable. This muscle is innervated by the median nerve.

The **flexor carpi ulnaris muscle** (Figs. 3-11A, 3-31, 3-36) arises from the upper half of the posteromedial margin of the ulna as well as the medial epicondyle of the humerus. Its tendon crosses the anteromedial aspect of the wrist and inserts on the pisiform, which in turn is connected via ligaments to the hamate and the fifth metacarpal. This muscle flexes and adducts the hand; therefore, its loss weakens both of these motions significantly. The flexor carpi ulnaris is the only superficial muscle that is innervated by the ulnar nerve.

The **flexor digitorum superficialis (sublimus) muscle** (Figs. 3-22, 3-31, 3-37) is positioned medially and deep to the other superficial muscles. Its fibers arise from the medial aspect of the proximal ulna and the anterior surface of the radius distal to the radial tuberosity in addition to the medial humeral epicondyle. The fibers converge to form a strong, flat muscle that joins a large, flat tendon. Individual tendons to each of the four medial digits are usually discernible at about the level of the wrist, but the one to the index finger is separable more proximally. The side-

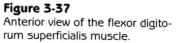

Figure 3-37
Anterior view of the flexor digitorum superficialis muscle.

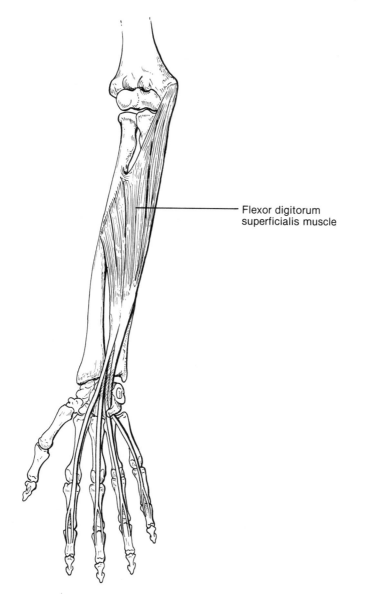

Flexor digitorum superficialis muscle

by-side arrangement of the tendons changes as they pass through the carpal tunnel so that those to the middle and ring fingers are ventral to those to the index and little fingers. Distal to the carpal tunnel the tendons diverge toward the digits. At the level of the proximal phalanx, each tendon splits around the deeper lying tendon of the flexor digitorum profundus muscle. The two terminal portions of each digital tendon then cross the PIP joint and insert on the ventral base of the middle phalanx.

The long digital flexors provide the strength for grasp. The flexor digitorum superficialis is the primary flexor at the PIP joints of the four medial digits. Typically, flexion at the PIP of the index finger can be controlled more individually than that of the other digits because of the longer individual tendon. This muscle can assist in flexion at the MP and wrist joints, but these are secondary activities. Complete flexion at the PIP joints requires a relatively short excursion of the flexor digitorum superficialis tendons. As a result, this muscle is greatly affected by the position of the wrist. Its ability to produce forceful flexion at the PIP joints is maximized when the hand is extended but greatly inhibited when the hand is flexed. The loss of this muscle is discussed on page 152. The flexor digitorum superficialis is supplied by the median nerve.

The **deep muscles** in the anterior compartment of the forearm consist of the **flexor digitorum profundus, flexor pollicis longus,** and **pronator quadratus muscles.** These muscles do not cross the elbow and thus arise from the ventral aspects of the radius, ulna, and interosseous membrane. Since neither their muscle bellies nor their tendons can be palpated, they can be tested only by evaluation of their functions.

The **flexor digitorum profundus muscle** (Figs. 3-22, 3-31, 3-38) occupies the medial two-thirds of the deep portion of the anterior compartment. From an origin on most of the anterior surface of the proximal two-thirds of the ulna and adjacent portion of the interosseous membrane, the fibers of this muscle join a strong, flat tendon well proximal to the wrist. The tendon to the index finger separates from the common tendon more proximally than any of the other tendons. The tendons pass through the carpal tunnel side-by-side and deep to the tendons of the flexor digitorum superficialis; the tendons then diverge toward their respective digits. Each digital tendon remains deep to the tendon of the flexor digitorum superficialis. Just proximal to the PIP joints the profundus tendons pass through the arches formed by the split superficialis tendons; they then cross both the PIP and DIP joints before inserting on the proximal bases of the distal phalanges. This muscle is the primary flexor at the DIP joints, but it can assist in producing flexion at the more proximal joints it crosses. As occurs with the flexor digitorum superficialis, the function of the flexor digitorum profundus muscle is significantly affected by the position of the wrist. Loss of this muscle is discussed on page 150. This muscle receives a dual innervation: The part to the index and middle fingers is supplied by the anterior interosseous branch of the median nerve, and the part to the ring and little fingers is supplied by the ulnar nerve.

The **flexor pollicis longus muscle** (Figs. 3-22, 3-31, 3-38) occupies the deep radial aspects of the anterior compartment. From an origin

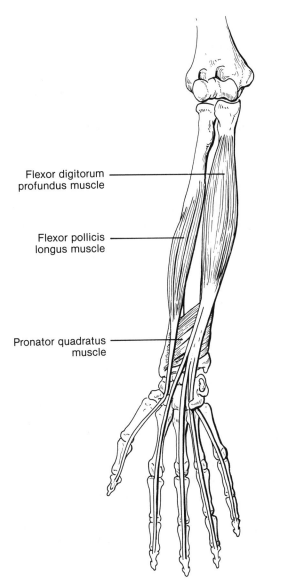

Flexor digitorum
profundus muscle

Flexor pollicis
longus muscle

Pronator quadratus
muscle

Figure 3-38
Deep muscles of the anterior compartment of the forearm.

on the ventral aspect of the middle half of the radius and adjacent part of the interosseous membrane, the fibers of this muscle descend along the radius and join the muscle's tendon, which passes through the carpal tunnel and inserts on the ventral base of the distal phalanx of the thumb. The tendon of this muscle passes around the trapezium and thus changes direction, a change that is necessary for the muscle to fulfill its function. This muscle flexes the IP joint of the thumb and provides virtually all of the force that is necessary for strong grasp involving the opposed thumb. Flexion of the thumb occurs in the coronal plane as opposed to the rest of the digits where flexion takes place in the sagittal plane; the thumb passes across the palm as it is flexed. Loss of the flexor pollicis longus greatly reduces the hand's ability to grasp with strength, but there is no loss of opposition per se, because that motion is produced primarily by intrinsic muscles. The anterior interosseous branch of the median nerve supplies this muscle.

The **pronator quadratus** (Figs. 3-22, 3-38) is a small, rectangularly shaped muscle that is found in the distal portion of the anterior compartment. Its fibers arise from the distal quarter of the anterior surface of the ulna, pass laterally and somewhat distally and then insert on the distal anterior surface of the radius. All muscles and/or their tendons in the anterior compartment pass superficial to this muscle. This muscle produces only pronation and is active whenever pronation occurs. The pronator teres muscle, the stronger pronator, becomes active when more pronation strength is required. Loss of the pronator quadratus obviously results in some reduction of the potential power of pronation, but that loss is less than that experienced if the pronator teres is lost. The pronator quadratus muscle is supplied by the median nerve, specifically its anterior interosseous branch.

Nerves of the anterior compartment of the forearm.   The **ulnar nerve** (Fig. 3-39) enters the forearm by passing posterior to the medial epicondyle of the humerus, where it occupies the ulnar nerve sulcus. This sulcus is transferred into the fibro-osseous "cubital tunnel" by a strong fibrous band that interconnects the medial epicondyle and the medial aspect of the olecranon. The cubital tunnel is thought to be a site of ulnar nerve entrapment, and, of course, the nerve is vulnerable to fractures of the medial epicondylar region of the humerus. The nerve enters the forearm by passing between the humeral and ulnar heads of origin of the flexor carpi ulnaris as it passes deep to the same muscle. It descends through most of the forearm deep to that muscle and to its tendon. The dorsal cutaneous branch arises 5 to 7 centimeters proximal to the wrist and passes dorsally to supply the skin of the dorsomedial hand. At the point where the tendon of the flexor carpi ulnaris muscle inserts on the pisiform, the ulnar nerve emerges from under the tendon, passing superficial to the deep part of the flexor retinaculum, lateral to the pisiform, and medial to the hook of the hamate. It is held in this superficial position by the investing fascia, which completes another fibro-osseous canal and thus an entrapment point that is called the "ulnar tunnel" or "Guyon's canal." At this point the nerve is superficially positioned and firmly fixed so it is vulnerable to laceration as well as blunt trauma, such as compression from hammering with the fist or from a bicycle's handlebar.

The **median nerve** (Fig. 3-39) enters the forearm by passing through the cubital fossa, deep to the bicipital aponeurosis. The sharp proximal edge of this aponeurosis is a potential entrapment point of the median nerve. In addition, with either a supracondylar fracture of the humerus or a dislocation of the elbow the median nerve may be compressed against the aponeurosis. The median nerve leaves the cubital fossa by passing between the two heads of origin of the pronator teres, where it also may be entrapped. Just distal to the pronator teres the nerve passes deep to the proximal border of the flexor digitorum superficialis muscle. This border, the "sublimis bridge," is fibrous and sharp and considered another

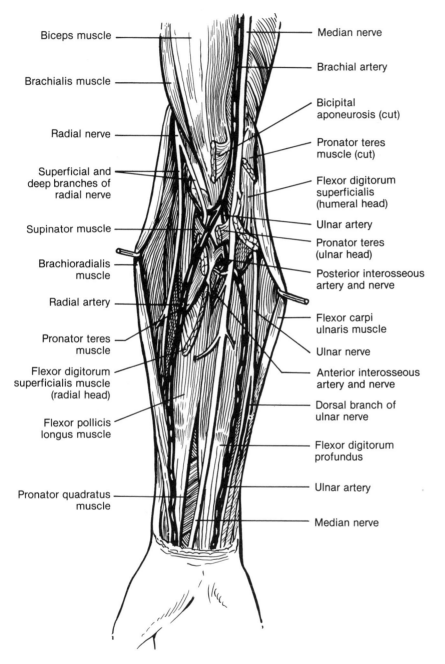

Biceps muscle

Brachialis muscle

Radial nerve

Superficial and deep branches of radial nerve

Supinator muscle

Brachioradialis muscle

Radial artery

Pronator teres muscle

Flexor digitorum superficialis muscle (radial head)

Flexor pollicis longus muscle

Pronator quadratus muscle

Median nerve

Brachial artery

Bicipital aponeurosis (cut)

Pronator teres muscle (cut)

Flexor digitorum superficialis (humeral head)

Ulnar artery

Pronator teres (ulnar head)

Posterior interosseous artery and nerve

Flexor carpi ulnaris muscle

Ulnar nerve

Anterior interosseous artery and nerve

Dorsal branch of ulnar nerve

Flexor digitorum profundus

Ulnar artery

Median nerve

Figure 3-39
Nerves and vessels of the anterior compartment of the forearm.

point of entrapment of the median nerve. The anterior interosseous nerve branches from the median nerve approximately 5 centimeters distal to the medial epicondyle, which is distal to the "sublimis bridge." This branch descends on the ventral aspect of the interosseous membrane and supplies the flexor digitorum profundus, the flexor pollicis longus, and the pronator teres. The integrity of the anterior interosseous nerve can be tested by forming a ring with the index finger and the thumb, that is, by approximating the pads of the index finger and the thumb. This branch has been reported entrapped by an accessory head of origin (Gantzer's muscle) of the flexor pollicis longus muscle. Distal to the anterior interosseous branch, the median descends on the deep surface of the flexor digitorum superficialis muscle. Proximal to the wrist the nerve is deeply located between the tendons of the palmaris longus and flexor carpi radialis muscles. The median nerve enters the hand by passing through the carpal tunnel, where it perhaps is the most commonly entrapped nerve in the body.

Blood vessels of the anterior compartment of the forearm.   The **brachial artery** (Figs. 3-7, 3-39) branches into its two terminal branches, the **radial** and **ulnar arteries,** in the cubital fossa. The **radial artery** passes laterally and then descends through most of the forearm deep to the brachioradialis muscle. Proximal to the wrist it is positioned just lateral to the tendon of the flexor carpi radialis muscle. As the artery approaches the wrist, it inclines dorsally, passing through the "**anatomic snuff box**" (Fig. 3-43) onto the dorsum of the hand. Just proximal to the wrist the superficial palmar branch arises and passes superficially into the palm of the hand.

Soon after its origin in the cubital fossa, the **ulnar artery** (Figs. 3-7, 3-39) gives rise to the short **common interosseous artery.** This artery passes medially toward the proximal border of the interosseous membrane, where it bifurcates into the **anterior** and **posterior interosseous arteries.** These arteries descend on their respective sides of the membrane, supplying the deeper structures in the anterior and posterior compartments. Distal to the origin of the common interosseous artery, the ulnar artery passes medially to a position that is deep to the flexor carpi ulnaris muscle. The artery descends through the forearm deep to that same muscle, and at the wrist is positioned just lateral to its tendon. It enters the hand with the ulnar nerve, passing superficially first lateral to the pisiform and then medial to the hook of the hamate. The common interosseous and proximal portions of the radial and ulnar arteries have recurrent branches that pass proximally across the elbow and form potential collateral arterial routes with the collateral branches of the brachial and deep brachial arteries of the arm.

Posterior Compartment of the Forearm

Since a number of the muscles in the posterior compartment are associated with the lateral epicondyle of the humerus, this compartment is lateral in the proximal forearm and posterior distally. The tendons of the muscles in this compartment cross the posterior and lateral aspects of the wrist. The major actions of these muscles are flexion of the forearm, extension of the hand and proximal phalanges, abduction of the thumb, and supination of the forearm. Every muscle in this compartment is innervated by the radial nerve. There is no large artery passing through this compartment but only the small and deeply positioned posterior interosseous artery.

Muscles of the posterior compartment of the forearm. Like those in the anterior compartment, the muscles in the posterior compartment are separated into superficial and deep groups. The superficial muscles consist of the **brachioradialis, extensor carpi radialis longus, extensor carpi radialis brevis, extensor digitorum, extensor digiti minimi,** and **extensor carpi ulnaris.** These muscles for the most part arise from the general area of the lateral epicondyle of the humerus and function both to extend the hand and the proximal phalanges of the four medial digits, and also to flex the forearm. The deep muscles are the **supinator, abductor pollicus longus, extensor pollicis longus, extensor pollicis brevis,** and **extensor indicis.** These muscles arise from the dorsal aspects of the radius, ulna, and interosseous membrane; and their tendons, with the exception of the supinator, pass across the dorsolateral aspect of the wrist. Their actions are supination of the forearm, extension of the proximal phalaynx of the index finger, and extension and abduction of the thumb.

The **brachioradialis muscle** (Figs. 3-11A, 3-22, 3-40) is different from the rest of the forearm muscles in that its major action is flexion of the forearm. This muscle is the most lateral and thus the most superficial in the superficial group; its origin is the most proximal from the lateral supracondylar ridge of the humerus. The muscle belly is positioned lateral to the radius and its fibers join a strong flat tendon in the middle third of the forearm. This tendon does not cross the wrist but rather inserts on the distal lateral aspect of the radius. The brachioradialis is a rather strong flexor of the forearm when the forearm is midway between pronation and supination. It also is capable of limited pronation and supination; that is, it can pronate from the position of full supination to the midposition and it can supinate from full pronation to the midposition. Loss of the brachioradialis does not affect useful pronation and supination but does weaken forearm flexion when the forearm is midway between supination and pronation. Still, there is no significant functional deficit. Atrophy of this muscle causes some flattening of the lateral aspect of the proximal forearm. The brachioradialis is innervated by the radial nerve.

The **extensor carpi radialis longus** and **extensor carpi radialis brevis muscles** (Figs. 3-11A, 3-33, 3-40) can be described together as they essentially form an anatomic and functional unit. They arise from the lateral epicondyle and supracondylar ridge of the humerus, the extensor carpi radialis longus extending more proximally than its mate. These muscles are positioned deep to the brachioradialis, and both join their tendons in the mid forearm. Their tendons occupy a common tendon sheath, with the tendon of the extensor carpi radialis brevis muscle being the deeper of the two. Proximal to the wrist the tendons diverge somewhat. The tendon of the extensor carpi radialis longus inserts on the dorsal base of the second metacarpal, and the tendon of the extensor carpi radialis brevis inserts on the dorsal base of the third metacarpal. These muscles are strong extensors and abductors of the hand. Their loss produces a profound weakness of both motions, and without these muscles active extension of the hand by intact muscles is weak and accompanied by significant adduction of the hand. Grasp also is weakened because strongly stabilized partial extension at the wrist is necessary for maximal

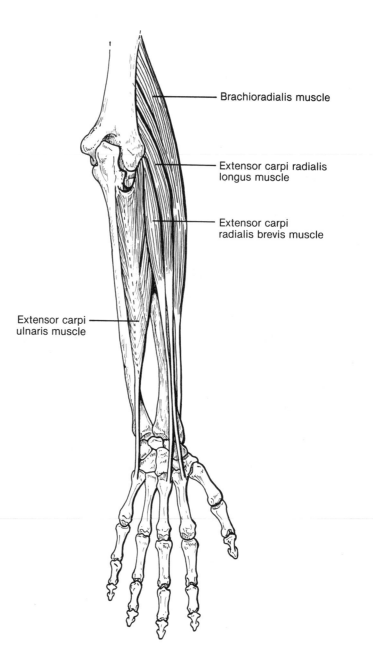

Brachioradialis muscle

Extensor carpi radialis longus muscle

Extensor carpi radialis brevis muscle

Extensor carpi ulnaris muscle

Figure 3-40
Superficial muscles of the posterior compartment of the forearm.

function of the long digital flexors. Atrophy of these muscles flattens the lateral aspect of the forearm. Both muscles are innervated by the radial nerve.

The **extensor digitorum** and **extensor digiti minimi muscles** (Figs. 3-11A, 3-33, 3-41) also can be discussed as a unit. In reality, the extensor digiti minimi is but the portion of the extensor digitorum that is some-what separated and associated only with the little finger. The overall mus-cle occupies the central portion of the posterior compartment. From its

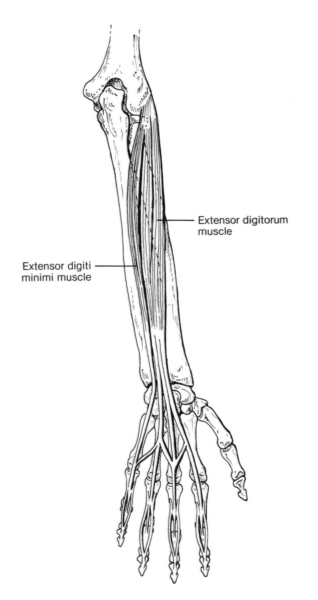

Extensor digitorum
muscle

Extensor digiti
minimi muscle

Figure 3-41
Extensor digitorum and extensor
digiti minimi muscles.

origin via the common extensor tendon on the lateral epicondyle of the
humerus, its muscle fibers form a broad flat muscle belly that is positioned
between the extensor carpi radialis brevis muscle laterally and the extensor carpi ulnaris muscle medially. The medial portion of the muscle, the
extensor digiti minimi, is separated and joins a tendon that extends only
to the little finger. Tendons to the index, middle, and ring fingers are
apparent proximal to the wrist. As the tendons pass through the dorsum
of the hand, they are variably interconnected. Almost always, the tendon
to the ring finger is connected to the tendon of the little finger just proximal to the MP joints. The tendon to each of the four fingers gives rise
to the extensor aponeurosis (expansion, hood) (Fig. 3-54). This tendi-

nous expansion covers the dorsum of each digit and is an integral part in the mechanics of the digit. The insertion of the extensor digitorum is unusual in that its tendon appears to attach to each of the phalanges. An insertion on the base of the proximal phalanx, however, is seldom definitive. Through extensions of the tendon, the central and lateral bands, the extensor digitorum very clearly inserts on the dorsal bases of the middle (central band) and distal (lateral bands) phalanges. However, the major action of the extensor digitorum is extension of the proximal phalaynx, and most anatomists agree that if the extensor digitorum extends the middle and distal phalanges, the extension is minimal. The loss of the extensor digitorum muscle is discussed on page 153. This muscle is supplied by the radial nerve.

The **extensor carpi ulnaris muscle** (Figs. 3-11A, 3-33, 3-40) is the most medial of the superficial muscles. In addition to its origin from the medial epicondyle of the humerus, it also arises from a line along the proximal half of the posterior aspect of the ulna. The proximal aspect of this muscle thus forms an arch that interconnects the ulna and the lateral humeral epicondyle. Its tendon inserts into the dorsomedial aspect of the base of the fifth metacarpal. The extensor carpi ulnaris both extends and adducts the hand. Loss of this muscle weakens extension of the hand and the hand is deviated toward the radial side. The loss of balanced extension appears to be more of a problem than the loss of strength. This muscle is innervated by the radial nerve.

The **deep muscles** in the posterior compartment of the forearm are the **supinator, abductor pollicis longus, extensor pollicis longus, extensor pollicis brevis,** and **extensor indicis.** With the exception of the supinator, these muscles are associated with the thumb and index finger. From origins on the ulna, radius, and interosseous membrane, the fibers of these muscles pass laterally as they descend. For the most part these muscles arise deep to the extensor digitorum muscle and emerge from its lateral border.

The **supinator muscle** (Figs. 3-22, 3-23, 3-42) is a short, flat muscle that is limited to the proximal half of the forearm. It arises from the lateral humeral epicondyle, a small ridge on the posterolateral surface of the ulna, and the intervening radial collateral ligament. Its fibers pass distally and laterally around the proximal aspect of the radius and insert on the anterolateral aspect of that bone. The supinator covers the proximal third of the posterior and lateral aspects of the radius. As the forearm is pronated, the supinator wraps further around the proximal radius; it unwraps as it contracts and thus produces supination. Loss of this muscle causes a definitive loss of the power of supination irrespective of the position of the forearm. The loss of supination power is measurable in the midrange of forearm flexion but is more obvious in full extension and full flexion of the forearm. This muscle is innervated by the radial nerve.

The **abductor pollicis longus muscle** (Figs. 3-23, 3-31, 3-42) is the most proximally arising muscle of the thumb. It arises from the posterior aspects of the radius, interosseous membrane, and ulna, just proximal to the midshaft region. Its fibers pass distally and laterally, passing superficial to the tendons of the extensor carpi radialis longus and brevis muscles.

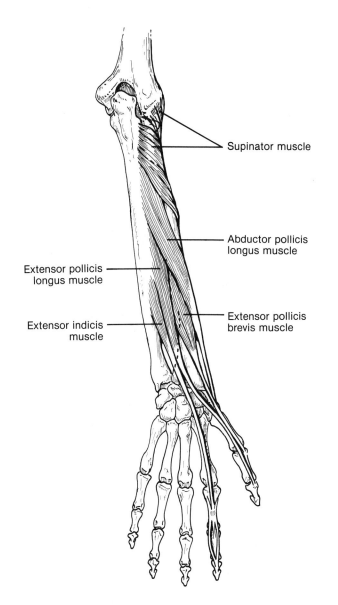

Figure 3-42
Deep muscles of the posterior compartment of the forearm.

Its tendon inserts on the ventral aspect of the base of the first metacarpal. Its primary actions are abduction, extension, and external rotation of the first metacarpal and, hence, the thumb. These motions are the reverse of those necessary for opposition of the thumb. It is important to note that the tendon of this muscle passes ventral to the flexion-extension axis of the wrist, and therefore the muscle is secondarily a flexor of the hand. This fact is of more significance surgically and relative to rehabilitation than it is in the normally functioning hand. Loss of this muscle does not produce a definitive functional loss since opening the hand (abducting and extending the thumb) to prepare for grasp is not substantially affected. This muscle is supplied by the radial nerve.

The **extensor pollicis longus muscle** (Figs. 3-23, 3-33, 3-42) arises just distal to the abductor pollicis longus, from the dorsal aspect of the ulna and adjacent interosseous membrane. Its relatively short muscle belly joins its tendon proximal to the wrist, and the tendon passes distally parallel to the radius. This tendon occupies the groove on the dorsal aspect of the radius just medial to the dorsal radial tubercle. At that tubercle, the tendon changes directions and passes laterally toward its insertion on the dorsal base of the distal phalaynx of the thumb. The point at which the tendon changes direction around the dorsal radial tubercle is significant because the tendon is vulnerable to trauma. At that point tendinitis is common, especially following trauma such as a Colles fracture. This muscle is the only extensor of the distal phalanx of the thumb. Its loss produces a flexion deformity of the IP of the thumb (due to the strong flexor pollicis longus) and an inability to "open the hand" to prepare for grasp. This muscle is innervated by the posterior interosseous branch of the deep radial nerve.

The **extensor pollicis brevis muscle** (Figs. 3-23, 3-33, 3-42) is the most distally arising of the extrinsic muscles of the thumb. From an origin on the distal posterior surfaces of the radius and adjoining interosseous membrane, its fibers pass laterally toward the base of the first metacarpal. Its tendon joins that of the abductor pollicis longus muscle, and the two tendons usually are enclosed in the same tendon sheath. The tendon of the extensor pollicis brevis passes along the lateral surface of the first metacarpal and inserts on the lateral aspect of the base of the proximal phalanx of the thumb. Loss of this muscle results in virtually no functional deficit. It is innervated by the posterior interosseous branch of the deep radial nerve.

The tendons of the extensor pollicis longus and brevis and the abductor pollicis longus muscles form the boundaries of the "anatomic snuff box" (Fig. 3-43). This depression is located on the dorsolateral aspect of the hand at the base of the thumb. The anterior border is formed by the tendons of the abductor pollicis longus and extensor pollicis brevis muscles; the posterior border is formed by the tendon of the extensor pollicis longus muscle; and the floor of the snuff box is the scaphoid. The radial artery passes through the snuff box, deep to its bounding tendons; and the superficial branch of the radial nerve passes across the snuff box in the subcutaneous tissue. Palpation of the uninjured scaphoid in the snuff box is uncomfortable; palpation of the fractured scaphoid produces considerable pain.

The **extensor indicis muscle** (Figs. 3-23, 3-42) arises from the distal aspect of the dorsal surface of the ulna. Its fibers are directed laterally, passing deep to the extensor digitorum muscle. Its tendon joins the medial aspect of the extensor digitorum tendon to the index finger. The tendon of the extensor indicis thus participates in the formation of the extensor expansion and the muscle functions in concert with the extensor digitorum. The presence of the extensor indicis enables the index finger to function more independently than the other three fingers, especially in finely controlled movements. Its presence, however, is not necessary for most everyday activities. This muscle is supplied by the posterior interosseous branch of the deep radial nerve.

Nerves of the posterior compartment of the forearm. The **radial nerve** (Figs. 3-39, 3-44) enters the forearm by crossing the elbow anteriorly and laterally, between the brachialis and brachioradialis muscles. At or about the level of the elbow the nerve splits into its **superficial** and **deep branches.** The superficial branch is a cutaneous nerve; the deep branch is a muscular nerve.

The **superficial radial nerve** (Figs. 3-43, 3-44) arises deep to the brachioradialis muscle and descends through most of the forearm deep to that muscle and its tendon. In the distal third of the forearm the nerve emerges from the posterior border of the tendon of the brachioradialis muscle and enters the subcutaneous tissue of the posterolateral forearm.

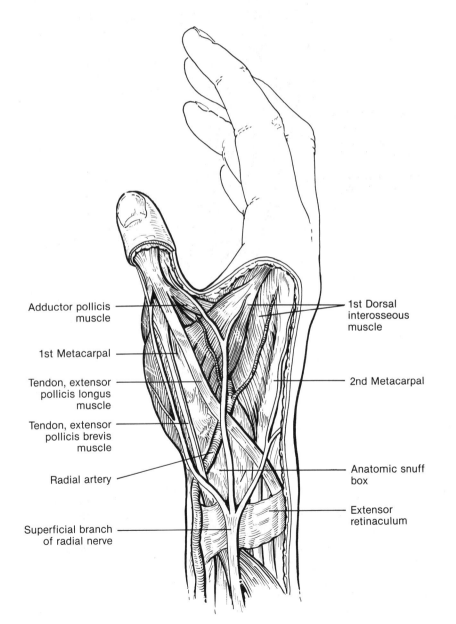

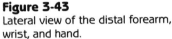

Figure 3-43
Lateral view of the distal forearm, wrist, and hand.

Adductor pollicis muscle

1st Metacarpal

Tendon, extensor pollicis longus muscle

Tendon, extensor pollicis brevis muscle

Radial artery

Superficial branch of radial nerve

1st Dorsal interosseous muscle

2nd Metacarpal

Anatomic snuff box

Extensor retinaculum

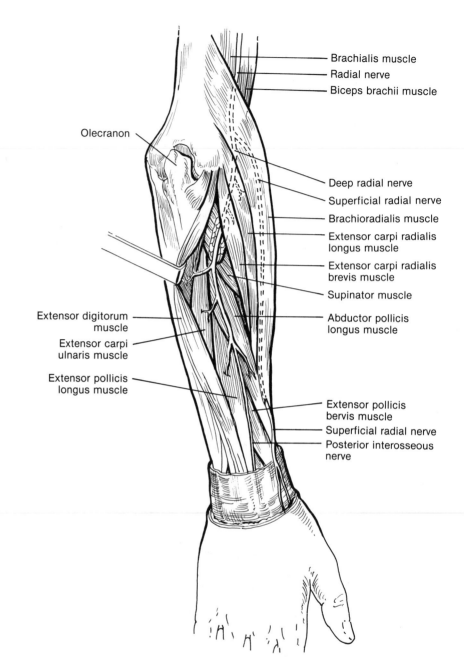

Brachialis muscle
Radial nerve
Biceps brachii muscle

Olecranon

Deep radial nerve
Superficial radial nerve
Brachioradialis muscle
Extensor carpi radialis longus muscle
Extensor carpi radialis brevis muscle
Supinator muscle
Abductor pollicis longus muscle

Extensor digitorum muscle
Extensor carpi ulnaris muscle
Extensor pollicis longus muscle

Extensor pollicis bervis muscle
Superficial radial nerve
Posterior interosseous nerve

Figure 3-44
Course of the radial nerve through the forearm.

The nerve descends across the wrist, splits into medial and lateral branches, and innervates the skin of the dorsolateral hand. Specifically, it supplies the skin of the dorsal aspect of the thumb, the index, middle, and lateral one-half of the ring fingers as far distally as the middle phalanx, and the corresponding portion of the hand. The loss of cutaneous sensibility resulting from a lesion of this nerve almost always includes the skin of the dorsal aspect of the first web space. The superficial branch of the radial nerve is most vulnerable to injury in the distal forearm and in the hand, where it is in a superficial position. It is vulnerable to laceration and to compression from casts, watchbands, heavy straps, and the like.

The **deep radial nerve** (Fig. 3-44) also begins at about the level of the elbow and deep to the brachioradialis muscle. This nerve is quite short (5–8 cm) because it divides into multiple muscular branches soon after it arises. From its origin the nerve inclines posteriorly and laterally, passing through the supinator muscle between its humeral and ulnar heads of origin as it wraps around the neck of the radius. The nerve typically emerges from the supinator muscle as multiple muscular branches. One of these branches, the **posterior interosseous nerve,** is considered the terminal portion of the deep radial nerve. This branch passes inferiorly on the posterior aspect of the interosseous membrane; it supplies the deeper muscles of the posterior compartment and ends by innervating the wrist joint. The deep radial nerve is most vulnerable to injury from its origin to the point where it emerges from the supinator muscle. Due to its multiple short branches and its course through the supinator, it is firmly fixed in its position. Although the nerve is usually separated from the radial neck by the supinator muscle, occasionally it is not, and thus is vulnerable to injury when the radial neck is fractured. The nerve may be stretched when the radius is dislocated distally. Either the proximal or distal borders of the supinator may be fibrous, or the nerve can be entrapped within the muscle.

Blood supply of the posterior compartment of the forearm. The **posterior interosseous artery** (Figs. 3-7, 3-39) is the only artery that descends in the posterior compartment. This small artery branches from the common interosseous branch of the ulnar artery in the proximal aspect of the anterior compartment. The posterior interosseous artery enters the posterior compartment by passing above the proximal border of the interosseous membrane and then descends on the posterior aspect of the interosseous membrane with the posterior interosseous nerve.

Carpal Tunnel

The ventral groove formed by the carpal bones is transformed into a tunnel or canal by the **deep part of the flexor retinaculum** (transverse carpal ligament) (Figs. 3-45, 3-46). This strong, fibrous band stretches from the pisiform and hook of the hamate medially to the tubercles of the scaphoid and trapezium laterally. From proximal to distal this canal is short, extending only the length of the two rows of carpal bones. The carpal canal is continuous distally with the central compartment of the hand; structures passing through the canal either enter the central compartment or go to the thumb.

The structures that enter the hand by passing through the carpal tunnel (Figs. 3-45, 3-46) are the tendons of the long digital flexor muscles and the median nerve. The tendons of the flexor digitorum profundus and superficialis muscles together with their tendon sheath, the ulnar bursa, occupy the majority of the canal. The tendons of the flexor digitorum profundus are positioned side-by-side dorsally and deeply; the ten-

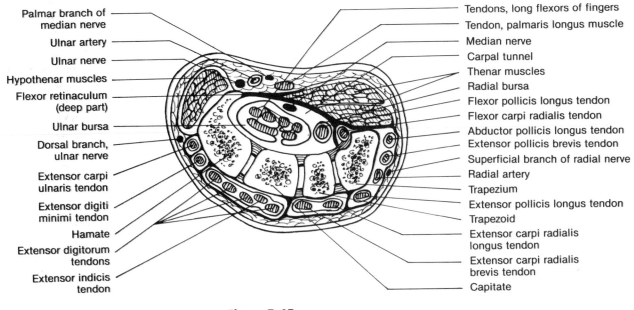

Palmar branch of
median nerve

Ulnar artery

Ulnar nerve

Hypothenar muscles

Flexor retinaculum
(deep part)

Ulnar bursa

Dorsal branch,
ulnar nerve

Extensor carpi
ulnaris tendon

Extensor digiti
minimi tendon

Hamate

Extensor digitorum
tendons

Extensor indicis
tendon

Tendons, long flexors of fingers

Tendon, palmaris longus muscle

Median nerve

Carpal tunnel

Thenar muscles

Radial bursa

Flexor pollicis longus tendon

Flexor carpi radialis tendon

Abductor pollicis longus tendon

Extensor pollicis brevis tendon

Superficial branch of radial nerve

Radial artery

Trapezium

Extensor pollicis longus tendon

Trapezoid

Extensor carpi radialis
longus tendon

Extensor carpi radialis
brevis tendon

Capitate

Figure 3-45
Cross section through the wrist at the level of the distal row of carpal bones.
The carpal tunnel is the area formed by the deep part of the flexor retinaculum and the carpal bones.

dons of the flexor digitorum superficialis are located more ventrally. The tendon of the flexor pollicis longus occupies the most radial portion of the canal and is enclosed by its tendon sheath, the radial bursa. The median nerve is the most ventral structure, located just deep to the deep part of the flexor retinaculum.

It is important to note that this canal is small and that the structures listed above are tightly packed in the canal. In addition, the borders of the canal are rigid and inflexible. As a result, either reduction of the size of the canal (by arthritis involvement of the intercarpal joints or dislocation of the lunate into the canal) or an increase in the size of any structures within the canal (due to tendonitis or synovitis) can cause mechanical compression of all structures within the canal. When compression occurs, the median nerve is the structure that usually is affected first, probably because it is the "softest" structure in the canal and thus the most susceptible to pressure. Compression of the median nerve in the carpal canal, the **carpal tunnel syndrome,** is probably the most common entrapment point of a nerve in the body. The symptoms resulting from this entrapment correspond to the distribution of the nerve distal to the canal and are discussed with the nerve injuries of the upper limb.

Relationships on the Anterior Aspect of the Wrist

All structures crossing the wrist cannot be palpated, but all structures can be definitively located. The superficial structures are easy to identify, and

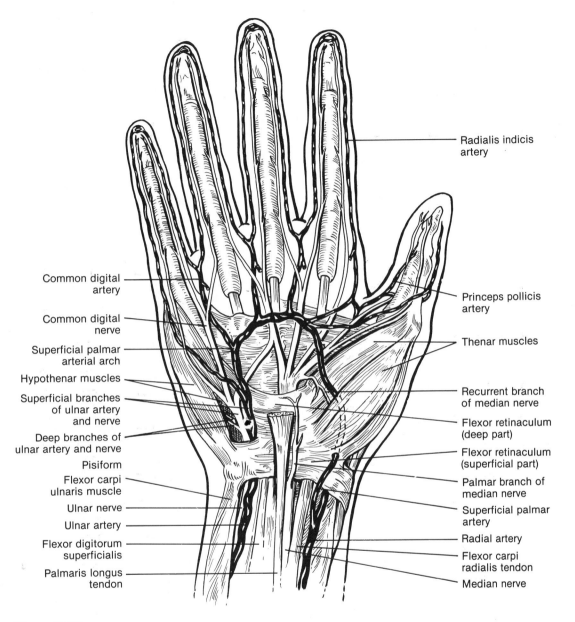

Radialis indicis artery

Common digital artery

Common digital nerve

Superficial palmar arterial arch

Hypothenar muscles

Superficial branches of ulnar artery and nerve

Deep branches of ulnar artery and nerve

Pisiform

Flexor carpi ulnaris muscle

Ulnar nerve

Ulnar artery

Flexor digitorum superficialis

Palmaris longus tendon

Princeps pollicis artery

Thenar muscles

Recurrent branch of median nerve

Flexor retinaculum (deep part)

Flexor retinaculum (superficial part)

Palmar branch of median nerve

Superficial palmar artery

Radial artery

Flexor carpi radialis tendon

Median nerve

Figure 3-46
Neurovascular structures of the ventral wrist and palm.

the positions of the rest are easily related to the former. Generally, two tendons stand out as they cross the midportion of the ventral aspect of the wrist (Fig. 3-46). The tendon of the flexor carpi radialis muscle is an important landmark and is positioned just lateral to the midportion of the wrist. When present, which is approximately 85 percent of the time, the tendon of the palmaris longus muscle is found immediately medial to that of the flexor capri radialis. The tendon of the palmaris longus is usually the more prominent but the smaller of the two, and it can be followed more distally. The interval between these two tendons marks the position of the median nerve, which is quite deep. In the absence of the palmaris longus muscle, the mass of tendons that is palpable medial to the tendon of the flexor carpi radialis belongs to the flexor digitorum superficialis muscle, and the median nerve is positioned medial to the tendon of the flexor carpi radialis muscle. The most medial tendon, that of the flexor carpi ulnaris muscle, can be followed directly to the pisiform. Proximal to the pisiform, the ulnar nerve is deep to this tendon, and the ulnar artery is lateral. Both the artery and nerve pass lateral to the pisiform. The radial artery is positioned lateral to the tendon of the flexor carpi radialis, but it does not cross the ventral aspect of the wrist. As a result, this artery must be palpated several centimeters proximal to the wrist.

Relationships on the Posterior and Lateral Aspects of the Wrist

The tendons that cross the dorsal and lateral aspects of the wrist (Figs. 3-43, 3-45, 3-47) are lashed to the distal aspects of the radius and ulna by the extensor retinaculum. This thickening of the investing (antebrachial) fascia is connected to the underlying bones by various septa that form compartments deep to the retinaculum through which the tendons pass. Each tendon or group of tendons is encased in a tendon sheath that facilitates the movement of the tendon(s) within the fibro-osseous compartments.

Most anatomists agree that there are six compartments across the dorsal aspect of the wrist. The most lateral compartment is on the radial side of the radius and contains the tendons of the abductor pollicis longus and extensor pollicis brevis muscles. The former tendon is easy to palpate; the latter must be palpated proximal to the base of the first metacarpal. The tendons of the extensor carpi radialis longus and brevis muscles occupy the second compartment, which is formed on that part of the dorsal aspect of the radius that is lateral to the dorsal tubercle of the radius. Although both of these tendons pass deep to the tendon of the extensor pollicis longus, they can be palpated as they cross the wrist and pass toward their respective insertions on the second and third metacarpals. The tendon of the extensor pollicis longus occupies the groove and compartment immediately medial to the dorsal radial tubercle. This tendon is readily palpable and visible as it changes its course around the tubercle. The fourth compartment is the largest and situated on the most medial part of the dorsal aspect of the radius. The tendons of the extensor digitorum and extensor indicis muscles pass through the compartment; those of the extensor digitorum are visible distal to the compartment. The tendon of the extensor digiti minimi occupies the fifth compartment, which is on the dorsal aspect of the ulna; and the tendon of the extensor carpi ulnaris is in the sixth compartment, situated on the medial aspect of the ulna. Both tendons are palpable, that of the extensor digiti minimi over the fifth metacarpal and that of the extensor carpi ulnaris distal to the ulnar styloid.

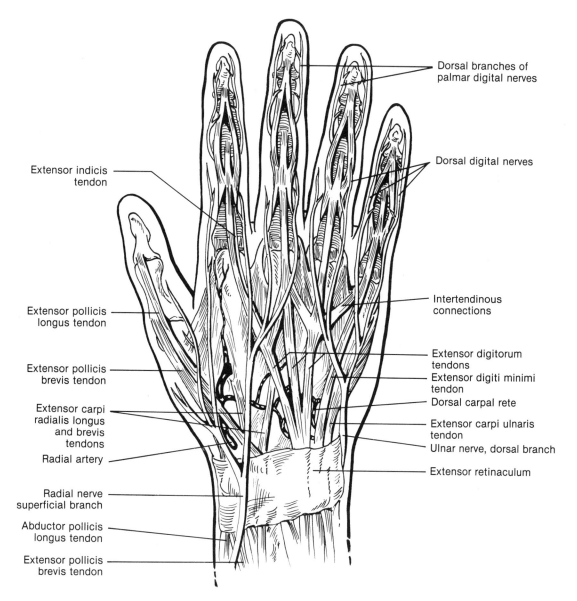

Extensor indicis tendon

Extensor pollicis longus tendon

Extensor pollicis brevis tendon

Extensor carpi radialis longus and brevis tendons

Radial artery

Radial nerve superficial branch

Abductor pollicis longus tendon

Extensor pollicis brevis tendon

Dorsal branches of palmar digital nerves

Dorsal digital nerves

Intertendinous connections

Extensor digitorum tendons

Extensor digiti minimi tendon

Dorsal carpal rete

Extensor carpi ulnaris tendon

Ulnar nerve, dorsal branch

Extensor retinaculum

Figure 3-47
Neurovascular structures of the dorsal wrist and hand.

Hand

Retinacular System of the Hand

The retinacular system of the hand consists of a number of connective tissue layers that hold the structures of the hand in place. This system enables the hand to be both efficient and versatile. The hand operates in two modes, one of strength and one of finely regulated and delicate dexterity. There are strong, thick fibrous layers and septa to hold the strength structures in place; there are thin layers for the finer structures. It is important to note that the skin of the palm is firmly attached to the underlying layers of connective tissue. The subcutaneous tissue (superficial fascia) is predominantly fat and forms an extensive fat pad, and the skin is firmly attached to the investing fascia by multiple septa that pass through the pad. As a result, the palmar skin is firmly fixed, a factor that greatly facilitates grasp.

The compartmentation of the hand is described briefly on page 54. The investing (antebrachial) fascia of the forearm continues into the hand as an investing stockinglike sheath. At the level of the distal forearm and wrist this fascia is thickened and reinforced by circumferential fibers to form the superficial part of the flexor retinaculum (volar carpal ligament) and the extensor retinaculum. The relationship between the superficial and deep parts of the flexor retinaculum (Fig. 3-46) is a bit confusing as they are continuous: The deep part is distal to the superficial part, and yet the deep part is at a different level (deeper) than the superficial part. With the exception of the palmar branch of the median nerve and variable superficial veins, the superficial part of the flexor retinaculum (volar carpal ligament) surrounds all structures that cross the ventral aspect of the wrist. The deep part of the flexor retinaculum (transverse carpal ligament) forms the ventral boundary of the carpal tunnel, and thus only those structures passing through the carpal tunnel are deep to that layer. The two retinacula are connected by an obliquely oriented layer of connective tissue; the structures passing between the two retinacula pass through this oblique layer. The deep flexor retinaculum is not a part of the investing fascia, but rather a separate and deeper layer of connective tissue.

In the palm the investing fascia (Figs. 3-48, 3-49) is thin medially (**hypothenar fascia**) and laterally (**thenar fascia**) and greatly thickened centrally as the **palmar aponeurosis.** The palmar aponeurosis fills the area between the thenar and hypothenar eminences and thus is narrow proximally but expands distally as its borders diverge toward the four medial digits. In the distal palm, several centimeters proximal to the MP joints, the single aponeurosis is replaced by digital slips to the index, middle, ring, and little fingers. These slips pass across the MP joints and contribute to the formation of the fibrous portions of the digital tendon sheaths. Proximal to the MP joints, the digital slips are interconnected by **transverse fasciculi**; at about the level of the MP joints the **superficial transverse metacarpal ligament** unites the slips. Proximally, the aponeurosis is continuous with the tendon of the palmaris longus muscle; if no muscle is present, the aponeurosis blends with the deep fascia. In the distal palm, variably developed septa extend from the deep aspect of the aponeurosis to the four medial metacarpals. The involvement of the palmar aponeurosis in **Dupuytren's contracture,** a shortening of connective tissue that leads to flexion contractures of predominantly the medial digits, is not clear. However, varying amounts of the aponeurosis and associated septa are commonly removed as part of the surgical treatment of the problem.

Two septa (Fig. 3-48) extend from the lateral and medial edges of the palmar aponeurosis, one to the first and the other to the fifth metacarpal.

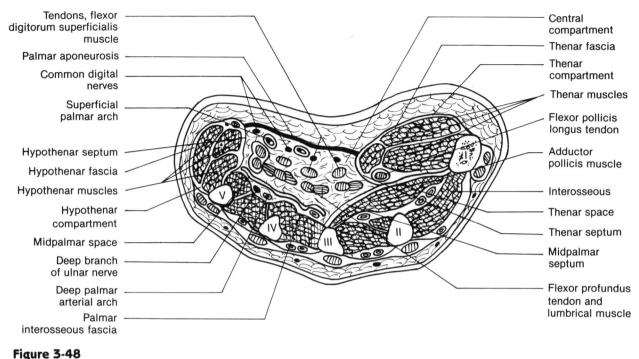

Figure 3-48
Cross section of the hand.

The **thenar septum** extends from the junction of the palmar aponeurosis and the thenar fascia to the first metacarpal; the thenar fascia and septum thus form a compartment associated with the first metacarpal, the thenar compartment. Similarly, the **hypothenar septum** and fascia form the hypothenar compartment. Deep in the palm the **palmar interosseous fascia** (adductor-interosseous fascia) stretches across the ventral aspects of the metacarpals and interossei muscles. This layer of fascia interconnects the first and fifth metacarpals, and attaches to the fourth and perhaps the third metacarpals as well. A third compartment in the palm, the central compartment, is bounded by the palmar aponeurosis ventrally, the thenar septum laterally, the hypothenar septum medially, and the palmar interosseous fascia dorsally (Fig. 3-48).

The deep fascia in the dorsum of the hand (Fig. 3-48) consists of layers superficial and deep to the long extensor tendons and the dorsal interosseous fascia. The **supratendinous fascia** is continuous with the extensor retinaculum and located superficial to the long extensor tendons; the **infratendinous fascia** is deep to the same tendons. These two layers blend together on either side of the long extensor tendons and are continuous with the periosteum of the second and fifth metacarpals. They thus form a potential space around the long extensor tendons. Trauma to the dorsum of the hand can lead to swelling that is limited to this space. The **dorsal interosseous fascia** interconnects adjacent metacarpals dorsal to the interossei muscles.

The **adductor-interosseous compartment** is the deepest compart-

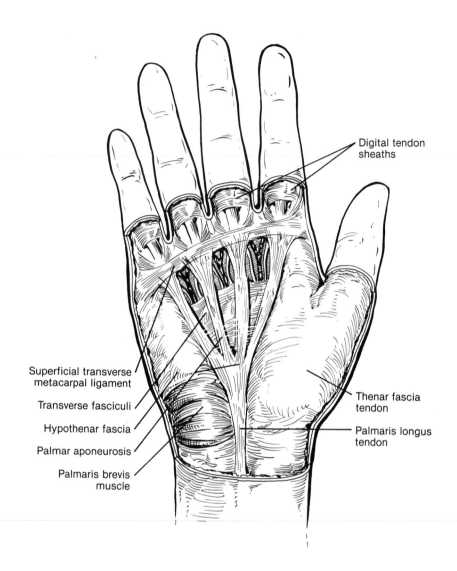

Digital tendon sheaths

Superficial transverse metacarpal ligament

Transverse fasciculi

Hypothenar fascia

Palmar aponeurosis

Palmaris brevis muscle

Thenar fascia tendon

Palmaris longus tendon

Figure 3-49
Superficial structures of the palm.

ment in the hand and essentially is situated between the metacarpals. It is bounded by the metacarpals and the dorsal and palmar interosseous fasciae.

Thenar Compartment

The thenar compartment (Fig. 3-48) contains three of the intrinsic muscles of the thumb (muscles that arise and insert within the hand) and the tendon of the flexor pollicis longus muscle. These intrinsic muscles form the thenar eminence of the hand. All of the thenar muscles are innervated by the **recurrent (thenar, motor) branch** of the median nerve.

The **abductor pollicis brevis muscle** (Figs. 3-31, 3-50) is the most superficial and ventrally positioned of the thenar muscles. It arises from the deep part of the flexor retinaculum and the trapezium, and inserts on the ventral aspect of the base of the proximal phalanx of the thumb. (The ventral aspect of the thumb is the same as the lateral aspects of the other digits.) As its name indicates, this muscle abducts the thumb or pulls it ventrally away from the hand.

The **flexor pollicis brevis muscle** (Figs. 3-31, 3-50) is more dorsal and partially deep to the abductor pollicis brevis. The fiber orientation of this muscle is similar to that of the abductor pollicis brevis; the flexor is simply more dorsal (deeper in the palm) and thus in position to flex the metacarpal and proximal phalanx of the thumb rather than produce abduction. Its fibers arise from the deep part of the flexor retinaculum and trapezium and insert on the ventromedial aspect of the base of the proximal phalanx of the thumb.

The **opponens pollicis muscle** (Figs. 3-31, 3-51) is the deepest of the three thenar muscles and covers the ventral aspect of most of the shaft of the first metacarpal. From an origin on the deep part of the flexor retinaculum and trapezium, its fibers pass laterally and distally and insert on a line along most of the ventral aspect of the shaft of the first metacarpal.

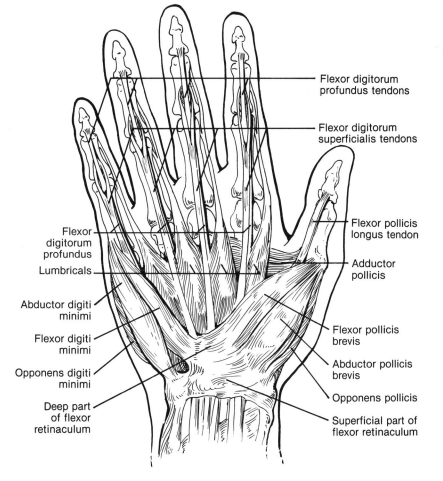

Figure 3-50
Superficial intrinsic muscles of the palm.

Flexor digitorum profundus tendons

Flexor digitorum superficialis tendons

Flexor pollicis longus tendon

Adductor pollicis

Flexor pollicis brevis

Abductor pollicis brevis

Opponens pollicis

Superficial part of flexor retinaculum

Flexor digitorum profundus

Lumbricals

Abductor digiti minimi

Flexor digiti minimi

Opponens digiti minimi

Deep part of flexor retinaculum

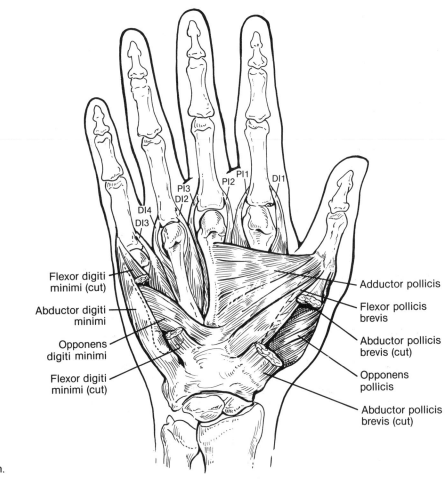

Figure 3-51
Deep intrinsic muscles of the palm.

This muscle's fibers are obliquely oriented relative to the shaft of the metacarpal and their contraction produces rotation of the bone, the essential ingredient of thumb opposition.

The recurrent branch of the median nerve (Fig. 3-46) branches from the median nerve at the distal end of the carpal tunnel. This branch passes laterally into the substance of the thenar muscles.

Hypothenar Compartment

The muscles in the hypothenar compartment are similar to those in the thenar compartment, but they move the fifth metacarpal very little because the fifth CM joint permits little motion. These muscles are innervated by the deep branch of the ulnar nerve.

The **abductor digiti minimi muscle** (Figs. 3-31, 3-50) is the most medial muscle of the compartment, extending from the pisiform to the medial aspect of the base of the fifth metacarpal. Its action is abduction of the fifth digit at the MP joint.

The **flexor digiti minimi muscle** (Figs. 3-31, 3-50) is positioned anteriorly and laterally. From an origin on the deep flexor retinaculum and the hook of the hamate, its fibers pass somewhat medially to their insertion on the medial aspect of the base of the fifth proximal phalanx. This muscle flexes the fifth digit at the MP joint.

The fibers of the **opponens digiti minimi muscle** (Figs. 3-31, 3-51) are oblique to the long axis of the fifth metacarpal. They arise on the hook of the hamate and insert along the medial aspect of the shaft of the fifth metacarpal. This muscle is an ideal position to rotate the fifth metacarpal; but since motion of that bone is limited, the opponens' action is limited to assisting in the "cupping" of the medial aspect of the hand.

The deep branches of the ulnar nerve and artery (Figs. 3-46, 3-52) pass through the hypothenar compartment between the abductor and

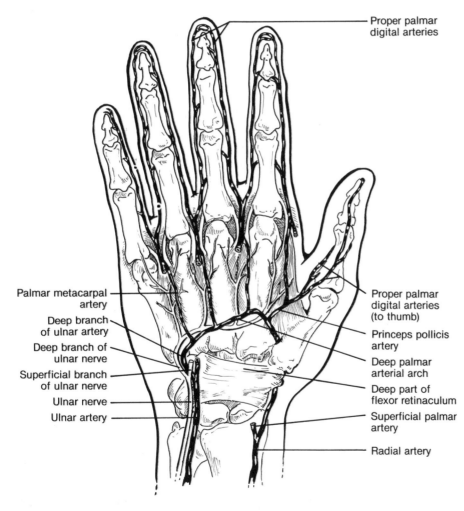

Proper palmar digital arteries

Palmar metacarpal artery

Deep branch of ulnar artery

Deep branch of ulnar nerve

Superficial branch of ulnar nerve

Ulnar nerve

Ulnar artery

Proper palmar digital arteries (to thumb)

Princeps pollicis artery

Deep palmar arterial arch

Deep part of flexor retinaculum

Superficial palmar artery

Radial artery

Figure 3-52
Neurovascular structures of the deep aspect of the palm.

flexor digiti minimi muscles. These structures arise just distal to the pisiform and pass deeply into the palm.

Central Compartment

The central compartment of the hand (Fig. 3-48) contains the tendons of the flexor digitorum superficialis and profundus muscles and the associated lumbrical muscles, the superficial palmar arterial arch and its branches, along with branches of the median and ulnar nerves.

The long digital flexor tendons pass through the center of this compartment, each pair of tendons passing toward the digit on which it acts. In each pair the superficialis tendon is ventral to the profundus tendon. The four **lumbrical muscles** (Fig. 3-50) are positioned on the radial sides of the tendons; each lumbrical arises from the profundus tendon on its medial side or from the two tendons between which it is positioned. The tendons of these small muscles pass distally and dorsally into the digits, where they insert into the extensor expansion; each inserts into both the central and lateral bands of that expansion. The functions of these muscles are discussed on page 145. The innervation of the lumbrical muscles is similar to that of the flexor digitorum profundus muscle in that the two lateral lumbricales are supplied by the median nerve, and the two medial, by the ulnar nerve.

In the proximal part of the central compartment, the superficial palmar arterial arch and the branches of the median and ulnar nerves are found in the interval between the palmar aponeurosis and the long digital flexor tendons. Distally, the branches of the superficial arch and the nerves are positioned between, rather than ventral to, the long flexor tendons.

Adductor-Interosseous Compartment

This compartment contains all of the interossei muscles and the adductor pollicis muscle. All of these muscles are innervated by the deep branch of the ulnar nerve, which together with the deep palmar arterial arch are embedded within the palmar interosseous fascia. Whether these structures are in the adductor-interosseous compartment, or in the central compartment, or neither is interesting but of questionable functional importance.

There are two sets of interossei, the **palmar** and **dorsal interossei muscles,** which are positioned between the metacarpals. These muscles are the major adductors and abductors of the digits, and, since the reference point for these motions is the middle finger, their locations and attachments relative to that finger determine those actions. Both groups of muscles are also integral parts of the flexion-extension balance of the digits.

The **palmar interossei muscles** (Figs. 3-31, 3-33, 3-51) are the adductors of the digits (the palmar adduct, abbreviated PAD), and are positioned to move the digits toward the middle finger. Since the thumb has its own adductor, there are three palmar interossei. They arise from the medial aspect of the second metacarpal and the lateral aspects of the metacarpals 4 and 5. These muscles pass distally and cross the MP joints dorsal to the deep transverse metacarpal ligament and then insert into the extensor aponeurosis (both the central and lateral bands) of their respective digits. An insertion on the base of the proximal phalanx is variable.

The **dorsal interossei muscles** (Figs. 3-31, 3-33, 3-51) are the abductors of the digits (the dorsal abduct, or DAB) and are positioned accordingly. Both the thumb and little finger have their own abductors and the middle finger must move medially and laterally away from its midposition reference point; consequently, there are four dorsal interossei. Each muscle has two heads of origin and arises from the adjacent sides of the metacarpals between which it is located. The muscles cross the MP joints and insert on the side of the base of the appropriate proximal phalanx and into the extensor aponeurosis (both the central and lateral bands). Specifically, the first dorsal interosseous inserts into the lateral aspect of the base of the second metacarpal; the second and third, into the lateral and medial aspects of the base of the third metacarpal; and the fourth, into the medial aspect of the base of the fourth metacarpal.

The **adductor pollicis muscle** (Figs. 3-31, 3-51) is the largest of the intrinsic muscles of the hand. Although it is an intrinsic muscle of the thumb, it is not located within the thenar compartment. It has two heads of origin, an oblique head from the lateral distal carpals and adjacent bases of the metacarpals and a transverse head from the shaft of the third metacarpal. It inserts on the ventromedial base of the proximal phalanx of the thumb. The only adductor of the thumb, it pulls the thumb toward the index finger.

Median Nerve

The median nerve (Fig. 3-46) enters the hand by passing through the carpal tunnel as the most ventral structure. At the distal end of the tunnel it separates into its terminal branches, the recurrent or muscular branch and multiple digital branches. The muscular branch passes laterally into the thenar compartment; although it may pass through some portion of the deep flexor retinaculum, it definitely passes through the thenar septum. This nerve is vulnerable to entrapment as it passes through either of these fibrous layers. Because of its superficial position in the thenar compartment, it is vulnerable to laceration. Its specific location is the halfway point along a line connecting the pisiform and the base of the first metacarpal.

The digital branches are of two types. A **common digital nerve** innervates the adjacent sides of two fingers. This nerve passes toward a web space where it divides into two **proper digital nerves.** Each proper digital nerve supplies the skin of one-half of the ventral (or dorsal) aspect of a digit. The digital branches of the median nerve are usually three proper branches to the thumb and radial side of the index finger, and two common branches to the web spaces between the index and middle and the middle and ring fingers. The proper digital nerve to the index finger and the common digital nerve to the index and middle fingers provide small branches to the first and second lumbrical muscles, respectively. The proper digital nerves have branches that pass dorsally in the distal aspects of the digits so they usually supply the skin of the entire digit distal to the DIP joint. The skin of the hand supplied by the median nerve includes the palmar aspects of the thumb, index, middle, and lateral half of the ring fingers, the distal dorsal aspects of the index, middle, and half of the ring fingers, and the corresponding part of the palm. The skin of the central palm is supplied by the palmar branch of the median, which arises proximal to the wrist and passes superficial to the carpal tunnel.

Ulnar Nerve

The ulnar nerve (Figs. 3-46, 3-52) is the major motor nerve of the hand. It enters the hand by passing superficial to the deep part of the flexor retinaculum and then passes, in succession, lateral to the pisiform and medial to the hook of the hamate. In this short part of its course the nerve is superficial to the deep part of the flexor retinaculum and piso-hamate ligament, and deep to the palmaris brevis muscle and the investing fascia. This fibro-osseous tunnel, in which the nerve and ulnar artery are firmly fixed, is the **ulnar tunnel** or **Guyon's canal.** The ulnar nerve separates into its superficial and deep branches while in this canal, and the main trunk or either of its branches is vulnerable to entrapment or injury from laceration or external compression (leaning on the handlebar of a bicycle) while in the canal.

The **superficial branch of the ulnar nerve** continues distally, and at the distal border of the palmaris brevis muscle, it branches into a proper digital nerve that supplies the medial aspect of the little finger and a common digital nerve that supplies the adjacent sides of the ring and little fingers. This superficial branch is essentially a cutaneous nerve, but it does innervate the small palmaris brevis muscle (Fig. 3-49).

After arising within the ulnar tunnel, the **deep branch of the ulnar nerve** (Figs. 3-46, 3-52) passes posteriorly into the hypothenar compartment between the abductor and flexor digiti minimi muscles, and then through the opponens digiti minimi muscle. It is vulnerable to entrapment as it crosses the distal edge of the pisohamate ligament and an occasional tendinous arch that may be associated with the hypothenar muscles. From the hypothenar compartment it passes laterally into the central compartment, where it is in company with the deep palmar arterial arch and embedded within the palmar interosseous fascia. The deep branch supplies the muscles in the hypothenar compartment, the two medial lumbricals, all of the interossei and ends by innervating the adductor pollicis muscle.

The skin of the posteromedial aspect of the hand, including the little and ulnar half of the ring fingers, is supplied by the dorsal cutaneous branch of the ulnar nerve (Fig. 3-47). This branch arises deep to the flexor carpi ulnaris, approximately 5 to 7 centimeters proximal to the wrist. It enters the subcutaneous tissue by passing between the tendon of that muscle and the ulna. It then crosses the medial aspect of the wrist as it passes to the dorsum of the hand.

Radial Nerve

The only part of the radial nerve that enters the hand is its **superficial branch** (Figs. 3-43, 3-44, 3-47). This nerve is completely cutaneous and enters the posterolateral aspect of the hand by passing across the anatomic snuff box and the tendon of the extensor pollicis longus muscle. Its branches supply the skin of the dorsolateral hand, specifically, the dorsal aspects of the lateral three and one-half fingers and corresponding part of the dorsum of the hand. The skin over the distal phalanges of the index, middle, and radial half of the ring fingers is supplied by the median nerve.

In the hand the superficial radial nerve is superficial throughout its course and is vulnerable to laceration. Since little separates the nerve from the underlying bones and it has little protection superficially, it also is vulnerable to extreme compression, as from a heavy strap or blunt trauma.

Summary of the Innervation of the Hand

The intrinsic muscles of the hand are innervated solely by the median and ulnar nerves. The muscular branch of the median supplies the muscles in the thenar compartment, and the two lateral lumbricals are innervated by the digital branches of the median. The superficial branch of the ulnar innervates only the palmaris brevis muscle, while the deep branch innervates all of the muscles in the hypothenar and adductor-interosseous compartments as well as the two medial lumbricals. It is important to note that there is variation in the innervation pattern just described although it cannot always be substantiated anatomically. Interconnections between the median and ulnar nerves in the hand (Fig. 3-46) are rather common, and more proximal communications (forearm and arm) have been reported in the literature. However, the presence of such connections does not ensure that variation in the innervation exists. This can be verified only by electrical stimulation studies or in the presence of peripheral nerve injuries.

The cutaneous innervation of the hand is provided by the median, ulnar, and superficial radial nerves. The ulnar nerve, through its dorsal cutaneous, palmar, and superficial branches, supplies the dorsal and ventral aspects of the little fingers and the medial half of the ring fingers and corresponding part of the palm and dorsum of the hand. Generally, the median nerve supplies the rest of the palmar skin, and the superficial radial nerve supplies the remaining skin of the dorsum of the hand. The median supplies the palm through its palmar cutaneous branch and the skin of the digits through its digital branches. These digital branches also supply the skin over the distal phalanges of the index, middle, and lateral half of the ring fingers. The area supplied by the superficial radial nerve includes the dorsum (lateral surface) of the thumb. Although this pattern of cutaneous innervation is generally true, variations do exist. These variations are more common dorsally, but dorsally or ventrally the variations usually involve the nerve supply to the middle and ring fingers.

Blood Supply of the Hand

The blood supply to the hand is provided by the radial and ulnar arteries, which together form a pair of arterial arches within the palm. Although both vessels participate in the formation of both arches, each arch is formed predominantly by one artery. The two arches are interconnected and have branches that supply the digits and other areas of the hand.

The **ulnar artery** (Figs. 3-7, 3-46, 3-52) enters the hand lateral to the ulnar nerve. The **deep palmar branch** arises just distal to the pisiform and accompanies the deep branch of the ulnar nerve through the hypothenar compartment and into the deep portion of the palm, where it completes the formation of the deep palmar arterial arch. Distal to the origin of the deep palmar branch, the ulnar artery becomes the **superficial palmar arterial arch.** This arch is formed in the central compartment between the palmar aponeurosis and the long digital flexor tendons at about the level of the palmar (medial) surface of the fully extended thumb. It usually is completed by the superficial palmar branch of the radial artery, which arises as the radial artery turns dorsally to cross the wrist. The superficial palmar artery passes through the thenar muscles and joins the superficial arch in the lateral aspect of the central compartment. This connection to the radial artery is not always present, and even when it is present, at times it is very small.

The main branches of the superficial arch (Fig. 3-46) are the digital branches. Like the nerves, the arteries to the digits are named "common" and "proper." The most constant branches are a proper digital to the medial side of the little finger and three common digitals that supply the adjacent sides of the little, ring, middle, and index fingers. The arteries to the thumb and lateral aspect of the index finger are typically branches of the radial artery, but they sometimes are branches of the superficial arch or of both the arch and the radial artery.

The **radial artery** (Figs. 3-7, 3-43, 3-46, 3-47, 3-52) enters the hand by passing posteriorly across the lateral aspect of the wrist and through the anatomic snuff box. Just distal to the tendon of the extensor pollicis longus muscle the artery reaches the interval between the first and second metacarpals, where it makes a sharp turn ventrally, passing between the two heads of the first dorsal interosseous muscle and into the deep palm. Once in the palm the radial artery becomes the **deep palmar arterial arch.** This arch is embedded in the palmar interosseous fascia approximately one finger's breadth proximal to the superficial arch. The deep arch is completed medially by the deep branch of the ulnar artery; the deep branch of the ulnar nerve accompanies the deep arch. The most lateral branch of the deep arch is the **princeps pollicis artery,** which divides into two branches that supply the thumb. The next branch is the **radialis indicis artery,** which supplies the radial side of the index finger. These two branches are quite variable relative to origin; either or both may arise from the superficial arch or from both arches. A variable number of **meta-carpal arteries** branch from the deep arch and join the common digital branches of the superficial arch in the distal aspect of the palm.

Both the radial and ulnar arteries have palmar and dorsal carpal branches. These branches unite on their respective surfaces of the carpus to form palmar and dorsal arches (rete) that are somewhat variable.

Bursae and Spaces of the Hand

In addition to the compartments of the hand, there are bursae (synovial tendon sheaths) associated with the long digital flexor tendons and a pair of spaces or clefts (really fascial planes). Fluid or inflammatory material can accumulate in these bursae and spaces and produce characteristic swellings in the hand.

The **radial bursa** (Figs. 3-45, 3-53A) is the tendon sheath of the flexor pollicis longus muscle. This sheath extends from the distal forearm (proximal to the carpal tunnel) to the insertion of the tendon. The **ulnar bursa** (Figs. 3-45, 3-53A) is the tendon sheath of the flexor digitorum profundus and superficialis muscles. It also begins proximal to the carpal tunnel and extends into the palm. That part associated with the tendons of the little finger typically extends to the insertions of those tendons. The rest of the sheath extends only into the palm; hence the tendons to the index, middle, and ring fingers are without tendon sheaths in the distal aspect of the palm. The radial and ulnar bursae occasionally communicate at the wrist.

The **thenar** and **midpalmar spaces** (Figs. 3-48, 3-53A) are found in the interval between the long digital flexor tendons and the adductor pollicis and interossei muscles. The term "space" is a clear misnomer because there are no actual spaces; they are fascial planes associated with the palmar interosseous fascia. A longitudinally oriented septum, the **mid-palmar septum,** attaches to the third metacarpal and separates this deep fascial plane into medial (midpalmar) and lateral (thenar) portions. These spaces extend distally to the MP joints and proximally to about the distal border of the carpal tunnel.

Long Digital Flexor Tendons and
Their Digital Tendon Sheaths

The tendons of the flexor digitorum superficialis and profundus muscles (Figs. 3-50, 3-53) enter the digits after passing through the palm, where the superficialis tendons are ventral to those of the profundus. At about the midshaft level of the proximal phalanx the superficial tendon splits and curves around the deeper profundus tendon. The two slips then come together and insert on the ventral base of the middle phalanx. The component fibers within the superficialis tendon are arranged so that tension on that tendon does not restrict the movement of the deeper tendon in any way. That is, the tendon of the flexor digitorum profundus slides freely through the tendinous arch irrespective of the position of the digit

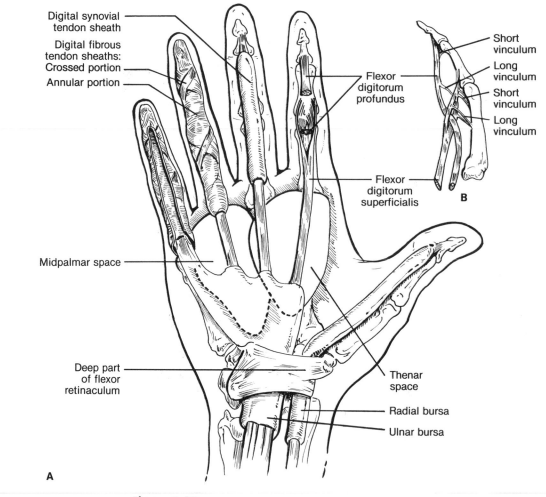

Figure 3-53

Ventral view of the hand (A) and lateral view of a digit (B) illustrating the bursae and spaces (A) and the insertions and tendon sheaths of the long digital flexor tendons (A, B).

or the amount of tension. The profundus tendon continues distally and attaches to the ventral base of the distal phalanx. Each tendon is connected to the phalanx proximal to its insertion by two or three vincula that conduct blood vessels to the tendons.

Each **digital tendon sheath** (Fig. 3-53A) is composed of an outer fibrous and a deeper synovial portion. The fibrous portion lashes the tendons to the ventral aspects of the phalanges while the synovial portion facilitates movement within the fibrous tunnel. With the exception of the little finger, the synovial portion of the sheath begins proximal to the MP joint and extends distally to the distal phalanx. This part of the sheath consists of two layers that form a closed space (really there is no actual space since the two layers are adjacent) around the tendons. The outer layer attaches to the walls of the fibrous tunnel; the inner layer is anchored to the tendons. During motion the two layers slide relative to one another.

The fibrous portions of the digital tendon sheaths are continuous with the digital slips of the palmar aponeurosis. The aponeurosis, however, forms only the most proximal portion of the sheath, which is in the area of the metacarpal head. The sheath extends distally to the base of the distal phalanx. The fibers of the sheath attach to the phalanges and palmar ligaments at the IP joints so the fibrous portion of the sheath is really a fibro-osseous tunnel. Those parts of the sheath along the bodies of the phalanges (annular portion) are thick and composed of parallel fibers that are perpendicular to the long axes of the bones. To facilitate motion, the sheath is thinner at the MP and IP joints and the component fibers are crossed (crossed portion). The annular portions are smaller in diameter than the crossed portions. This difference is significant when changes occur in the size of either the tendon or the sheath. For example, an increase in the size of a tendon (or reduction in the diameter of the sheath) can interfere with the tendon's motion within the sheath. In this situation the tendon enlargement usually gets stuck proximal to the narrow part of the sheath. That is, it gets stuck in the crossed portion, and the finger is flexed because the digital flexors are stronger than the extensors. The resulting condition is called a **trigger finger.**

The Extensor Aponeurosis

The expansion and/or specializations of the tendons of the extensor digitorum (and extensors indicis and digiti minimi) muscle have several names: **extensor aponeurosis, extensor hood, extensor mechanism** (Fig. 3-54). This aponeurosis covers most of the dorsum of the four medial digits; the lumbricales and interossei insert into it, and various ligaments contribute to its formation. An understanding of this system is essential to the understanding of the posture and mechanics of these digits. The components described in this account are those most involved in the function of the digits.

As the tendons of the extensor digitorum (and associated muscles) cross the MP joints they have variable attachments to the dorsal bases of the metacarpals and they expand on both sides of the joints, forming what is properly called the extensor hood. This hood attaches ventrally to the capsule of the joint (palmar ligament) and the deep transverse metacarpal ligament and serves as attachment sites for the tendons of the interossei and lumbrical muscles. Tension on the extensor tendon extends the proximal phalanx by pulling the extensor hood proximally and, if present, through its direct attachment to the proximal phalanx.

Distal to the MP joint the extensor tendon splits into three tendinous bands that continue distally. The single **central band** passes across the dorsal aspect of the proximal phalanx and the PIP joint and then attaches to the dorsal aspect of the base of the middle phalanx. The two **lateral bands** diverge medially and laterally around the PIP and then converge as they near the DIP joint; they cross the dorsal aspect of that joint and then attach to the dorsal aspect of the base of the distal phalanx. It is

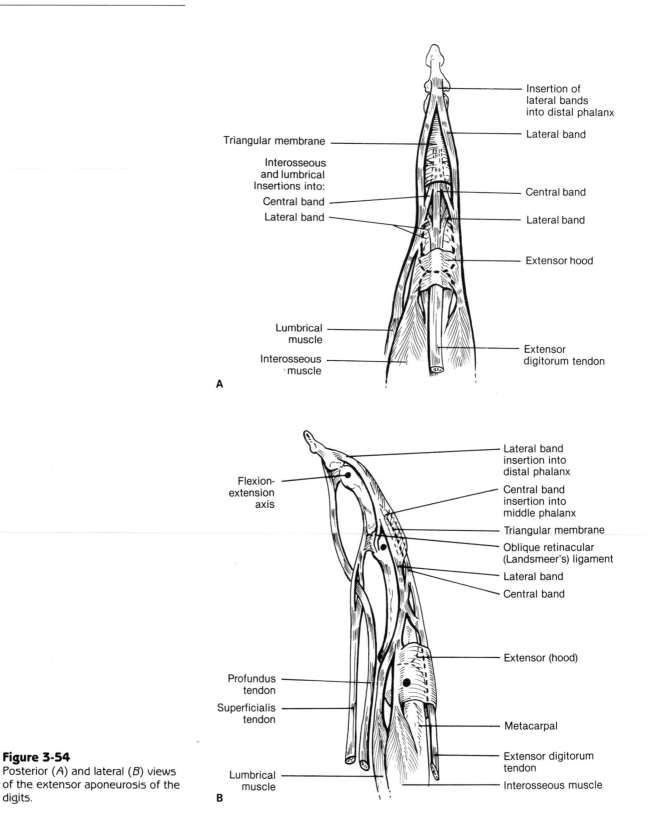

Insertion of
lateral bands
into distal phalanx

Lateral band

Triangular membrane

Interosseous
and lumbrical
Insertions into:

Central band

Lateral band

Central band

Lateral band

Extensor hood

Lumbrical
muscle

Interosseous
muscle

Extensor
digitorum tendon

A

Lateral band
insertion into
distal phalanx

Flexion-
extension
axis

Central band
insertion into
middle phalanx

Triangular membrane

Oblique retinacular
(Landsmeer's) ligament

Lateral band

Central band

Extensor (hood)

Profundus
tendon

Superficialis
tendon

Metacarpal

Extensor digitorum
tendon

Lumbrical
muscle

Interosseous muscle

B

Figure 3-54
Posterior (*A*) and lateral (*B*) views
of the extensor aponeurosis of the
digits.

important to note that the central band passes dorsal to the flexion-extension axis of the PIP joint and the lateral bands pass dorsal to the flexion-extension axis of the DIP joint.

The lumbrical and interossei (dorsal and palmar) muscles are an important part of the extensor mechanism, and the tendons of each of these muscles insert into the central and lateral bands. The tendons of both the lumbrical and interossei muscles pass ventral to the flexion-extension axis of the MP joint, and thus they are flexors of the proximal phalanx. The tendons of the lumbricales are positioned more ventrally than those of the interossei, so the lumbricales are the major flexors for the initial degrees of flexion. As the proximal phalanx is flexed, however, the tendons of the interossei become relatively more ventral and thus stronger flexors. By virtue of the lumbrical and interossei insertions into the central band, they are extensors of the middle phalanx; by virtue of their insertions into the lateral bands, they extend the distal phalanx. The combined action of the lumbrical and interossei muscles, then, is simultaneous flexion of the proximal phalanx and extension of both the middle and distal phalanges. This is the skill position of the hand (as used in writing) and it is regulated by the small intrinsic muscles of the hand.

To ensure correct function of the extensor mechanism, all components must be held in their exact positions. This is accomplished by an intricate network of fibrous bands that includes the extensor hood, triangular membrane, and retinacular ligament. As discussed above, the **extensor hood** (Fig. 3-54) is associated with the MP joint and is thus the most proximal of the supporting elements of the extensor mechanism. This hood stabilizes the lumbrical and interossei tendons and provides the mechanism by which the extensor digitorum extends the proximal phalanx.

The **triangular membrane** (Fig. 3-54) interconnects the lateral bands across the dorsal aspect of the PIP joint. In addition to forming a protective connective tissue hood over the joint, it holds the lateral bands in place, preventing them from moving anteriorly.

The **retinacular ligament** (Fig. 3-54B) is in the area of the PIP and consists of two parts. The **transverse part** is thin and superficial and does not have a major supporting function. The **oblique part of the retinacular ligament (Landsmeer's ligament)** is a strong cord that attaches to the lateral bands distal to the PIP joint. From that attachment the ligament passes proximally and ventrally, and attaches to the lateral aspect of the proximal phalanx. These ligaments prevent the lateral bands from sliding dorsally. Landsmeer's ligaments also unite the PIP and DIP joints functionally. As the distal phalanx is flexed, these ligaments transmit a force across the flexor aspect of the PIP joint, and the middle phalanx is flexed. Conversely, as the middle phalanx is extended, these same ligaments transmit an extensor pull across the DIP joint, and the distal phalanx is extended. In other words, the distal phalanx cannot be flexed without the middle phalanx also being flexed, nor can the middle phalanx be extended without the distal phalanx also being extended. However, if Landsmeer's ligaments are a bit slack, the lateral bands can slide dorsally and the PIP joint can be "locked" in extension. Then, the distal phalanx can be flexed while the middle phalanx is extended.

Static and Dynamic Balances Affecting the Fingers

The position of each of the segments of the finger, whether at rest or during motion, is determined by the balance between the various flexor and extensor forces across the MP, PIP, and DIP joints. Likewise, loss of any of these forces results in characteristic deformities and functional losses. Certain of these forces are static in that they are produced by ligaments; others are dynamic because they result from muscle action. An appreciation of these forces facilitates the understanding of the normal motion of the hand and is essential to understanding the static deformities and active losses that result from peripheral nerve injuries as well as destruction of static supports.

Normal forces. Figure 3-54B summarizes both the muscular and ligamentous forces that affect the joints of the fingers. On the ventral surface of the digit, the flexor digitorum profundus muscle is the only force at the DIP joint, and it contributes to the flexor forces at both the PIP and MP joints. The flexor digitorum superficialis is the primary force at the PIP, and it contributes to the palmar force at the MP joint. Flexor force at the MP joint is provided by the lumbrical and interossei muscles as well as from the two long digital flexors. Although the flexor force across the MP joint is provided by multiple muscles, the amount of that force varies considerably and is largely dependent on the position of the wrist. The long digital flexor muscles are strong but function through a limited range of motion. As a result, their action is greatly affected by the positions of the joints more proximal to their primary sites of action. Each can produce strong and full motion at its primary site of action, but both the force and range of motion either can provide at more proximal joints decreases sharply as flexion occurs at each of the primary joints. The force in a strong grasp occurs at the DIP and PIP joints, and, if the hand is extended, at the MP joints as well. Flexion of the proximal phalanges by the lumbricales and interossei occurs when the hand is performing delicate maneuvers. The only static force on the flexor side of the digit is provided by the oblique part of the retinacular ligament across the PIP joint.

That the overall force on the flexor side of the digits exceeds that on the extensor side is apparent when observing the resting position of the hand. There is flexion of all phalanges and it typically is greater on the ulnar side of the hand.

The only extensor force across the MP joint is the extensor digitorum muscle; and if that muscle provides any force across the PIP and DIP joints, it is minimal. At both the PIP and DIP joints the major muscular force is provided by the lumbrical and interossei muscles. The oblique portion of the retinacular ligament is a static support across the extensor aspect of the DIP joint, and the triangular membrane is a static support across the PIP joint.

Deformities resulting from loss of static balance.   Changes in the forces across these joints obviously occur when muscle function is lost, but also can result from destruction of the tendons per se or from changes in their positions secondary to destruction of their connective tissue supports. Such destruction commonly results from inflammatory joint disease such as rheumatoid arthritis.

Destruction of the oblique portion of the retinacular ligament results in a dorsal displacement of the lateral band. Loss of the oblique ligament removes a flexor force across the PIP joint, and the resulting dorsal displacement of the lateral band increases the force on the extensor side of the joint. The net result is an imbalance of force in favor of the extensor side, which in turn pulls the middle phalanx into extension. The extension at the PIP joint causes an increase in the tension in the tendons of both the flexor digitorum profundus and superficialis muscles, which produces passive flexion of the distal and proximal phalanges. The resulting posture of the digit is referred to as a **swan neck deformity.**

Destruction of the soft structures dorsal to the PIP joint produces a different deformity. Loss of the central band releases the lumbrical and interossei (and extensor digitorum if any exists) force across that joint, and loss of the triangular membrane permits the lateral bands to slide ventrally. Force across the extensor side of the joint is reduced; if the ventral displacement of the lateral band is sufficient (ventral to the flexion-extension axis), virtually all extensor force is lost and force may be added to the flexor aspect. In either case the balance of power shifts toward the flexor side of the PIP joint, and flexion at that joint results. The passive tension in the flexor digitorum profundus and superficialis muscles is reduced with resulting extension of the distal and proximal phalanges. The **boutonniere (buttonhole) deformity** results.

Nerve Injuries of the Upper Limb

This section begins with a comparison of peripheral and segmental patterns of innervation of the upper limb, followed by a discussion of the more common nerve injuries of the upper limb. The consideration of each lesion will include the static deformity, the mechanism behind that deformity, and the active or dynamic loss. It is important to note that in most injuries the static deformity and dynamic loss are exactly opposite. For example, a patient with a radial nerve deficit has a flexed hand or a wrist drop (static deformity) and is unable to extend the hand (active loss). Where appropriate, injury of the same nerve at different levels is considered.

Segmental Versus Peripheral Innervation of the Upper Limb

Segmental innervation is based on those muscles and areas of skin that are innervated by fibers from a single spinal cord segment. In the limbs, through a somatic plexus, the fibers from a single spinal cord segment are distributed to multiple peripheral nerves and thus combined with fibers from other segments to innervate muscles. As a result, the motor symptoms resulting from a lesion of a single spinal nerve are widespread, and individual muscles are weakened but not completely paralyzed. Cutaneous nerve fibers from a single spinal cord segment also are distributed to multiple peripheral nerves, but these nerves innervate adjacent skin areas, which collectively are called a **dermatome.** As a result, injury of a single spinal nerve results in a definitive and circumscribed (dermatomal) loss of cutaneous sensibility.

The dermatomes of the upper limb (Fig. 3-55) are

C4   point of the shoulder
C5   lateral aspect of the arm
C6   lateral aspects of the forearm and hand, and the thumb and
        index finger
C7   middle finger
C8   ring and little fingers, medial aspects of the hand and wrist
T1   medial aspect of the forearm
T2   medial aspect of the arm

The segmental muscular (motor) innervation of the upper limb is

C5,C6   all intrinsic muscles of the shoulder (abduction and ex-
            ternal rotation of the arm)
            anterior compartment of the arm (flexion and supina-
            tion of the forearm; biceps brachii reflex)
C6,C7(8)   pronators of the forearm
C7(6,8)   posterior compartment of the arm (extension of the
            forearm; triceps brachii reflex)
            superficial muscles in the posterior compartment of the
            forearm (extension of the hand and proximal pha-
            langes)
C8(7,T1)   anterior compartment of the forearm (flexion of the
            hand and fingers)
C8,T1   intrinsic muscles of the hand (adduction and abduction
            of the fingers, digital flexion at the MP joints and
            extension at the PIP and DIP joints, opposition of
            the thumb)

Peripheral innervation is based on those groups of muscles and areas of skin innervated by a specific peripheral nerve. In the upper limb such a nerve is a major terminal nerve (radial) of the brachial plexus or a smaller branch (long thoracic) of the plexus proper. In either case, a group of muscles (or single muscle) and area(s) of skin (if the nerve has cutaneous branches) are supplied solely by that nerve; destruction of that nerve produces complete paralysis of the muscles and a total loss of cutaneous sensibility in the prescribed area.

In either the upper or lower limb, a preplexus injury (spinal nerve) leads to a segmental loss and a postplexus injury (radial nerve) to a peripheral loss. Lesions of the plexus itself produce mixed symptoms. For example, injury of the superior trunk would be similar to injury of both the C5 and C6 spinal nerves; a lesion of the posterior cord would be the same as a lesion involving both the radial and axillary nerves; a lesion of the lateral cord would involve all of the musculocutaneous nerve and part of the median.

Ulnar Nerve

It is practical to consider injury to the ulnar nerve at two levels, not only because the resulting symptoms are somewhat different but also because the nerve is commonly injured at these levels. Injury of the nerve as it enters the hand, where it passes through the ulnar tunnel, is considered a "low" injury. A "high" injury occurs at or proximal to the elbow.

A **low ulnar nerve injury** results in loss of the muscles and cutaneous areas innervated by the superficial and deep branches. The paralyzed muscles are the adductor pollicis, all interossei, the two medial lumbricals, and the muscles of the hypothenar compartment. The cutaneous loss is limited to the palmar aspects of the little finger and ulnar half of the ring finger, and skin over the hypothenar eminence. There is no dorsal cutaneous loss because the dorsal cutaneous branch arises proximal to the injury site.

The static deformity is aptly named the incomplete claw hand. The essential ingredient in the production of a claw hand is the loss of the interossei and/or lumbrical muscles. This loss creates the imbalance that creates the deformity. Significant flexor force across the MP joint and the primary extensor force across both the PIP and DIP joints are lost. At the MP joint the unopposed extensor digitorum muscle pulls the proximal phalanx into hyperextension. This positional change increases the passive stretch on the tendons of both the flexor digitorum profundus and superficialis muscles and thus the flexor force across the DIP and PIP joints. The combination of reduced extensor force and increased passive stretch across the flexor side causes passive flexion at both the DIP and PIP joints. Loss of both the interossei and lumbrical muscles causes a more pronounced claw than loss of either interossei or lumbricals alone. Since the two lateral lumbricals are intact in a low ulnar nerve injury, the claw is more pronounced in the little and ring fingers and the term "incomplete claw" is used. The loss of the adductor pollicis and hypothenar muscles usually does not cause a noticeable change in the posture of the hand. The motor loss accompanying this injury is limited to the hand. There is an inability to adduct and abduct the fingers as well as to adduct the thumb. (Adduction of the thumb is approximation of its posterior aspect and the palmar aspect of the index finger.) Opposition of the thumb is somewhat weakened by the loss of the adductor pollicis, and opposition of the little finger is lost. Although a patient with this type of nerve injury can make a fist, he or she can do so only in a clumsy manner. The median nerve can be considered the "skill nerve" because it innervates most of the muscles associated with the thumb and index finger. The ulnar is then the "power nerve" because it innervates most of the muscles of the medial

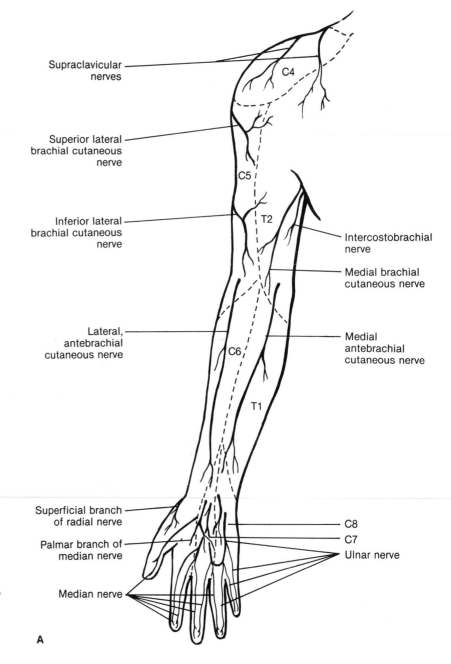

Supraclavicular nerves

Superior lateral brachial cutaneous nerve

Inferior lateral brachial cutaneous nerve

Lateral, antebrachial cutaneous nerve

Superficial branch of radial nerve

Palmar branch of median nerve

Median nerve

C4

C5

T2

C6

T1

Intercostobrachial nerve

Medial brachial cutaneous nerve

Medial antebrachial cutaneous nerve

C8

C7

Ulnar nerve

A

Figure 3-55
Anterior (A) and posterior (B) views of the upper limb indicating both the peripheral and segmental (dermatomal) patterns of cutaneous innervation.

side of the hand. This is true only to a point because with a low ulnar nerve lesion the ability to perform skilled activities, such as writing, is limited.

The additional losses that accompany a **high ulnar nerve lesion** are the flexor carpi ulnaris and the ulnar half of the flexor digitorum profundus muscles, and the cutaneous sensibility on the dorsomedial aspect of

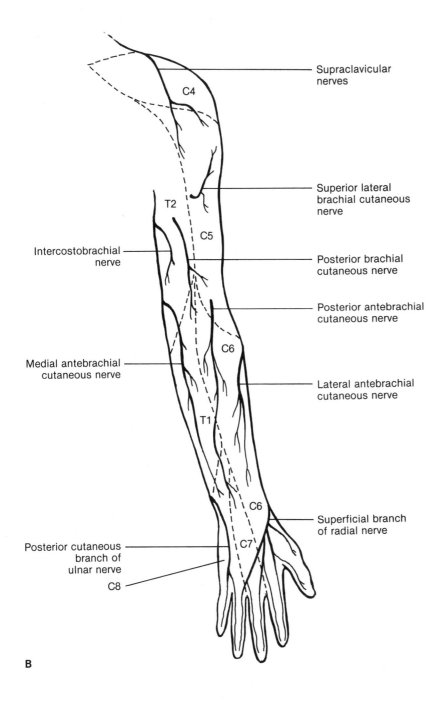

Supraclavicular
nerves

C4

Superior lateral
brachial cutaneous
nerve

T2

C5

Intercostobrachial
nerve

Posterior brachial
cutaneous nerve

Posterior antebrachial
cutaneous nerve

C6

Medial antebrachial
cutaneous nerve

Lateral antebrachial
cutaneous nerve

T1

C6

Superficial branch
of radial nerve

Posterior cutaneous
branch of
ulnar nerve

C7

C8

B

the hand and wrist. The static deformity of the hand is somewhat less pronounced than that of the low lesion because the claw position of the little and ring fingers is less severe. This is due to the loss of the flexor force of the flexor digitorum profundus muscle; the imbalance is less severe, and the middle and distal phalanges of the little and ring fingers are thus less flexed. The hand may be slightly extended and deviated radially due to loss of the flexor carpi ulnaris muscle. There are additional motor deficits. Making a fist is more difficult because of the loss of the ulnar half of the flexor digitorum profundus, and flexion at the wrist is weakened and accompanied by some radial deviation.

Median Nerve

Consideration of lesions of the median nerve also include "low" (wrist) and "high" (proximal to the elbow) levels. An example of a **low median nerve lesion** is a carpal tunnel syndrome. The common and proper digital branches and the motor branch are involved; the muscles in the thenar compartment and the two lateral lumbricals (index and middle fingers) are paralyzed. The sensory loss is restricted to the palmar aspects of the medial three and one-half digits and the dorsal skin over the distal phalanges of the same fingers. There is no loss of sensation on the majority of the midpalm because the palmar branch of the median nerve arises proximal to the palm and does not pass through the carpal tunnel.

The static deformity involves the thumb, index, and middle fingers. Since the two lateral lumbricals are lost, the index and middle fingers exhibit a partial but quite noticeable claw deformity. The thumb is derotated, partially flexed (the flexor pollicis longus is intact), and adducted; thus the thumb nail of this "simian hand" is in the same plane as those of the other digits, and the thumb is fixed against the lateral aspect of the index finger. The thenar eminence is flattened. The major active or dynamic loss is opposition of the thumb. Strong grasp utilizing the flexor pollicis longus is possible (if the thumb is positioned so it can grasp), but true opposition and subsequent skilled activities are not. Skilled activities utilizing the index and middle fingers are clumsy.

A **high median nerve lesion** involves the majority of the muscles in the anterior compartment of the forearm. Only the flexor carpi ulnaris and the ulnar half of the flexor digitorum profundus muscles are spared. Because the palmar branch also is included, the sensory loss includes the midpalm as well as the digits.

The static deformity is quite characteristic. There is a slight claw of the index and middle fingers, but it is less than that of the low injury because the passive flexor force of neither of the long digital flexors is present. The index finger typically is straighter than the middle, perhaps due to the autonomy of the flexor digitorum profundus tendon to that finger. The posture of the relaxed ring and little fingers is the usual partial flexion at all joints. The partially extended index and middle fingers, the flexed ulnar fingers, and the extended simian thumb (the flexor pollicis longus is lost) combine to form the "sign of the papal benediction." Since both pronators and the flexor carpi radialis are lost, the hand is statically supinated and may be deviated medially.

The dynamic loss with this type of lesion is significant. Flexion of the ring and little fingers is weak; flexion of the thumb, index, and middle fingers is virtually zero. Flexion of the hand is weak and accompanied by adduction. Pronation is possible only to about the midpoint between pronation and supination (brachioradialis) and best accomplished with the forearm flexed to about 90 degrees. Overall, the hand is virtually useless.

The situation is aggravated by the lack of pronation because many skilled activities are performed with the hand between pronation and the mid-position.

Combined Median and Ulnar Nerves

The most dramatic losses of hand function that result from peripheral nerve injuries are secondary to combined median and ulnar nerve involvement. With a **low median-ulnar nerve injury** (wrist level), all intrinsic muscles of the hand are denervated. There is an "intrinsic minus" deformity that consists of a complete claw hand. All lumbricals and interossei are lost and the passive force of the long digital flexor tendons is completely intact. The thumb is in a simian position. With the possible exception of the midpalmar region (assuming the median nerve involvement is in the carpal tunnel), cutaneous sensation is lost on the entire palmar surface of the hand and the dorsal distal aspects of the lateral digits. The dynamic loss is characterized by an extremely clumsy hand that is capable of crude grasp via the long flexors of the fingers and thumb. However, precision movements of any digits are virtually impossible.

A **high median-ulnar nerve lesion** (proximal to the elbow) causes a loss of all intrinsic muscles of the hand as well as all muscles in the anterior compartment of the forearm. The claw deformity of the digits, however, is considerably less severe than that of a combined low median-ulnar lesion. The major reason is the paralysis of the long digital flexor muscles that removes the passive force on the flexor side of the PIP and DIP joints. In addition, there is a static extension at the wrist that reduces the tension in the extensor digitorum tendons, which in turn causes less extension of the proximal phalanges. The thumb position is the same as that in the low median-ulnar lesion except it is extended. The sensory loss is expanded and includes the dorsomedial aspect of the hand. Functionally, making a fist, grasp, and precision motions simply are not possible. Flexion of the digits, via passive tendon action of the long digital flexor muscles, can be caused and crudely regulated by extension of the hand. This motion, however, is not at a functional level. Flexion at the wrist, albeit weak, can be produced by the abductor pollicis longus muscle. Overall, this is the most debilitating peripheral nerve injury that affects the function of the hand per se.

Radial Nerve

This discussion is based on a lesion in the axilla, which means that all structures and areas innervated by the radial nerve are lost. Specifically included are all muscles in the posterior compartments of the arm and forearm and the skin of the posterolateral arm, posterior forearm, and posterolateral hand. The presence of a static deformity is dependent on the position of the upper limb. With the limb at the side little is apparent. When the forearm is flexed and pronated the hand flexes ("wrist drop") because all wrist extensors and long digital extensors are lost. The thumb is adducted due to the loss of the abductor pollicis longus. A static deformity is seldom apparent at the elbow because the limb is either dependent or resting on something most of the time.

The major dynamic losses obviously are extension at the elbow, wrist, thumb, and MP joints. The loss of wrist extension reduces the force of grasp because extension at the wrist increases the mechanical advantage of the long digital flexor muscles. Loss of the thumb extensors and its long abductor is not particularly detrimental to the thumb's role in grasp; however, the thumb must be moved (extended) passively before it can grasp.

The radial nerve is most commonly injured as it passes around the midshaft region of the humerus. Injury at that point can be misleading because several muscular branches to the triceps brachii muscle and one or two cutaneous branches arise proximal to the injury. With an injury at that level it is important to check the viability of the wrist flexors because the triceps are, at least partially, intact. In addition, the sensory loss may well be limited to the dorsolateral hand.

Musculocutaneous Nerve

Loss of the musculocutaneous nerve results in a profound weakness of forearm flexion and supination, and a loss of cutaneous sensibility on a portion of the lateral aspect of the forearm. Without the muscles in the anterior compartment of the arm, only the brachioradialis and the superficial muscles in the anterior compartment of the forearm can flex the forearm, and only the supinator and brachioradialis muscles can supinate. As a result, useful forearm flexion is virtually lost and supination, especially with the forearm flexed approximately 90 degrees, is greatly weakened. Statically, the forearm is pronated and extended.

Axillary Nerve

Injury of the axillary nerve causes a small sensory loss in the upper lateral arm and paralysis of only two muscles, the deltoid and teres minor. The overall usefulness of the upper limb, however, can be affected significantly because positioning of the hand is limited. The major loss is abduction of the arm. Beyond the small amount produced by the supraspinatus muscle, abduction at the shoulder is not possible. For hand activities other than those in which the forearm is supported on a table or desk, some amount of abduction at the shoulder and shoulder stabilization are necessary. In the standing position there would be no apparent deformity because the upper limb normally hangs at the side. The rounded contour of the shoulder, however, would be flattened and more angular. Neither the sensory loss nor the loss of the teres minor muscle is significant.

Lesions of the Brachial Plexus

The **superior trunk of the brachial plexus** is vulnerable to injury from varying causes, ranging from the compression caused by a heavy backpack to the traction of a breech birth, whereby the head and shoulder are forcibly separated. In either case all nerve fibers in the ventral rami of spinal nerves C5 and C6 are involved (Erb–Duchenne palsy). The upper limb is fixed in adduction and medial rotation at the shoulder and extension and pronation of the forearm, the "waiter's tip" position. This position simply reflects the imbalance produced by the denervated muscles. All intrinsic muscles of the shoulder and thus all humeral abductors and lateral rotators are lost. The strong medial rotators of the humerus, the latissimus dorsi and the pectoralis major muscles, are unopposed. The muscles in the anterior compartment of the arm, the major flexors of the forearm and the strongest supinator, also are lost. The active loss is devastating in that the abduction and external rotation of the humerus are not possible, and flexion and supination of the forearm are greatly weakened. The hand remains completely functional, but it cannot be positioned and stabilized universally. Loss of cutaneous sensibility involves the lateral aspects of the arm and forearm.

The **inferior trunk of the brachial plexus** is the usual nerve bundle involved in the thoracic outlet syndrome. Since the inferior trunk is composed of fibers from spinal cord segments C8 and T1, the motor symptoms result from the loss of the intrinsic muscles of the hand and of muscles in the anterior compartment of the forearm, and the sensory loss is restricted to the medial hand and forearm. In this situation the hand can be moved to almost any position, but its usefulness is greatly impaired. The hand is fixed in abduction and extension, the fingers are extended at the MP joints and flexed at both IP joints (a mild claw hand), and the thumb is derotated. A general rule regarding the segmental innervation of the forearm muscles is that the lateral muscles (in both the anterior and posterior compartments) are supplied by higher segments of the brachial plexus than the medial muscles. As a result, the adductors and medial flexors of the hand are more affected than the abductors and lateral flexors. Loss of the lumbrical and interossei muscles produces a claw hand deformity. However, loss of the long digital flexors makes this deformity less severe than if those forearm muscles were intact (see ulnar and median nerve injuries). The derotated thumb is the direct result of the loss of the opponens pollicis muscle. This nerve lesion results in a virtually useless hand in that delicate movement, thumb opposition, and strong grasp are not possible.

Lower Limb

Organization of the Lower Limb

Although the anatomy of the upper and lower limbs is similar in a number of respects, the functional demands placed on the limbs are considerably different, and the structure of each reflects these differences. Whereas a major function of the upper limb is the positioning and stabilization of the hand, the functions of the lower limb are weight bearing and propulsion. The lower limb must accommodate the weight of the body in a variety of circumstances—such as, when walking, running, climbing stairs and ladders—and it must provide a soft landing and forceful push-off during ambulation. The muscles and bones are large, and the articulations, for the most part, reflect the strenuous functional demands.

The discussion of the lower limb follows much the same order as that of the upper limb. The regions are discussed from proximal to distal with a full consideration of each region. The major exception to the sequence is the discussion on the basic principles of gait, at the beginning of the chapter just after the section on the organization of the limb. The purpose of including gait is not to provide a detailed treatise but rather to provide a basic understanding so muscle and joint actions, along with muscular deficits, can be discussed in a meaningful context. The courses of the vessels and nerves are followed through each region, with special attention given to the potential injury points of the nerves. Nerve injuries are discussed at the end of the chapter.

Regions and Nomenclature

The lower limb consists of three segments, the thigh, leg, and foot, that are joined by articulations and connected proximally to the trunk. The bony **pelvis,** or **pelvic girdle,** is the base or foundation to which the lower

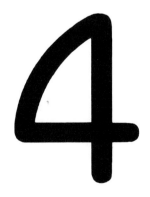

limb is anchored, and the **hip** is the general region of the **hip joint.** The junctional regions associated with the hip are the **gluteal region** posterolaterally and the **inguinal region** and **femoral triangle** anteriorly. The segment of the lower limb between the hip and knee is the **thigh.** Since the thigh contains a single bone, the femur, the term **femoral** denotes areas of the thigh or structures within the thigh. The **knee,** or **genu,** joins the thigh and leg; the posterior aspect of the knee is the **popliteal region.** The **leg,** or **crural region,** is the segment between the knee and ankle; its posterior aspect is the **calf,** or **sural region.** The ankle, or **talocrural region,** joins the leg and foot. The **foot** is the **pes.** It is separated from posterior to anterior into the **calcaneal, tarsal,** and **metatarsal regions.** The **great toe** is the **hallux;** the **small toe** is the **digiti minimus.**

Compartmentation of the Lower Limb

Like the upper limb, the lower limb is encased in an investing fascia that combines with intermuscular septa and other connective tissue structures to separate the various segments of the limb into compartments. These compartments are generally anterior and posterior and somewhat similar to those of the upper limb. However, the lower limb undergoes a rotation during development that results in the anterior positioning of the original posterior compartments. Very early in development the ventral aspects of both limbs (the palmar surface of the hand and the plantar surface of the foot) face anteriorly. That orientation of the upper limb is maintained throughout development. The lower limb, however, undergoes both an actual rotation and a positional change. The actual rotation is about 90 degrees of medial rotation in the region of the hip or proximal thigh; and the positional change is a combination of adduction and extension at the hip. The end result is a medial rotation of approximately 180 degrees; thus, the posterior compartments of the lower limb are similar (to some degree at least) to the anterior compartments of the upper limb. Certain structures, such as the sartorius muscle and the ischiofemoral ligament, curve medially around the femur and may reflect this change in position. The muscles in the anterior compartments of the upper limb and posterior compartments of the lower limb are innervated by nerves derived from the anterior divisions of the brachial and lumbosacral plexuses, respectively, and vice versa. The general actions of these muscle groups are also similar.

The investing fascia (**fascia lata**) of the thigh (Fig. 4-1A) is thickened laterally by the **iliotibial tract (band)** that extends from the anterior aspect of the iliac crest to the lateral tibial condyle. This fascia lata is interconnected to the femur by the anteromedially positioned **medial intermuscular septum** and the posterolateral **lateral intermuscular septum.** The resulting **anterior** and **posterior compartments** are positioned anterolaterally and posteromedially, respectively. The muscles in the anterior compartment are the extensors of the leg and assist in flexion of the thigh, and are innervated by the femoral nerve. The posterior compartment contains both the posterior and medial femoral muscles. The posterior femoral muscles, or hamstrings, both flex the leg and extend the thigh. They are supplied predominantly by the tibial portion of the sciatic nerve. The medial femoral muscles are located in the medial aspect of the posterior compartment. These muscles are the adductors of the thigh and for the most part are innervated by the obturator nerve.

The leg (Fig. 4-1B) is similar to the forearm in having two bones and an interosseous membrane. The locations and shapes of the compartments, however, do not change, because the bones are fixed and there are no motions similar to pronation and supination. The investing **crural fascia** blends with the periosteum of the subcutaneous tibia and is interconnected to the fibula by both the **anterior** and **posterior intermuscular septa.** The **anterior compartment** is positioned anterolaterally and defined by the tibia, interosseous membrane, and the anterior intermuscular septum. The muscles in this compartment are the dorsiflexors and invertors of the foot and the extensors of the toes. These muscles are supplied by the deep peroneal nerve. The small **lateral compartment** is limited by the anterior and posterior intermuscular septa; its muscles evert and plantar flex the foot and are innervated by the superficial peroneal nerve. The muscles in the large **posterior compartment** are separated into superficial and deep groups by the **transverse intermuscular septum,** but all are supplied by the tibial nerve. These muscles plantar flex and invert the foot, and also flex the toes.

The compartmentalization of the foot (Fig. 4-1C) appears similar to that of the hand, and to a degree it is. There is a compartment associated with the small toe and a deep one between the metatarsals, and the muscles are generally similar to those in the hand. However, other compartments defined by fibrous septa do not exist in the foot, so the muscles are usually described in layers. The layers and the muscles forming each of these layers are described with the detailed description of the foot on page 237. The medial muscles associated with the large toe flex and abduct that toe, and are innervated by the medial plantar nerve. Those muscles in the compartment of the little toe flex and abduct that toe, and are innervated by the lateral plantar nerve. The muscles in the central plantar area, similar to the central compartment of the hand, flex the toes and adduct the great toe and are supplied by both the medial and lateral plantar nerves. The deep muscles between the metatarsals, the interossei, abduct and adduct the toes and are supplied by the lateral plantar nerve. The foot differs from the hand in that it has dorsal intrinsic muscles. These muscles extend the toes and are innervated by the deep peroneal nerve.

Superficial Structures

The superficial structures of the limb are found superficial to the investing fascia and include the superficial set of veins (Fig. 4-2) and the cutaneous nerves (Fig. 4-47). As in the upper limb, there are two major superficial veins, both of which originate from a venous network on the dorsum of the foot. The **great saphenous vein** appears on the medial aspect of the dorsum of the foot and passes proximally along the anteromedial aspect of the leg. It crosses the anterior aspect of the ankle where it is consis-

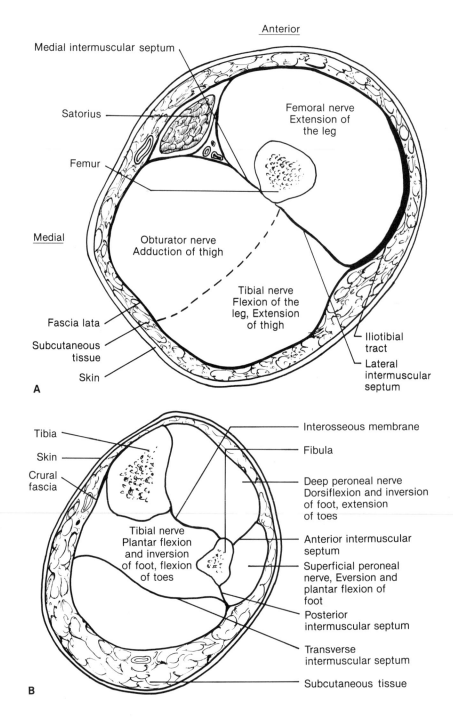

Anterior

Medial intermuscular septum

Satorius

Femur

Medial

Femoral nerve
Extension of
the leg

Obturator nerve
Adduction of thigh

Tibial nerve
Flexion of the
leg, Extension
of thigh

Fascia lata

Subcutaneous
tissue

Skin

Iliotibial
tract

Lateral
intermuscular
septum

A

Tibia

Skin

Crural
fascia

Interosseous membrane

Fibula

Deep peroneal nerve
Dorsiflexion and inversion
of foot, extension
of toes

Tibial nerve
Plantar flexion
and inversion
of foot, flexion
of toes

Anterior intermuscular
septum

Superficial peroneal
nerve, Eversion and
plantar flexion of
foot

Posterior
intermuscular septum

Figure 4-1
Cross sections through the thigh
(*A*), leg (*B*), and foot (*C*), indicating
the compartments of each.

Transverse
intermuscular septum

Subcutaneous tissue

B

tently positioned about 2 centimeters lateral to the medial malleolus and
commonly utilized for venous cutdown. This vein crosses the medial aspect of the knee and then passes proximally toward the femoral triangle,
where it joins the femoral vein. The **small saphenous vein** begins on the
lateral aspect of the foot, passes inferior to the lateral malleolus, and then

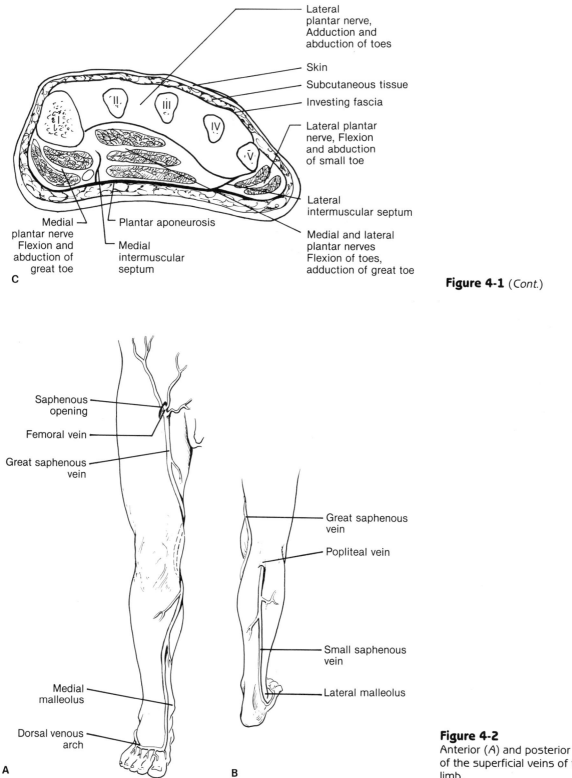

Lateral
plantar nerve,
Adduction and
abduction of toes

Skin

Subcutaneous tissue

Investing fascia

Lateral plantar
nerve, Flexion
and abduction
of small toe

Lateral
intermuscular septum

Medial and lateral
plantar nerves
Flexion of toes,
adduction of great toe

Medial
plantar nerve
Flexion and
abduction of
great toe

Plantar aponeurosis

Medial
intermuscular
septum

C

Figure 4-1 (*Cont.*)

Saphenous
opening

Femoral vein

Great saphenous
vein

Medial
malleolus

Dorsal venous
arch

A

B

Great saphenous
vein

Popliteal vein

Small saphenous
vein

Lateral malleolus

Figure 4-2
Anterior (*A*) and posterior (*B*) views
of the superficial veins of the lower
limb.

ascends along the posterior aspect of the leg toward the popliteal fossa, where it joins the popliteal vein. The cutaneous innervation of the lower limb is summarized on page 245.

Gait

The following account of gait is separated into two parts: the static and dynamic phases, or standing and walking. The discussion of each part includes the effects of gravity on the various segments of the lower limb and the anatomic structures that counteract and overcome those gravitational forces to maintain the upright posture and produce forward motion of the entire body. The functional deficits that result from muscular loss are covered with the discussions of the individual muscles or muscle groups and in the nerve injury section at the end of the chapter. Abnormal gait patterns resulting from pain, joint pathology, and diseases of the central nervous system are not covered in this book.

General Principles

Understanding the effect of gravity on the body as a whole, and more particularly on each weight-bearing segment, is paramount to the study of gait. When the body is considered as a single unit and in the upright position, its **center of gravity** or **mass** (Fig. 4-3) is situated approximately

Figure 4-3
Lateral view of the skull, vertebral column, pelvis, and lower limb, indicating the relationship of these various parts of the skeleton to the line of gravity.

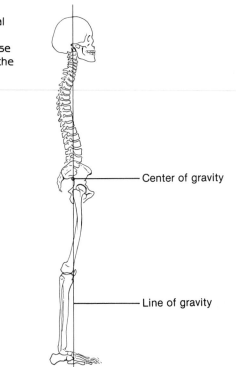

— Center of gravity

— Line of gravity

just anterior to the second sacral vertebrae. The pull of gravity on the body as a whole and on each of its individual segments parallels a line that passes through the center of gravity and is projected toward the center of the earth. If this **line of gravity** (Fig. 4-3) were to pass through the center of each segment (leg, thigh, pelvis) and the center of each link (joint) between segments, there would be equilibrium and no force would be needed to maintain the position of each of the segments. If, however, the line of gravity is anterior or posterior, or medial or lateral to a given segment or joint, some type of force is necessary to counteract gravitational forces and maintain the vertical alignment of that segment. In the body these forces are provided by ligaments and muscles.

The effect of gravity on any specific segment is dependent on where the line of gravity falls relative to the joint below that segment; the segment moves toward that line. For example, if the line is anterior to a joint, the segment above that joint has a tendency to move anteriorly. The force necessary to counteract that tendency must be provided by ligaments posterior to the joint or by muscles that can prevent forward motion of the segment.

It is convenient to use the knee joint and the quadriceps femoris muscle to illustrate the action of muscles as they counteract gravity during weight bearing. The quadriceps is defined as the extensor of the leg. However, for most of us this muscle seldom extends the leg as in kicking a football. Most often, during weight bearing, it prevents flexion at the knee. During the weight-bearing phase of gait the knee is almost always bent (flexed) and the gravitational forces tend to produce even more flexion. These forces are counteracted by the quadriceps, which undergoes a lengthening contraction and thus prevents flexion at the knee. In the usual descriptions of muscle actions the insertion is the movable attachment. During weight bearing the distal attachments of the muscles in the lower limb are fixed because the foot is on the ground, and the proximal attachments are thus movable. In this case the thigh is the movable segment, and its movement is prevented by the quadriceps muscle.

Paralysis of a muscle or group of muscles typically produces characteristic postural changes during weight bearing. When a muscle or group of muscles that counteracts gravity is paralyzed, the body usually compensates by leaning toward the loss. In the case of a paralyzed quadriceps muscle the body leans anteriorly above the knee. This maneuver moves the center of gravity of the body anteriorly and hence the line of gravity well anterior to the knee joint. In this position there is full extension at the knee, which is maintained by the posterior ligaments of the joint. During standing such compensatory changes in position typically are subtle, but during ambulation, they are usually exaggerated and more obvious to the observer.

The first requirement to maintain the upright position is that the line of gravity enter the floor within the **base of support.** During quiet standing this is the area between the feet, or more specifically, the area between the great toes and the heels, and between the lateral borders of the feet. As long as the line of gravity enters the floor within those boundaries, the individual can maintain the upright position with no external assistance—that is, without holding onto or leaning against something or someone. When the line of gravity enters the floor outside of these boundaries, independent equilibrium is not possible on a prolonged basis.

The second requirement for maintenance of the upright posture is the vertical alignment and maintenance of the weight-bearing segments of the lower limb and the vertebral column. Each segment is connected to adjacent segments through articulations, and gravity acts on a segment at its articulations. When the limb is weight bearing (the foot is on the ground), the movement of a segment by gravity occurs at the lower joint. For example, the thigh is connected to the pelvis through the hip joint and to the leg through the knee joint. With the foot on the ground, gravitational forces causing movement of the thigh produce movement at the knee. For maintenance of the upright posture each segment must be either in equilibrium (the line of gravity must pass through the center of the segment and its lower joint) or the gravitational forces must be overcome. In quiet standing and during walking, equilibrium of any specific segment seldom occurs, and if it does, it is only transient. As a result, ligamentous and/or muscular support is necessary virtually at all times.

Standing

As stated on page 35, in quiet standing the line of gravity intersects the vertebral column at its junctional regions: occipitocervical, cervicothoracic, thoracolumbar, and lumbosacral. Therefore, little support other than the ligaments of the vertebral column is necessary to maintain the vertical alignment. As soon as motion occurs, this equilibrium is lost and gravitational forces must be overcome.

During quiet standing the line of gravity passes through neither the center of any of the segments nor the interconnecting joints of the lower limb. This line passes anterior to both the ankle and the knee joints, and posterior to the hip (Fig. 4-3). As a result, support is needed at each joint to maintain the vertical alignment of the segments of the limb.

Since the line of gravity passes anterior to the ankle joint, there is a tendency for the leg to move anteriorly (dorsiflexion) at the ankle. This motion is resisted by the plantar flexors of the foot—the soleus and the gastrocnemius muscles. Since the foot is fixed, the soleus and gastrocnemius are able to pull the leg posteriorly. During quiet standing there is a small amount of sway; and as the body sways anteriorly the plantar flexors become more active. If the body were to sway posteriorly enough to move the line of gravity behind the ankle, the dorsiflexors would become active.

There is virtually no muscular activity at the knee during quiet standing. The line of gravity passes slightly anterior to the joint, so there is a tendency for the femur to move anteriorly (extension occurs at the knee). As the femur is extended, the knee is supported by the posterior aspect of the joint capsule and probably the anterior cruciate ligament. Neither the hamstrings nor the quadriceps are active unless the amount of sway is sufficient to necessitate their support. This inactivity in the quadriceps femoris muscle can be verified by passive movement of the patella.

The line of gravity passes posterior to the hip joint, so the tendency is for the pelvis and trunk to lean posteriorly. In quiet standing this movement is easily resisted by the strong iliofemoral and ischiofemoral ligaments, both of which tighten as the thigh is extended. Balance at the hip, however, is tenuous because the line of gravity passes only slightly posterior to the very slippery articular surfaces of that joint. Any appreciable sway elicits appropriate activity in either the flexors (iliopsoas) or extensors (hamstring and gluteus maximus muscles) of the thigh. During standing the consideration of balance is limited essentially to motion that could occur in the sagittal plane because both feet are on the ground. This is **sagittal balance.** During gait a considerable amount of time is spent on only one foot, thus side-to-side (**coronal**) balance is important, particularly at the hip.

Gravity and Gait

During standing the center of gravity is stationary or moves only slightly from front to back and side to side. During walking, the center of gravity obviously moves anteriorly, but it also moves both vertically and laterally. Both of these directional changes in the position of the center of gravity reflect the directional changes of the body as a whole. Both of these movements circumscribe a repeating sinusoidal curve, and the flatter the curve in either direction, the more efficient the gait pattern.

The force for the forward propulsion of the body is derived from the foot pushing off the ground and the ground pushing back. The force from the ground, the **ground reaction,** is transferred proximally through the lower limbs. The location of the ground reaction force relative to each of the joints and segments of the lower limb can be used to analyze the mechanics of gait much as the line of gravity was used in normal standing. Since there is constant motion and shifting of weight, the effects of gravity on each segment of the lower limb change during gait. The position of the ground reaction relative to the segments of the lower limb changes continuously.

Gait Cycle

The **gait cycle** (Fig. 4-4) is one complete revolution of gait, beginning with the heel strike of one foot and extending to the subsequent heel strike of the same foot. During this cycle the limb has both weight-bearing and non-weight-bearing periods; and as a result, the gait cycle is separated into the **stance phase,** which occupies approximately 60 percent of the cycle, and the **swing phase,** which accounts for the remaining 40 percent.

During the stance phase the major function of the lower limb obviously is bearing weight. Since this is the only period of contact with the ground, this is the only time that the push-off necessary for forward propulsion can occur. Although the stance phase can be subdivided a number of ways, the major activities occur at three points. **Heel strike** signifies the beginning of the gait cycle and the stance phase and indicates

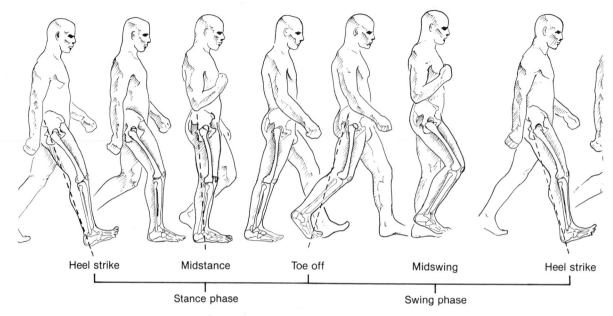

Heel strike   Midstance   Toe off   Midswing   Heel strike

Stance phase   Swing phase

Figure 4-4
The phases of one complete gait cycle of the right lower limb. The broken line represents the ground reaction.

the beginning of weight bearing as the heel strikes the floor. **Midstance** occurs approximately halfway through the weight-bearing phase; during this period the body weight is directly over (superior to) the supporting limb. **Heel-off** is the final portion of the stance phase and represents the point at which the body is propelled forward.

During the swing phase, the non-weight-bearing phase, the major objectives are moving the limb rapidly forward to position it for the next heel strike and shortening its length as it swings through. Initially the limb **accelerates** to catch up with the rest of the body. At midswing it must be shortened maximally as it passes the supporting limb (which is at midstance). Finally, the limb **decelerates** as it is positioned and prepared to assume the body weight at heel strike.

There is a short period during the gait cycle when both lower limbs are weight bearing, and the stance phases of the two limbs overlap. This period of **double support** encompasses approximately one-quarter of the cycle and occurs at heel strike of one limb and heel-off of the other. The length of the period of double support is inversely related to the speed of walking, and ceases to exist during running.

Muscle Activity During Gait

The position of the ground reaction during the stance phase of gait is indicated in Fig. 4-4. Similar to the line of gravity during quiet standing, the position of the ground reaction during gait indicates how gravity affects each segment of the lower limb. As in standing, a segment moves (rotates around its lower joint) toward the ground reaction and unwanted motion must be counteracted by mucles or ligaments. Gait differs from quiet standing regarding the magnitude of the gravitational forces. Since there is momentum in addition to the straight downward gravitational forces, the muscular activity necessary to counteract those forces must be considerably greater than that needed while standing.

At heel strike the body comes to a crash landing. Not only does the limb suddenly become weight bearing, but it also experiences a definite lag in its forward progression; that is, its forward momentum is slowed. As a result, there is a tendency for the various lower limb segments to continue their anterior motion. The ankle is in the neutral position, but the ground reaction passes considerably posterior to that joint so that there is a strong tendency for the foot to slap the floor, moving forcibly into plantar flexion. This plantar flexion is prevented and controlled by a strong lengthening contraction of the muscles in the anterior compartment of the leg, specifically the tibialis anterior muscle. The ground reaction is also well posterior to the slightly flexed knee joint and the force tends to increase that flexion. Almost full extension at the knee is maintained by a strong contraction of the quadriceps femoris muscle. Since there is a small amount of flexion at the knee, the lower limb is somewhat flexible and allows a "soft" landing; it would be rigid if the knee were fully extended. The hip is partially flexed and the ground reaction passes anterior to that joint, so the trunk tends to fall anteriorly (flexion at the hip). Forward rotation of the pelvis is prevented by both the hamstring and gluteus maximus muscles, and flexion of the vertebral column is counteracted by the erector spinae muscles.

At midstance the body weight is directly superior to the supporting limb. The ankle is slightly dorsiflexed and the ground reaction passes anteriorly, so the leg tends to move anteriorly (dorsiflexion of the foot). Dorsiflexion is prevented, the leg held vertically, by the plantar flexors (gastrocnemius and soleus muscles). The knee is slightly flexed, and the ground reaction passes posterior. The tendency for that flexion to increase is controlled by the extensors of the knee. The hip is very close to full extension so the ligaments of the hip joint are taut and resisting further extension. The ground reaction passes posterior to the hip joint and thus holds the hip in extension because the ligaments are taut. Since midstance occurs during single support, all body weight is on the supporting limb. The superincumbent weight enters the pelvis through the lumbosacral junction, which is medial to the hip joint and the weight-bearing foot. As a result, there is a tendency for the pelvis to tilt or drop toward the non-weight-bearing side. The pelvis remains relatively level, however, and is held in that position by a strong contraction of the gluteus medius and minimus muscles (which prevent adduction at the hip joint) of the weight-bearing side.

Heel-off occurs during the final moments of the stance phase and provides the important push against the ground that generates the forward propulsion of gait. The ankle is plantar flexed, and the ground reaction passes anterior to the joint. The muscles in the posterior compartment of the leg, the gastrocnemius and soleus, undergo the very strong shortening contraction that provides the push-off. The ground reaction passes posterior to the flexed knee, so the quadriceps are active and thus prevent further flexion at the knee. Since the body weight is being transferred to the opposite lower limb, this point of the gait cycle is within the period of double support. As a result, a strong contraction of the quadriceps is not needed. The hip is fully extended, and the ground reaction is posterior. Although the ligaments of the joint resist extension at the joint, the hip flexors (mainly the iliopsoas) are active to prevent further extension and prepare for the acceleration portion of the swing phase.

The limb supports no weight during the swing phase. The muscle's major tasks are to move the limb rapidly forward and shorten it so it can pass under the pelvis. To accomplish this, most of the muscles undergo shortening contractions. The shortening of the limb occurs primarily at the knee and ankle as the hamstrings flex the leg and the tibialis anterior dorsiflexes the foot. This shortening is maximal at midswing. The forward movement of the limb is the result of a strong contraction of the iliopsoas, which flexes the thigh and moves it rapidly forward. In preparation for

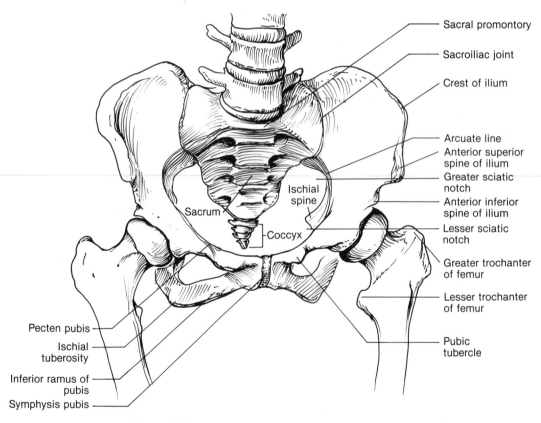

Figure 4-5
Anterior and slightly lateral view of the pelvis, lower lumbar vertebrae, and proximal portions of the femurs.

heel strike the hip extensors become active as they slow the forward swing of the limb and prepare to prevent hip flexion at the moment of impact; the quadriceps and hamstring muscles contract simultaneously so the limb is both firm and yet flexible at impact; and the contraction of the tibialis anterior becomes stronger to prevent plantar flexion at impact.

Bony Pelvis

The bony pelvis, or **pelvic ring** (Figs. 4-5, 4-6), is composed of the sacrum and the two **ossa coxae,** or **hip bones.** Each os coxae is joined to the sacrum through a **sacroiliac joint,** and the ossa coxae are united anteriorly at the **symphysis pubis.** This ring is extremely stable; thus displacement of a portion of the pelvis occurs only if there are two points of injury, that is, two fractures or two joint dislocations, or a fracture and a dislocation.

Each os coxae is irregularly shaped and formed by the fusion of three bones, the **ilium, ischium,** and **pubis** (Figs. 4-7, 4-8). The expanded and flattened superior aspect is the ilium; the heavy posterior and inferior portion is the ischium; and the anteromedial aspect is the pubis. The three bones fuse in the region of the acetabulum, which is the deep, inferolaterally directed socket of the hip joint. Inferiorly, portions of the ischium and pubis surround the opening called the **obturator foramen.**

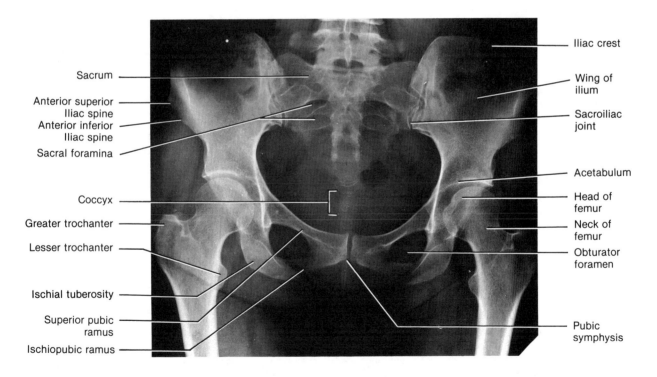

Figure 4-6
Anteroposterior radiograph of the pelvis, lumbosacral junction, and the hip joints.

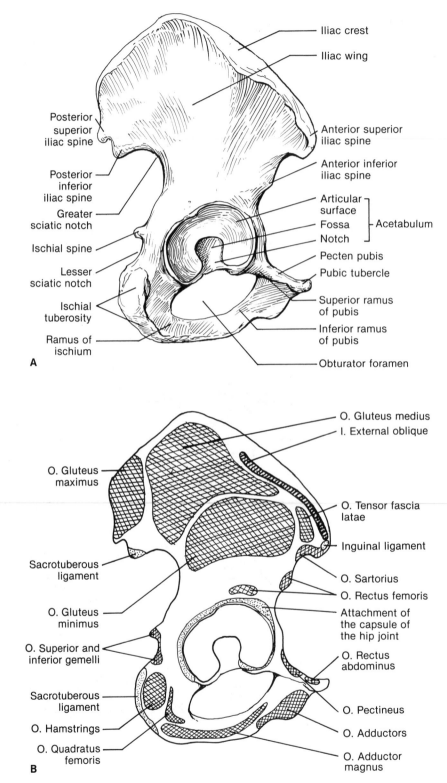

Iliac crest

Iliac wing

Posterior superior iliac spine

Anterior superior iliac spine

Anterior inferior iliac spine

Posterior inferior iliac spine

Articular surface

Greater sciatic notch

Fossa — Acetabulum

Notch

Ischial spine

Pecten pubis

Lesser sciatic notch

Pubic tubercle

Ischial tuberosity

Superior ramus of pubis

Inferior ramus of pubis

Ramus of ischium

Obturator foramen

A

O. Gluteus medius

I. External oblique

O. Gluteus maximus

O. Tensor fascia latae

Inguinal ligament

Sacrotuberous ligament

O. Sartorius

O. Rectus femoris

O. Gluteus minimus

Attachment of the capsule of the hip joint

O. Superior and inferior gemelli

O. Rectus abdominus

Sacrotuberous ligament

O. Pectineus

O. Hamstrings

O. Adductors

O. Quadratus femoris

O. Adductor magnus

B

Figure 4-7
Lateral views of the os coxae indicating the component bones and their prominences (A) and the locations of muscle attachments (B). The areas of origin are indicated by crosshatch, the insertions by parallel lines.

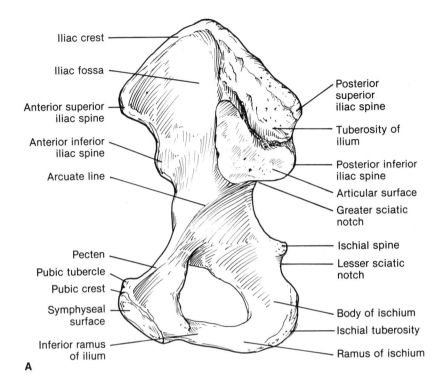

Iliac crest

Iliac fossa

Anterior superior iliac spine

Anterior inferior iliac spine

Arcuate line

Pecten

Pubic tubercle

Pubic crest

Symphyseal surface

Inferior ramus of ilium

A

Posterior superior iliac spine

Tuberosity of ilium

Posterior inferior iliac spine

Articular surface

Greater sciatic notch

Ischial spine

Lesser sciatic notch

Body of ischium

Ischial tuberosity

Ramus of ischium

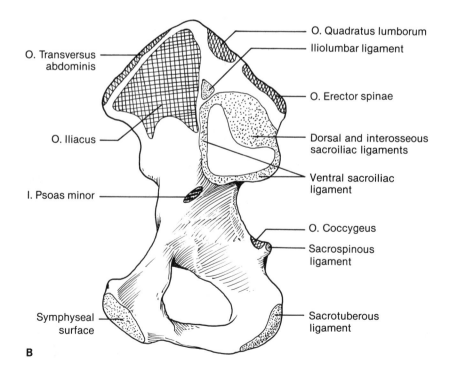

O. Transversus abdominis

O. Iliacus

I. Psoas minor

Symphyseal surface

B

O. Quadratus lumborum

Iliolumbar ligament

O. Erector spinae

Dorsal and interosseous sacroiliac ligaments

Ventral sacroiliac ligament

O. Coccygeus

Sacrospinous ligament

Sacrotuberous ligament

Figure 4-8
Medial views of the os coxae indicating the component bones and their prominences (*A*) and the locations of muscle attachments (*B*). The areas of origin are indicated by crosshatch, the insertions by parallel lines.

The **ilium** (Figs. 4-7, 4-8) consists of the flattened **wing** superiorly and the **body** inferiorly. The wing is oriented obliquely about midway between the sagittal and coronal planes. The upper rim of the wing, the **iliac crest,** is thickened and palpable throughout its length. It ends anteriorly in the prominent **anterior superior iliac spine,** and posteriorly in the **posterior superior iliac spine.** The **anterior inferior iliac spine** and **posterior inferior iliac spine** are inferior to their respective superior spines. The medial aspect of the wing consists of the concave anterior **iliac fossa** and the large, posteriorly located **iliac tuberosity.** The smooth **auricular surface,** which is the articular surface that participates in the formation of the sacroiliac joint, is positioned anterior and inferior to the iliac tuberosity. The prominent **arcuate line** begins at the anterior aspect of the auricular surface and passes anteriorly and inferiorly toward the superior ramus of the pubis. The entire lateral aspect of the iliac wing is the **gluteal surface.** Several prominent ridges, the **gluteal lines,** separate the attachments of the gluteal muscles and cross this surface. The lateral aspect of the body of the ilium forms the heavy superior portion of the acetabulum.

The **ischium** (Figs. 4-7, 4-8) is composed of the heavy, vertically oriented **body** and the smaller, anteromedially directed **ramus.** The superior aspect of the body forms the posterior portion of the acetabulum, and the inferior aspect is the **ischial tuberosity.** The **ischial spine** projects posteromedially and separates the **greater sciatic notch** above from the **lesser sciatic notch** below. The ischial ramus projects anteromedially and somewhat superiorly from the inferior aspect of the ischial body and fuses with the inferior ramus of the pubis.

The **pubis** (Figs. 4-7, 4-8) consists of a medial **body** and **superior** and **inferior rami,** which project, respectively, superolaterally and inferolaterally. The posterior aspect of the superior ramus forms the anterior portion of the acetabulum and fuses with both the ilium and ischium. The inferior ramus fuses with the ramus of the ischium; the combination of the two rami is commonly called the **ischiopubic ramus.** Both the superior and inferior rami of the pubis partially bound the obturator foramen. The medial aspect of the pubic body presents the **symphyseal surface** that attaches to the disk between the two pubic bones. The elevation on the superior aspect of the body is the **pubic tubercle.** Projecting medially from that tubercle is the **pubic crest**; projecting superolaterally along the superior aspect of the superior ramus is the ridge referred to as the **pecten** of the pubis.

The **acetabulum** is formed on the lateral aspect of the os coxae by portions of all three component bones. The articular surface of this socket is shaped like a horseshoe with its open end directed inferiorly and anteriorly. The deep central area of the socket (**acetabular fossa**) and its open end (**acetabular notch**) are nonarticular surface.

The **pelvic inlet** or rim is formed by the sacral promontory, the arcuate line of the ilium, the pecten of the pubis, and the superior aspects of the body of the pubis and the pubic symphysis (Fig. 4-5). This border separates the **false pelvis** above from the **true pelvis** below. This inlet is oriented obliquely between the coronal and transverse planes but is usually closer to the coronal plane. The false pelvis is not a separate cavity but is continuous with the abdominal cavity and thus part of the single abdominopelvic cavity. There is no physical separation between the abdominal and pelvic cavities; there simply is the imaginary plane of the pelvic inlet.

Male and Female Pelves

The differences in the male and female pelves reflect the differences in the functional demands placed upon them. The female pelvis must accommodate childbearing, while that of the male is constructed for speed and strength. Generally, the male pelvis is heavier, the muscle attachments are more pronounced, and the overall shape is more vertical and conical than that of the female. The angle of the subpubic arch is approximately 70 to 75 degrees in the male and 90 to 100 degrees in the female. The pelvic inlet is larger in women, and it tends to be oval or round as opposed to the usual triangular shape in men. In the man the iliac wings are rather vertical; in the woman they flare laterally and thus increase the size of the false pelvis. The male pelvic canal is long and tapered, while the female pelvic canal has parallel sides and is shorter. In addition, in women the ischial spines are shorter, directed more posteriorly, and farther apart.

Articulations of the Pelvis

Even though the **sacroiliac joints** are synovial joints, they permit very little motion and even fuse in a large number of people during later life. In addition, an extremely heavy network of ligaments binds the two bones together. However, there is potential for actual movement, and this motion may have significant clinical implications. This articulation is formed between similarly shaped articular surfaces on the medial aspect of the ilium (**auricular surface**) and the lateral aspect of the sacrum (Figs. 4-8, 2-7). These articular surfaces are not flat but somewhat curved, and they correspond to each other; since they are held tightly together, the unevenness of the surfaces actually resists movement. Oriented obliquely, these surfaces slope medially from above downward. This orientation presumably stabilizes the sacroiliac joints and resists motion, because the wedge-shaped sacrum is forced against both ilia during weight bearing. The joint cavity is surrounded by strong ligaments. The **ventral sacroiliac ligament** interconnects the anterior and inferior aspects of the two bones. Posteriorly, there are large, roughened areas that are interconnected by the massive **interosseous sacroiliac ligament,** which is surrounded peripherally by the **dorsal sacroiliac ligament.** Other ligaments, situated farther from the joint, also provide stabilization. The **sacrotuberous ligament** extends from the ischial tuberosity to the sacrum, and the **sacrospinous ligament** interconnects the ischial spine and the sacrum. Both of these ligaments resist anterior and inferior rotation of the sacral promontory relative to the ilia, the direction in which the superincumbent weight tends to move the sacrum. The **iliolumbar ligament** extends from the transverse process of the fifth lumbar vertebrae to the medial aspect of the ilium.

The minimal motion that occurs at this joint appears to be a gliding motion that consists of rotation of the sacrum relative to the ilia; the sacrum rotates in the sagittal plane around a transverse axis so that its promontory moves either anteriorly and inferiorly or posteriorly and superiorly. In addition, the sacrum may be able to slide superiorly and inferiorly. The amount of motion is related to both sex and age. It is greater in women than in men and is particularly free around the time of parturition. The motion is greatest in the earlier decades of life and tends to disappear during the fourth decade in men and the fifth decade in women. By the sixth decade the joint has ankylosed in most men and in about one-third of women. This general decline in motion is likely related to degenerative changes, such as those due to osteoarthritis, that occur in a high percentage of both sexes.

The **pubic symphysis** (Figs. 4-5, 4-6) is a cartilaginous articulation that unites the bodies of the pubic bones. The fibrocartilaginous disk that connects the two bones is strong and reinforced superiorly and inferiorly by the **superior pubic** and **arcuate pubic ligaments,** respectively. Other than around the time of parturition, virtually no motion occurs at this articulation.

Transfer of Weight Across the Pelvis

In both the standing and sitting positions weight passes through the bones of the pelvis. During standing, weight obviously must pass from the vertebral column to the femur (Figs. 4-5, 4-6). The weight passes inferiorly across the lumbosacral junction into the sacrum and then laterally across the sacroiliac articulation to the ilium. The weight continues anteriorly and inferiorly through the thickest part of the ilium, which is marked by the arcuate line. This line leads directly to the heavy superior aspect of the acetabulum, which is the major weight-bearing portion of that socket. At that point the weight is transferred to the head of the femur.

During sitting the weight-bearing points are the ischial tuberosities. After passing across the sacroiliac articulation, the weight is transferred inferiorly through the body of the ischium to the ischial tuberosity. This same bony prominence becomes the major weight-bearing surface for most patients who have above-knee amputations. An above-knee prosthesis is designed so the ischial tuberosity rests on the major weight-bearing portion of the prosthesis during standing.

Hip Region

Although there is no specific anatomic term for the entire junctional area between the trunk and lower limb, the area consists of the gluteal region posterolaterally and the inguinal region and femoral triangle anteriorly. The term "hip region" generally denotes the hip joint, but in this discussion it includes the entire junctional area: the lumbosacral plexus, hip joint, gluteal region, and the anterior muscles of the hip. The femur is included as well, because it participates in the formation of the hip joint and provides attachments for most of the muscles of the hip.

Lumbosacral Plexus

Branches of the **lumbosacral plexus** (Fig. 4-9) innervate the lower limb, the perineum, and the skin of the buttock and the lower anterolateral abdominal wall. This plexus is formed by the ventral rami of spinal nerves L1 through S4 in much the same manner as the brachial plexus—there are fusions and splittings before the terminal peripheral nerves are formed. However, the study of this plexus need not be as detailed as that of the brachial plexus. First, the lumbosacral plexus is considerably less vulnerable to injury because it is positioned very deeply, where it is protected, and the limited mobility of the hip joint greatly reduces the potential for stretching injuries of the plexus. Second, the formation of the plexus occurs over a very short distance; therefore, its organization is difficult to dissect and resolve. As a result, the specific location and relationships of the plexus together with the terminal nerves should be emphasized.

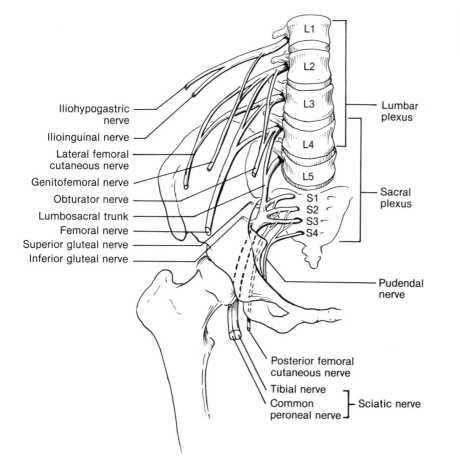

Figure 4-9
Anterior view of the lumbosacral plexus.

The lumbosacral plexus is a combination of two separate plexuses: the **lumbar** and **sacral plexuses,** which are separated physically and supply different parts of the lower limb. They are, however, interconnected by a large nerve trunk and share one segment of origin. They are considered separately simply to facilitate discussion.

The **lumbar plexus** (Fig. 4-9) is derived from spinal cord segments L1–L4, along with a variable but usual contribution from segment T12. This plexus is formed within the substance of the psoas major muscle (which is positioned lateral to the bodies of the lumbar vertebrae); and the terminal nerves that arise from the plexus emerge from various parts of that muscle. The psoas muscle is enclosed within a firm fascial envelope; therefore a collection of material, such as inflammatory material or blood, may cause pressure on the plexus itself or the proximal parts of its branches. The initial portions of the branches of this plexus are retroperitoneal and thus fixed in place. As a result, they may be compressed against the posterior body wall by a space-occupying lesion. The components of the plexus also are vulnerable to entrapment by a shortened psoas muscle, because as the muscle lengthens, the nerves may be compressed more than normally.

The small branches of the upper part of the lumbar plexus, the **subcostal, iliohypogastric,** and **ilioinguinal nerves,** innervate portions of the lower anterolateral abdominal wall and the proximal thigh. The **genitofemoral nerve** passes along the anterior aspect of the psoas major and supplies the **cremasteric muscle** of the spermatic cord as well as a small cutaneous area of the proximal thigh. The **lateral femoral cutaneous nerve** (L2, L3) emerges from the lateral aspect of the psoas and passes laterally across the iliac fossa. It then usually passes through the iliotibial tract, where it is vulnerable to entrapment. The result of such entrapment is meralgia paraesthetica, or paresthesia over the lateral thigh.

The major branches of the lumbar plexus are the **femoral** and **obturator nerves.** The femoral nerve, formed by the posterior branches of ventral rami L2–L4, emerges from the lateral aspect of the psoas major muscle just proximal to the inguinal ligament. This nerve supplies the muscles in the anterior compartment of the thigh. The **saphenous nerve,** the continuation of the femoral nerve, passes into the leg to supply the skin of the medial aspects of the knee, leg, and foot. The obturator nerve, formed by the anterior branches of ventral rami L2–L4, emerges from the medial side of the psoas major muscle and then enters the pelvis and the medial aspect of the thigh. This nerve innervates the medial femoral muscles and the skin of the distal medial thigh. It is important to note that this nerve also supplies both the hip and knee joints, an important point clinically because it is thought to mediate referred pain from the hip to the knee and vice versa.

The **sacral plexus** (Fig. 4-9) is formed on the posterolateral wall of the pelvis on the ventral aspect of the piriformis muscle. The internal iliac artery and vein are medial to this plexus, and branches of both intermingle with those of the plexus. The plexus is formed by fibers from spinal cord segments L4–S4. The fibers from segments L4 and L5 form a large trunk, the **lumbosacral trunk,** that enters the pelvis by crossing the pelvic brim just lateral to the sacral promontory. The ventral rami of spinal nerves S1–S4 pass ventrally through their respective ventral sacral foramina and then laterally into the plexus. This plexus appears as a giant triangular mass with its widest dimension medially where the contributing trunks converge to form the plexus; its apex is directed inferolaterally where all of the nerve trunks appear to come to an apex and disappear (exit from the pelvis) through the greater sciatic foramen. Since this is a somatic plexus and thus innervates the body wall and lower limb, most of its branches have very short pelvic courses and therefore exit from the pelvis soon after they are formed.

The **superior** (L4–S1) and **inferior** (L5–S2) **gluteal nerves** branch from the superolateral aspect of the plexus. Both of these nerves pass through the greater sciatic foramen, one above and one below the piriformis muscle, and into the gluteal region, where they supply the gluteal muscles. A number of short nerves, each named by the muscle it supplies, branch from the plexus and innervate the nearby short external rotators of the thigh. The **posterior femoral cutaneous nerve** (S1–S3) enters the gluteal region by passing through the greater sciatic foramen and passing inferior to the piriformis muscle. It supplies the skin of the posterior thigh and popliteal region.

The largest branch of the sacral plexus is the **sciatic nerve,** which is really two nerves, the **tibial** and **common peroneal,** wrapped in a common connective tissue sheath. This nerve appears to be the continuation of the sacral plexus as it exists from the pelvis through the greater sciatic foramen. Generally, the tibial and common peroneal nerves separate in the distal aspect of the thigh. The tibial nerve (L4–S3) supplies most of the posterior femoral muscles and all of the muscles in the posterior compartment of the leg and the plantar aspect of the foot. The common peroneal (L4–S2) nerve innervates the muscles in the anterior and lateral compartments of the leg and the dorsal intrinsic muscles of the foot. Branches of these nerves supply the skin of the lateral half of the leg along with the plantar and dorsal aspect of the foot, except its posteromedial aspect.

Femur

The **femur** (Figs. 4-10, 4-11) is the largest bone in the body and the only bone in the thigh. Both its proximal and distal aspects are large, with the proximal head offset from the shaft and joined to it by a **neck.** The bone's long shaft is slightly bowed anteriorly.

The rounded **head** of the femur is large and slightly greater in shape than a hemisphere. As a result, its diameter laterally is somewhat less than its maximal diameter. The entire surface of the head is articular surface with the exception of the centrally located **fovea.** The **neck** of the femur is short and joins the head with the proximal aspect of the femoral shaft at the **trochanteric region.** Although the angle between the long axes of the neck and shaft (angle of inclination) is quite variable, it averages approximately 125 to 130 degrees and is usually greater in the man. The lesser angle in the woman presumably is one of the contribut-

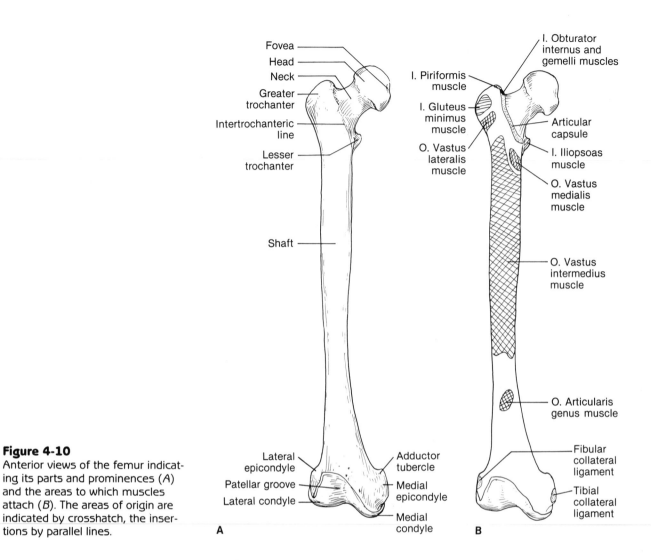

Figure 4-10
Anterior views of the femur indicating its parts and prominences (*A*) and the areas to which muscles attach (*B*). The areas of origin are indicated by crosshatch, the insertions by parallel lines.

A

B

ing factors to the greater incidence of femoral neck fracture in women. The shaft of the femur is twisted medially, creating a difference between the longitudinal axis of the femoral neck and the axis (line) through the center of the two femoral condyles. This **angle of torsion (declination),** although quite variable, is usually close to 15 degrees.

The trochanteric region of the femur is the expanded proximal portion of the shaft. The **greater trochanter** is the large, laterally placed prominence that extends superior to the junction of the femoral neck. The **lesser trochanter** is positioned medially and inferiorly and is directed posteromedially so only a small portion is visible in a normal anteroposterior radiograph (Fig. 4-6). Anteriorly, the **intertrochanteric line** extends inferomedially from the greater trochanter to a point below the lesser trochanter. Posteriorly, the large **intertrochanteric crest** stretches between the trochanters, and the obvious fossa medial to the superior aspect of this crest is the **trochanteric fossa.**

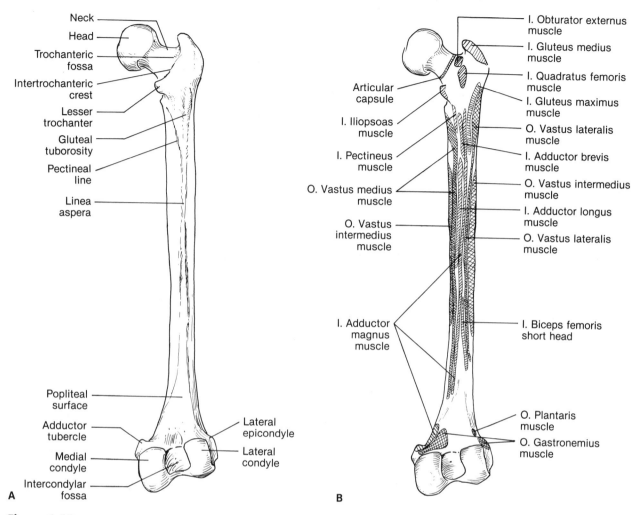

Neck
Head
Trochanteric fossa
Intertrochanteric crest
Lesser trochanter
Gluteal tuborosity
Pectineal line
Linea aspera
Popliteal surface
Adductor tubercle
Medial condyle
Intercondylar fossa
Lateral epicondyle
Lateral condyle

A

Articular capsule
I. Iliopsoas muscle
I. Pectineus muscle
O. Vastus medius muscle
O. Vastus intermedius muscle
I. Adductor magnus muscle

I. Obturator externus muscle
I. Gluteus medius muscle
I. Quadratus femoris muscle
I. Gluteus maximus muscle
O. Vastus lateralis muscle
I. Adductor brevis muscle
O. Vastus intermedius muscle
I. Adductor longus muscle
O. Vastus lateralis muscle
I. Biceps femoris short head
O. Plantaris muscle
O. Gastronemius muscle

B

Figure 4-11
Posterior views of the femur indicating its parts and prominences (A) and the areas to which muscles attach (B). The areas of origin are indicated by cross-hatch, the insertions by parallel lines.

The shaft of the femur is smooth and presents few distinguishing characteristics. In cross section it is rounded anteriorly, but posteriorly it has a flattened surface. This flat surface is the vertically oriented **linea aspera** that extends the entire length of the femoral shaft. The medial and lateral edges of the linea aspera are roughened and provide the points of attachment for several of the muscles that attach to the femoral shaft. Proximally, the medial edge diverges medially, provides attachment for the pectineus muscle (the **pectineal line**), and spirals around the medial aspect of the femur where it is continuous with the intertrochanteric line. The lateral edge of the proximal part of the linea aspera extends toward the greater trochanter where it is usually markedly roughened as the **gluteal tuberosity.** Distally, the two edges of the linea aspera diverge toward the femoral condyles (the **medial** and **lateral supracondylar lines**) and define the **popliteal** or **supracondylar surface** of the bone.

The distal portion of the femur is quite large and contains articular surfaces that articulate with both the tibia and the patella. The large **medial** and **lateral condyles** are the distal articular surfaces of the femur; both of these surfaces extend posteriorly well beyond the femoral shaft. The medial condyle extends more distally than the lateral, thereby compensating for the obliquity of the femoral shaft relative to the vertical tibia. Anteriorly, the two articular surfaces join to form a vertical groove in which the patella rides. The lateral lip of this groove is larger than the medial and is one of the structural features that resists lateral movement of the patella when the leg is extended. Distally and posteriorly, the two condyles are separated by the **intercondylar fossa.** The nonarticular areas superior to both condyles are the **medial** and **lateral epicondyles** with the medial extending superiorly as far as the prominent **adductor tubercle.**

The blood supply to the proximal part of the femur (Fig. 4-14), to the head and neck, is particularly important because of its vulnerability when the femoral neck is fractured. A branch of the obturator artery enters the femoral head through the ligament of the head of the femur and supplies a variable, but generally small, portion of the bone adjacent to the fovea. The head and neck of the femur are supplied predominantly by branches of the medial and lateral femoral circumflex arteries. These branches (**retinacular arteries**) pass proximally along the neck of the femur, where they are tethered to the bone by the synovial portion of the joint capsule. Since these vessels are held against the bone, they are vulnerable to injury when the femoral neck is fractured. Further, the blood (provided by the nutrient arteries) that supplies the shaft typically does not extend proximally into either the neck or the head. As a result, loss of blood supply from the retinacular vessels may well result in a greatly reduced rate of healing or simply preclude any healing.

Hip Joint

The **hip joint** (Figs. 4-12 through 4-14) is formed between the head of the femur and the acetabulum. In many ways its basic structure is similar to that of the shoulder joint; however, its structure and the nature of its supports reflect the functional demands necessitated by its weight-bearing function. This joint is intrinsically stable and vulnerable to pathology that generally involves the bones of the joint rather than the soft tissue that supports and surrounds the joint.

The large head of the femur fits rather snugly into the deep acetabular socket of the os coxae. The two articular surfaces almost coincide, except the socket is not quite deep enough to accommodate the entire head, and the acetabulum is incomplete centrally and inferiorly. The fovea of the head of the femur is adjacent to the nonarticular surface of the acetabulum. The heaviest part of the acetabulum is its superior aspect, which accommodates weight during standing.

The strong fibrocartilaginous **acetabular labrum** is attached firmly to the rim of the acetabulum. The labrum forms an entire circle, and a

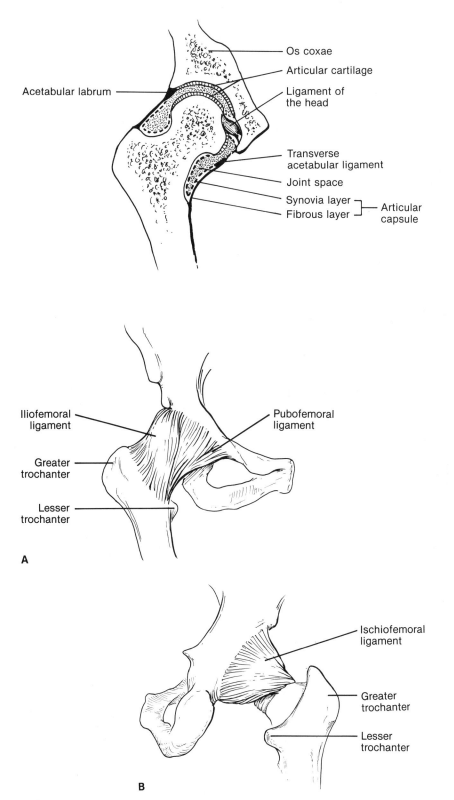

Os coxae

Articular cartilage

Acetabular labrum

Ligament of
the head

Transverse
acetabular ligament

Joint space

Synovia layer ⎤
Fibrous layer ⎦ Articular
capsule

Figure 4-12
Coronal section through the hip
joint indicating the positions of the
synovial and fibrous portions of the
joint capsule and the extent of the
joint cavity.

Figure 4-13
Anterior (A) and posterior (B) views
of the joint capsule and extracapsular ligaments of the hip joint.

Iliofemoral
ligament

Pubofemoral
ligament

Greater
trochanter

Lesser
trochanter

A

Ischiofemoral
ligament

Greater
trochanter

Lesser
trochanter

B

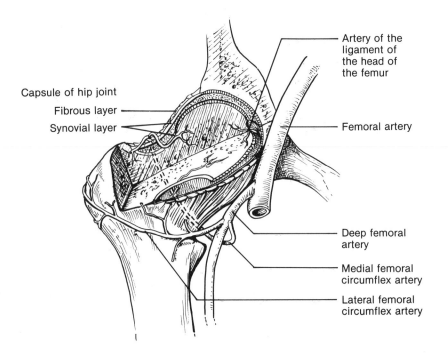

Capsule of hip joint
Fibrous layer
Synovial layer

Artery of the
ligament of
the head of
the femur

Femoral artery

Deep femoral
artery

Medial femoral
circumflex artery

Lateral femoral
circumflex artery

Figure 4-14
Anterior view of the hip joint with
the anterosuperior aspect of the
proximal part of the femur
removed. Note the relationship of
the terminal arterial branches to the
joint capsule.

portion of it, the **transverse acetabular ligament,** bridges the acetabular notch. This labrum increases the congruency between the two articular surfaces as it extends distally to the edge of the articular surface of the femoral head. The diameter of the circle formed by the labrum is actually less than the greatest diameter of the femoral head; as a result, the labrum grips the head and holds it in the acetabulum. Thus, dislocation of the femoral head must be accompanied by a tear or significant stretch of the acetabular labrum.

The **ligament of the head of the femur** (Fig. 4-12) extends from the acetabular notch to the fovea of the head of the femur. Although this intra-articular ligament appears to be in an ideal position to reinforce the hip joint, it is not sufficiently taut during the normal range of motion to provide significant support. Its major function apparently is to convey a small artery to the head of the femur.

The **capsule** (Figs. 4-12 through 4-14) of the hip joint is typical of the synovial joint in that it has fibrous and synovial components that form a closed joint space. However, the capsule is atypical because it extends distally along the femoral neck, well beyond the edge of the articular surface of the head of the femur. The fibrous and synovial portions of the capsule are not coextensive. The fibrous portion attaches proximally to the labrum and adjacent part of the os coxae. It extends distally and attaches to the medial aspect of the greater trochanter superiorly, the intertrochanteric line anteriorly, just superior to the lesser trochanter inferiorly, and approximately two-thirds of the way distally along the neck of the femur posteriorly. As a result, the entire femoral neck is intracapsular anteriorly but only about two-thirds is intracapsular posteriorly. The synovial portion of the capsule attaches to the lip of the acetabulum and the labrum, and then lines the fibrous portion of the capsule. At the points where the fibrous capsule attaches to the femur, the synovial layer reflects proximally along the neck of the femur and extends to the edge of the articular surface of the femoral head. The synovial portion of the capsule is attached rather firmly to the neck of the femur. The result of this capsular construction is a joint space that extends distally along the neck of the femur, enclosing the entire neck anteriorly and approximately two-thirds of the neck posteriorly. The synovial membrane forms a tube that attaches to the edges of the fovea of the femoral head and the acetabular fossa, and thus surrounds the ligament of the head of the femur. This ligament, like other intracapsular ligaments, is between the fibrous and synovial layers of the capsule and not bathed in synovial fluid.

The courses of the blood vessels that supply most of the head and neck of the femur (Fig. 4-14) and their vulnerability are discussed on page 180. Since a portion of the posterior aspect of the femoral neck is extracapsular, blood vessels crossing that area of the bone are not firmly anchored to the bone and are less vulnerable to femoral neck fracture than those passing deep to the synovial portion of the joint capsule.

The fibrous portion of the joint capsule is reinforced by three strong ligaments (Fig. 4-13). These ligaments extend from the component bones of the os coxae to the distal attachment of the fibrous capsule. Although they are extracapsular ligaments, they blend with the joint capsule and are not always easily defined. The **iliofemoral ligament** is a very strong ligament that covers the anterior aspect of the joint. From a superior attachment to the anterior inferior iliac spine and adjacent part of the body of the ilium, its fibers diverge as they pass inferiorly and attach to the intertrochanteric line of the femur. This ligament may resemble an inverted Y; hence the eponym **Y ligament of Bigelow.** This ligament tightens as the femur is extended; in fact, it prevents extension beyond zero degrees. Its strength is sufficient to support the body's weight above the hips so a person with no hip musculature, such as a paraplegic or a child with muscular dystrophy, can position his or her trunk posterior to the flexion-extension axes of the hips and maintain the upright position. The **ischiofemoral ligament** attaches proximally to the body of the ischium. Its fibers pass anteriorly, superiorly, and laterally as they spiral around the superior aspect of the neck of the femur and then attach to the medial aspect of the greater trochanter and the upper aspect of the intertrochanteric line. This ligament tightens as the femur is extended; and since its femoral attachment is considerably lateral to its ischial attachment, the femoral head is "screwed into" the acetabulum as the femur is extended. The **pubofemoral ligament** crosses the lower anterior aspect of the joint, extending from the body and superior ramus of the pubis to the inferior aspect of the intertrochanteric line and adjacent portion of the femoral neck. This ligament limits abduction of the femur.

The extracapsular ligaments of the hip, particularly the iliofemoral and ischiofemoral ligaments, play a major role in the stability of the joint. They are taut when the femur is extended and support the most weight, and thus provide the greatest support when it is most needed. These ligaments provide the least amount of support, though, when the thigh is flexed, and the majority of the hip joint dislocations occur. Most traumatic dislocations of the hip are posterior and commonly occur when an individual is sitting, as when driving an automobile, and there is a strong proximally directed force on the femur.

As with the shoulder, the potential directions for motions at the hip are virtually unlimited but are described relative to the cardinal planes of the body. In addition, the amount of each motion is relatively restricted because of the construction of the joint. **Flexion** and **extension** occur in the sagittal plane, flexion as the femur moves anteriorly, and extension as the femur moves posteriorly. The question of whether the femur can be "hyperextended"—extended beyond the coronal plane—is an academic one. I believe it cannot and that apparent hyperextension of the femur is in reality motion in the lumbar portion of the vertebral column. The femur can be **abducted, adducted, circumducted,** and **rotated.** Rotation of the femur is not longitudinal rotation of the bone around an axis through its shaft because the head is offset from the shaft. The axis of rotation passes through the head of the femur and enters the shaft at about the midthigh level. Rotation occurs around this axis rather than the shaft.

The major flexor of the femur is the iliopsoas muscle; both the gluteus maximus and hamstring muscles are strong extensors. Abduction is produced by the gluteus medius and minimus, and adduction is a function of the medial femoral muscles. A muscle's capacity to rotate the femur is dependent on its relationship to the axis of rotation rather than the location of its attachment to the femur. The gluteus maximus is the strongest lateral rotator; the gluteus medius and tensor fascia lata rotate the femur medially. Other muscles, particularly some of the adductors, can produce either medial or lateral rotation, depending on whether the femur is flexed or extended.

Gluteal Region

The **gluteal region** is the junctional region between the posterior and lateral aspects of the thigh and trunk. The general contours of this area are formed predominantly by the gluteal muscles, which also have important functions in gait. A group of smaller muscles, collectively called the short external rotators of the thigh, is positioned deep to the gluteus maximus muscle. All muscles in this area interconnect the os coxae and the femur and are innervated by branches of the sacral plexus.

The **gluteal muscles** are the **gluteus maximus, gluteus medius, gluteus minimus,** and **tensor fasciae latae.** The **gluteus maximus** (Figs. 4-7B, 4-11B, 4-15) is the largest of the gluteal muscles and forms the entire buttock region. It arises from the posterolateral aspect of the ilium, the posterior aspects of the sacrum and coccyx, and the sacrotuberous ligament. From this wide origin its fibers pass inferiorly and laterally toward an equally extensive insertion into the iliotibial tract and on the gluteal tuberosity of the upper posterior aspect of the femur.

The gluteus maximus is both a strong extensor and an external ro-

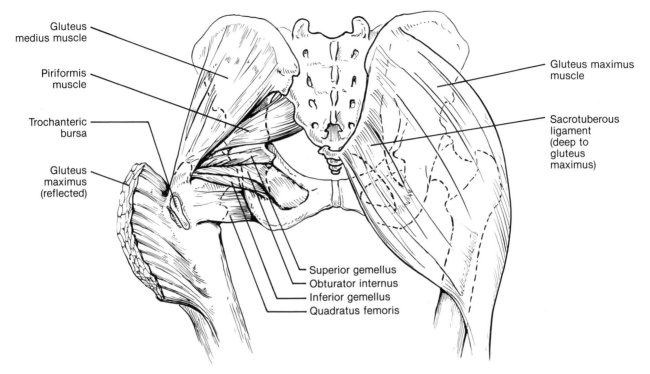

Gluteus medius muscle

Piriformis muscle

Trochanteric bursa

Gluteus maximus (reflected)

Gluteus maximus muscle

Sacrotuberous ligament (deep to gluteus maximus)

Superior gemellus
Obturator internus
Inferior gemellus
Quadratus femoris

Figure 4-15
Posterior view of the gluteal region showing the gluteus maximus (*on the right*) and deeper muscles (*on the left*).

tator of the femur. With the foot on the ground this muscle can produce extension at the knee through the iliotibial tract. During gait the gluteus maximus is active at heel strike, when it prevents hip flexion. Loss of this muscle results in a flattened contour of the buttock and a postural change during quiet standing because the trunk is positioned more posteriorly than normal. At heel strike, the trunk is thrown noticeably posteriorly. In addition, there is difficulty in activities such as rising from a sitting position and climbing stairs. The gluteus maximus is innervated by the inferior gluteal nerve.

The **gluteus medius** and **minimus muscles** (Figs. 4-7B, 4-11B, 4-15, 4-16) are the lateral muscles of the gluteal region and fill the interval between the iliac crest and greater trochanter of the femur. Both muscles are somewhat triangular with rather wide origins and narrow insertions. The gluteus medius is superficial to the gluteus minimus and arises from a large portion of the upper lateral aspect of the wing of the ilium. The origin of the gluteus minimus is from the lateral aspect of the wing of the ilium, but it is inferior to that of the gluteus medius. The fibers of both muscles converge as they pass toward their insertions on the greater trochanter of the femur. These two muscles are the main abductors of the femur and function during the stance phase of gait to keep the pelvis from dropping on the nonstance side, thus preventing adduction at the hip. A

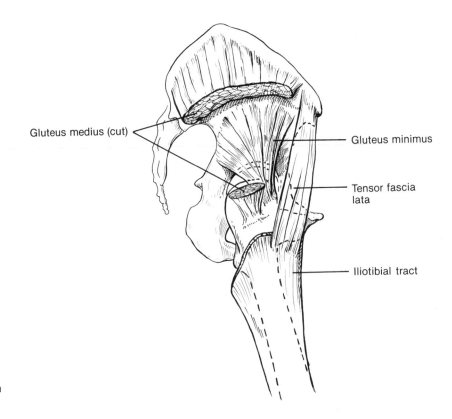

Gluteus medius (cut)

Gluteus minimus

Tensor fascia lata

Iliotibial tract

Figure 4-16
Lateral view of the gluteus medius
and minimus, and tensor fascia lata
muscles.

unilateral loss of these muscles may or may not be apparent during quiet standing, because a person can stand on both feet with little trouble. However, standing on only the involved lower limb is accompanied by a laterally bent trunk over the supporting limb (a positive Trendelenberg sign). Similarly, during gait the trunk is thrown laterally at heel strike to maintain the upright position. Both the gluteus medius and minimus are supplied by the superior gluteal nerve.

The **tensor latae muscle** (Figs. 4-7B, 4-16) is the most anterior of the gluteal muscles and is located within the upper portion of the iliotibial tract. This muscle arises from the anterior-most part of the iliac crest. Its fibers descend vertically and insert into the anterior portion of the iliotibial tract approximately one-third of the way down the thigh. In reality, the iliotibial tract is the tendon of the tensor fasciae latae, and its bony insertion is the lateral tibial condyle. This muscle contributes to both flexion and internal rotation of the thigh but is a major force of neither. Loss of this muscle produces neither a noticeable static nor functional deficit. The tensor fasciae latae is innervated by the superior gluteal nerve.

Most of the **short external rotators of the thigh** (Figs. 4-7B, 4-11B, 4-15) are located deep to the gluteus maximus muscle. The fibers of these muscles generally pass horizontally; they are all innervated by small branches of the upper portion of the sacral plexus; and from superior to inferior they include the **piriformis, superior gemellus, obturator inter-**

nus, **inferior gemellus,** and **quadratus femoris.** The **piriformis muscle** is an important landmark in the plane that is deep to the gluteus maximus, because the neurovascular structures passing from the pelvis to the gluteal region are either above or below this muscle. From an origin on the deep or ventral aspect of the sacrum its fibers pass anterolaterally through the greater sciatic foramen, which the muscle fills; its fibers insert on the medial aspect of the greater trochanter of the femur.

The **obturator internus muscle** (Figs. 4-15, 4-17) also extends from the pelvis into the gluteal region and passes through the lesser sciatic foramen. From an origin on the deep aspect of the rim of the obturator foramen its fibers converge as they pass posteriorly to join the tendon. This tendon glides around the smooth bony anterior wall of the lesser sciatic foramen before inserting into the medial aspect of the greater trochanter of the femur.

Both the **superior** and **inferior gemelli muscles** (Figs. 4-7B, 4-15, 4-17) are closely related to the obturator internus tendon; in fact, they occasionally obscure that tendon. These muscles arise, respectively, from the ischial spine and tuberosity and join the tendon of the obturator internus as it inserts into the greater trochanter.

The **quadratus femoris muscle** (Figs. 4-7B, 4-11B, 4-15, 4-17) is a strong, rectangular muscle that is located totally outside of the pelvis and partially deep to the gluteus maximus. From an origin on the lateral aspect of the body of the ischium, the fibers of this muscle pass laterally

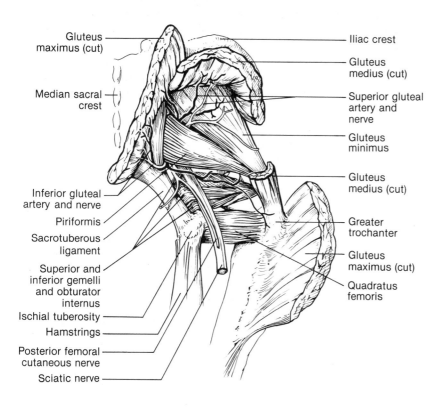

Figure 4-17
Posterior view of the neurovascular structures of the gluteal region.

and insert on the central aspect of the posterior intertrochanteric region of the femur.

The **sciatic, posterior femoral cutaneous, superior gluteal,** and **inferior gluteal nerves** (Fig. 4-17) are the large nerves of the gluteal region. The **sciatic nerve** passes through the gluteal region but innervates no structures in that area. It enters the gluteal region by passing through the greater sciatic foramen and inferior to the piriformis muscle. Initially it passes obliquely and laterally, but then it descends vertically between the gluteus maximus and the short external rotators; its vertical course is about midway between the ischial tuberosity and the greater trochanter of the femur. It enters the posterior thigh as it passes the inferior border of the gluteus maximus muscle. The nerve is vulnerable to entrapment or other injury at several points in this region. In approxmiately 15 percent of the population part or all of the nerve passes through the piriformis muscle, predisposing it to entrapment (**piriformis syndrome**). The nerve is also vulnerable as it crosses the lower bony edge of the greater sciatic notch. Also, it passes posterior to the hip joint, where it can be stretched by a posteriorly dislocated femoral head. And, throughout its course in this region, it is vulnerable to injury during a gluteal injection.

The **inferior gluteal nerve** (Fig. 4-17) enters the gluteal region by passing through the greater sciatic foramen and inferior to the piriformis muscle. It then passes directly into the gluteus maximus so its overall length is quite short.

The **superior gluteal nerve** (Fig. 4-17) enters the gluteal region by passing through the greater sciatic foramen and superior to the piriformis muscle. It then passes anteriorly between the gluteus medius and minimus muscles and ends anteriorly in the tensor fascia latae muscle.

The course of the **posterior femoral cutaneous nerve** (Fig. 4-17) parallels that of the sciatic through the gluteal region. It continues its vertical course as it descends through the posterior thigh and provides cutaneous branches to the skin of the posterior thigh and proximal posterior calf.

Both the **superior** and **inferior gluteal arteries** (Fig. 4-17) are branches of the internal iliac artery. Each of these vessels accompanies the nerve of the same name into and through the gluteal region and provides the blood supply to the same structures.

Anterior Hip Muscles

The **iliopsoas muscle** (Figs. 4-8B, 4-10B, 4-18) is positioned deeply in both the abdomen and the thigh. Although this muscle can be considered as two, the **psoas major** and **iliacus muscles,** it is really a single muscle that has two large and distinctly different origins and a single insertion. Its origins are from both the lumbar part of the vertebral column and the os coxae. The psoas major portion arises from the anterolateral aspects of the lumbar vertebral bodies and transverse processes; it frequently arises from the twelfth thoracic vertebra as well. The iliac portion arises from most of the medial aspect of the wing of the ilium (iliac fossa). The fibers of the two heads converge as they descend deep to the inguinal ligament

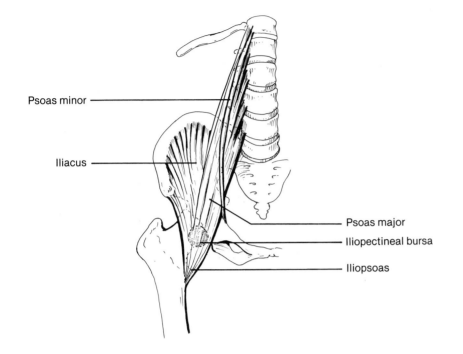

Psoas minor

Iliacus

Psoas major

Iliopectineal bursa

Iliopsoas

Figure 4-18
Anterior view of the iliopsoas and
psoas minor muscles.

and anterior to the hip joint. The single insertion is by means of a strong
tendon to the lesser trochanter of the femur. Both bellies of the muscle
are innervated by fibers derived from the second, third, and fourth lumbar
spinal cord segments. The psoas portion receives direct branches from the
lumbar plexus (which is formed within the muscle), and the iliac portion
receives branches from the femoral nerve.

The variable **psoas minor muscle** (Fig. 4-18) is positioned on the
anterior aspect of the psoas major muscle, extending from the twelfth
thoracic and first lumbar vertebrae to a point on the arcuate line of the
ilium. It is usually innervated by fibers from upper lumbar spinal cord
segments; and since it does not cross the hip joint, it has no role in
motion at that joint. Any potential function is thus limited to the vertebral column. However, its considerable variability (it is present approximately 40 to 50 percent of the time) and small size make its functional
importance questionable.

The iliopsoas is the major flexor of the thigh, providing both a full
range of motion and most of the strength of flexion. Its role in other
motions at the hip appears minimal, and it is probably of no functional
importance. With the femur fixed a shortening contraction of this muscle
produces an anterior and inferior pull on the lumbar vertebrae, which
can result in an increase in the lumbar curve (extension of the lumbar
spine). If this occurs in the supine position with extension at both the
hips and knees, as in performing a sit-up with the thighs and legs extended, the lumbar extension is likely to be even more marked because
that position lengthens the iliopsoas and thus makes its contraction more
efficient. Loss of the iliopsoas muscle results in a profound loss of thigh

flexion. During gait, this loss is manifest predominantly during the swing phase, because there is a reduction in the initial acceleration and the thigh cannot be flexed to shorten the limb. A unilateral loss of this muscle may also contribute to the formation of scoliosis as the normal symmetrical pull of both muscles (left and right) on the vertebral column is lost.

The iliopsoas muscle is separated from the anterior aspect of the hip joint by the **iliopectineal bursa** (Fig. 4-18). This bursa communicates with the synovial cavity of the hip joint in a small percentage of adults (approximately 5–10 percent) and can become inflamed to cause an **iliopectineal bursitis.** The symptom is usually pain upon motion or palpation; the pain typically is localized just below the middle portion of the inguinal ligament.

Surface Anatomy of the Hip Region

The **anterior superior iliac spine** (Fig. 4-5) is palpable as the most prominent bony landmark in the inferolateral aspect of the abdominal wall, and the **anterior inferior iliac spine** is inferior and slightly medial to the superior spine. The **pubic bodies** and **symphysis** are in the midline at the most inferior aspect of the abdomen; the prominence at the lateral aspect of each pubic body is the **pubic tubercle.** The diagonal line interconnecting the pubic tubercle and anterior superior iliac spine marks the position of the **inguinal ligament.** Most of the **iliac crest** is easily felt as it is followed posteriorly from the anterior superior iliac spine to the **posterior superior iliac spine,** which is marked by a definitive dimple in the skin. The very prominent **greater trochanter of the femur** is easily located well inferior to the middle of the iliac crest; and the **gluteus medius** and **minimus muscles** account for most of the soft tissue bulk between these two bones. Anteriorly in this interval (generally inferior to the anterior superior iliac spine) the **tensor fasciae latae muscle** can be palpated.

Posteriorly, the major contour of the buttock region is formed by the **gluteus maximus muscle**; the gluteal fold, however, does not correspond to the inferior border of that muscle. Inferiorly and medially the large **ischial tuberosity** is easily palpable, and passing anteriorly and medially from that prominence, the **ischial** and **inferior pubic rami** can be followed to the body of the pubis.

Bones of the Leg

Although both the **tibia** and **fibula** (Figs. 4-19, 4-20) are the bones of the leg, the tibia bears virtually all of the weight that is transmitted from the thigh to the foot. The tibia is the only bone of the leg involved in the formation of the knee joint; it also presents the major weight-bearing surface at the ankle joint. The tibia and fibula are interconnected by two articulations and an interosseous membrane in much the same way as the radius and ulna; the relationship between the two bones, however, is essentially fixed; therefore, no motion similar to pronation and

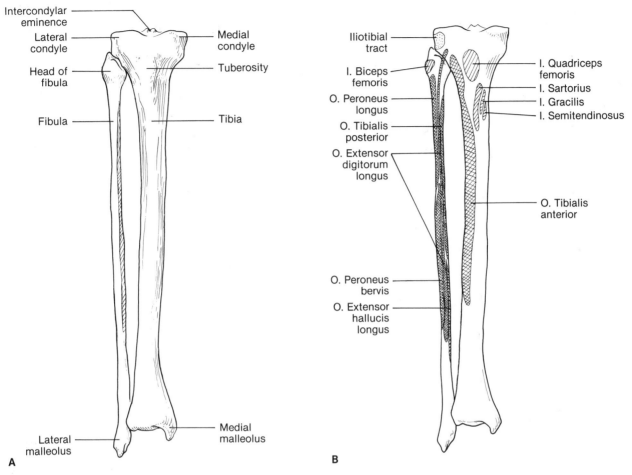

Intercondylar eminence
Lateral condyle
Head of fibula
Fibula
Medial condyle
Tuberosity
Tibia
Lateral malleolus
Medial malleolus

A

Iliotibial tract
I. Biceps femoris
O. Peroneus longus
O. Tibialis posterior
O. Extensor digitorum longus
O. Peroneus bervis
O. Extensor hallucis longus
I. Quadriceps femoris
I. Sartorius
I. Gracilis
I. Semitendinosus
O. Tibialis anterior

B

Figure 4-19
Anterior views of the tibia and fibula demonstrating their parts and prominences (*A*) and the areas of muscle attachment (*B*). The areas of origin are indicated by crosshatch, the insertions by parallel lines.

supination is available. The **proximal** and **distal tibiofibular joints** unite the proximal and distal portions of the bones.

The proximal tibiofibular joint is a synovial joint that is reinforced by anterior and posterior ligaments between the two bones. The distal union is usually a fibrous joint that also is reinforced by strong anterior and posterior tibiofibular ligaments. Both articulations are strongly fortified by the **interosseous membrane.**

The **tibia** (Figs. 4-19, 4-20) is the larger and longer of the two bones, and the majority of the strong muscles that control the knee joint attach to this bone. Its proximal end is expanded and flattened, forming the horizontal **tibial plateau.** This plateau is formed by two articular surfaces, the **medial** and **lateral tibial condyles,** that are separated by the nonarticular **intercondylar area.** The intercondylar area contains a centrally positioned **intercondylar eminence,** which further separates the intercon-

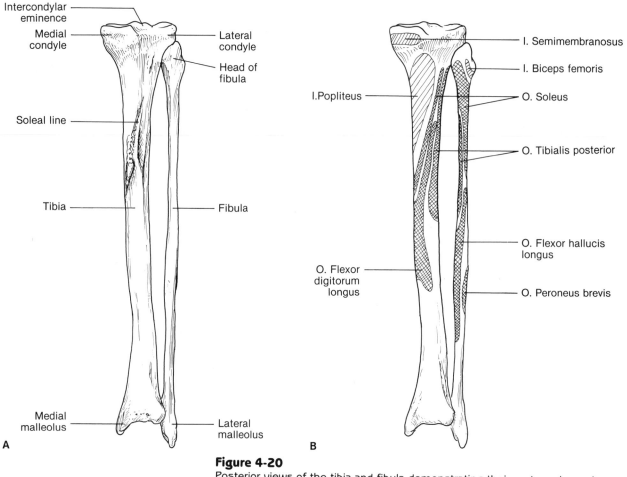

Intercondylar eminence

Medial condyle

Soleal line

Tibia

Medial malleolus

A

Lateral condyle

Head of fibula

Fibula

Lateral malleolus

I. Semimembranosus

I. Biceps femoris

O. Soleus

O. Tibialis posterior

O. Flexor hallucis longus

O. Peroneus brevis

I. Popliteus

O. Flexor digitorum longus

B

Figure 4-20
Posterior views of the tibia and fibula demonstrating their parts and prominences (A) and the locations of muscular attachments (B). The areas of origin are indicated by crosshatch, the insertions by parallel lines.

dylar area into anterior and posterior sections. The shaft of the tibia is roughly triangular in cross section and has a sharp anterior border that extends throughout most of its length. The prominent **tibial tuberosity** is positioned at the upper end of the anterior border and several centimeters below the tibial plateau. Posteriorly on the proximal half of the shaft, the obliquely oriented **soleal line appears** as a ridge across the bone. The distal end of the bone presents a flattened articular surface and a medial extension, the **medial malleolus,** that is covered with articular surface on its lateral aspect. Laterally, the **fibular notch** accommodates the fibula, and posteriorly there is a series of grooves that house the tendons of the deep posterior muscles of the leg.

The **fibula** (Figs. 4-19, 4-20) provides muscle attachments and participates in the formation of the ankle joint. The expanded proximal **head** of the fibula presents a flattened medial surface that articulates with the tibia. The head tapers to a rather fragile shaft that presents various borders to which muscles attach. Inferiorly the shaft expands to form the **lateral malleolus,** which is covered by articular surface on its medial aspect and extends somewhat more distally than the medial malleolus.

Knee Joint and Patella

The knee is formed between the femur and the tibia. Although it is supported against displacement in all directions by strong ligaments, the knee relies primarily on the large anterior and posterior muscles of the thigh for its stability. This joint permits a large range of motion; and throughout a large percentage of that range, it must accommodate forces that can greatly exceed the weight of the body. The freedom of motion, the extreme forces, and the construction of the joint make it vulnerable to traumatic injury and degenerative disease, perhaps more so than any other joint in the body. The knee is particularly vulnerable to injury when the foot is planted on the ground.

Patella

The patella (Fig. 4-26), the largest sesamoid bone in the body, is partially embedded within the tendon of the quadriceps femoris muscle. This bone is generally triangular in shape with its apex directed distally. Its posterior aspect is covered with articular cartilage and presents a vertical ridge that occupies the groove between the femoral condyles, forming the **patellofemoral joint.** As the leg is flexed and extended, the patella slides along the groove in the femur. Its presence is thought to be especially important in full extension at the knee because the patella positions the quadriceps tendon anteriorly and thus increases the obliquity of the tendon's pull. Removal of this bone frequently results in difficulty obtaining full extension of the leg.

Articular Surfaces of the Knee Joint

Both the femur and the tibia have a pair of **articular surfaces** (Figs. 4-10, 4-11, and 4-21 through 4-23), the shapes of which are quite disparate. The **medial** and **lateral femoral condyles** are convex from anterior to posterior and joined by a vertically oriented anterior groove that accommodates the patella. The curves of both condyles are such that they are relatively flat distally but become increasingly curved as they are followed posteriorly. The articular surfaces of the tibia, the **medial** and **lateral tibial condyles,** are generally horizontally oriented and slightly concave. At no point in the range of motion are there large areas of contact between the two sets of condyles. The greatest amount of bony contact occurs when the knee is in full extension and the flattest portions of the femoral condyles are adjacent to the tibial condyles. As the leg flexes, the areas of contact become smaller and smaller. Generally, during flexion and extension at the knee, the tibial condyles slide around the femoral condyles. Only toward full extension is there a small amount of rocking motion, a point-to-point contact between the two articular surfaces.

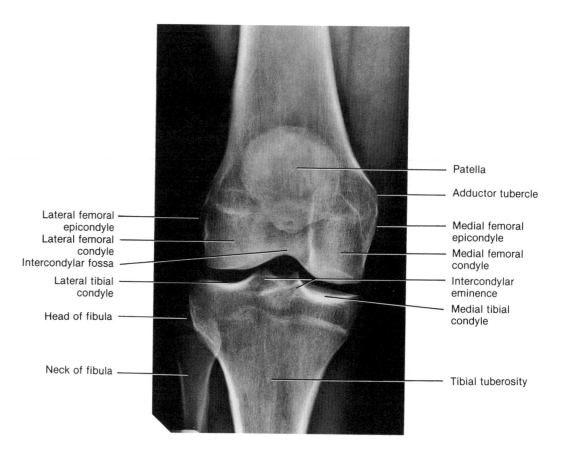

Patella

Adductor tubercle

Lateral femoral epicondyle

Medial femoral epicondyle

Lateral femoral condyle

Medial femoral condyle

Intercondylar fossa

Lateral tibial condyle

Intercondylar eminence

Head of fibula

Medial tibial condyle

Neck of fibula

Tibial tuberosity

Figure 4-21
Anteroposterior radiograph of the knee.

Menisci

The congruency between the femoral and tibial condyles is improved by the **medial** and **lateral menisci** or **semilunar cartilages** (Fig. 4-24). These intra-articular disks are typical in that they are composed of fibrocartilage, yet they are atypical in that they are not true disks but are **C**-shaped. The ends (horns) of each disk are directed toward the intercondylar area where they attach. (These are the only direct bony attachments of either meniscus.) Each disk is wedge-shaped in cross section; the apices of the wedges are directed toward the center of the articular surfaces. During motion at the knee the menisci are "deformed." Specifically, they are deformed posteriorly during flexion and anteriorly during extension. Although each disk is generally **C**-shaped, there are specific differences in their shapes and attachments that have functional significance. The lateral meniscus is more symmetrical than the medial in that the width of its anterior and posterior horns is about the same. The width of the posterior horn of the medial meniscus is typically greater than that of its anterior horn; as a result, the posterior horn is between the medial femoral and tibial condyles during a large percentage of knee flexion. Several anatomic features render the medial meniscus less movable than the lat-

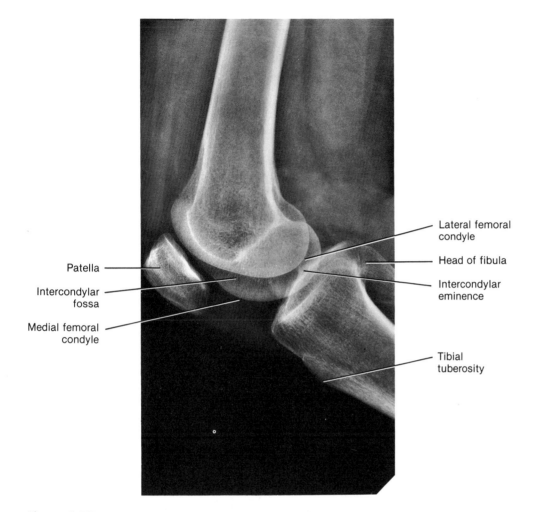

Patella

Intercondylar
fossa

Medial femoral
condyle

Lateral femoral
condyle

Head of fibula

Intercondylar
eminence

Tibial
tuberosity

Figure 4-22
Lateral radiograph of the knee.

eral (Fig. 4-24). First, the medial cartilage is **C**-shaped, whereas the lateral is more of a complete circle, so the horns of the medial meniscus and their central attachments are farther apart than those of the lateral meniscus. As a result the lateral meniscus is more deformable than the medial. Second, although both cartilages are attached to the fibrous portion of the joint capsule, the medial is firmly attached to the medial collateral ligament, whereas the lateral meniscus is totally separated from the lateral collateral ligament. Third, the lateral meniscus is attached to the popliteus muscle; therefore, contraction of that muscle moves the cartilage.

There are several theories regarding why the medial meniscus is more commonly injured than the lateral. Its wide posterior horn and relative immovability are implicated in a number of these theories. Such injuries commonly occur when the foot is planted on the ground and the knee is somewhat flexed. In that position the posterior horn is usually positioned between the medial femoral and tibial condyles; so when the causative

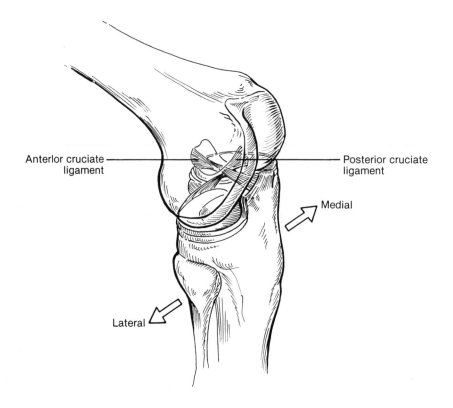

Figure 4-23
Anterolateral view of the knee illustrating the location and orientation of the cruciate ligaments.

force occurs, the cartilage is caught between the bones and vulnerable to injury.

Cruciate Ligaments

The **anterior** and **posterior cruciate ligaments** (Figs. 4-23, 4-24) provide anteroposterior stability to the knee. Their common name, "cruciate," describes their relationship to one another. Their positional names are

Figure 4-24
Superior view of the tibial plateau indicating the locations of the menisci and major ligaments of the knee. The area enclosed by the broken line corresponds to the area of the joint space.

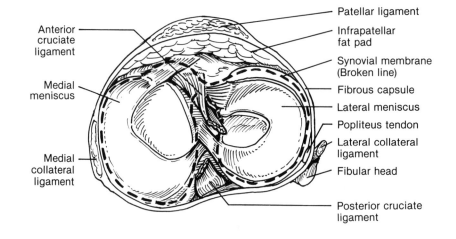

based on the locations of their tibial attachments. These ligaments are positioned in the intercondylar area, and like all intra-articular ligaments, are between the fibrous and synovial portions of the joint capsule.

The **anterior cruciate ligament** attaches to the anteromedial aspect of the intercondylar area of the tibia. From that point the ligament is directed posteriorly, superiorly, and laterally to an attachment on the medial aspect of the lateral femoral condyle. With the foot planted on the ground the anterior cruciate resists posterior movement of the femur on the tibia. (If the tibia is not bearing weight, this ligament resists anterior movement of the tibia on the femur.) The attachments, fiber orientation, and function of the **posterior cruciate** are the reverse of those of the anterior cruciate. Its tibial attachment is to the posterior intercondylar area of the tibia. From that point it passes superiorly, anteriorly, and medially, passing posterior to the anterior cruciate, to attach to the lateral aspect of the medial femoral condyle. With the foot fixed, the posterior cruciate resists anterior movement of the femur on the tibia.

The integrity of any ligament is best tested when it is most taut and thus providing maximal support. Although there is considerable discussion regarding the position in the range of motion where each cruciate is most taut, there is general agreement that both ligaments are quite tense throughout the range of motion and at no point is either ligament slack. There are manual tests for these ligaments with the knee in either flexion or extension. Both ligaments can be tested with the thigh fixed, the leg flexed, and the muscles of the thigh relaxed. The ligaments are tested by grasping the tibia and trying to slide it anteriorly and posteriorly; excessive anterior movement (an anterior drawer sign) may indicate a stretched or torn anterior cruciate, and a posterior drawer sign may indicate a posterior cruciate injury. The integrity of the anterior cruciate may be more critically evaluated by employing Lachman's test, which tests the ligament with the leg slightly flexed and thereby eliminates some of the criticisms of the drawer test.

Collateral Ligaments

The **tibial (medial)** and **fibular (lateral) collateral ligaments** (Figs. 4-24, 4-25) provide medial-lateral stability at the knee. The shapes and sizes of these ligaments are quite different, as is the amount of functional support they provide. The tibial collateral ligament is a broad, flat tendon that has rather extensive attachments to both the femur and tibia, attaching to most of the medial femoral epicondyle and to the tibia as far inferiorly as the tibial tuberosity. This ligament is a strong thickening of the fibrous portion of the joint capsule, and it attaches firmly to the medial meniscus. Since the force that causes most knee injuries comes from the lateral side, the tibial collateral ligament is much more commonly injured than the fibular collateral ligament. The fibular collateral ligament is a strong but relatively small ropelike structure that extends from the lateral femoral epicondyle to the head of the fibula. This ligament is positioned well lateral to the joint and attaches to neither the joint capsule nor the lateral meniscus. Both collateral ligaments are taut when the knee is extended

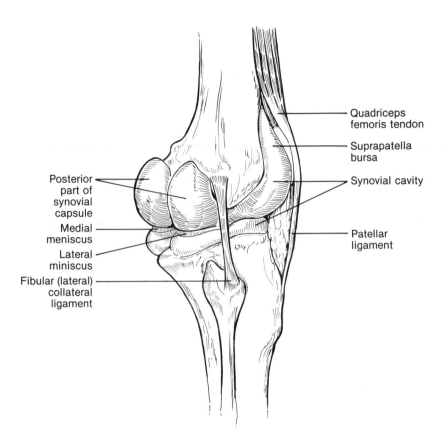

Figure 4-25
Posterolateral view of the knee joint indicating the extent and subdivisions of the synovial cavity.

and relaxed during flexion. As a result, rotation of the tibia is possible when it is flexed but not when it is extended.

Articular Capsule

The **joint capsule** of the knee joint is large and complicated; also, the synovial and fibrous portions are not coextensive. In very general terms the fibrous part of the capsule surrounds the entire knee and attaches to the femur and tibia at the edges of the articular surfaces. The synovial layer generally lines the fibrous capsule, but it reflects away from that part of the capsule centrally so the intercondylar area is not part of the synovial cavity.

The **fibrous portion of the joint capsule** (Fig. 4-24) is far from simple. Anteriorly, it is formed by the tendon of the quadriceps femoris muscle, the patella, and the patellar ligament, and on either side of these structures by the medial and lateral patellar retinacula. These retinacula, in turn, are partially formed by fibrous extensions from the vastus medialis and lateralis muscles. The remainder of the fibrous capsule—medially, laterally, and posteriorly—consists of fibrous tissue that stretches between the edges of the articular surfaces of the two bones. The medial aspect of the capsule is reinforced by the tibial collateral ligament.

The **synovial cavity** (Figs. 4-24, 4-25) of the knee is generally horseshoe-shaped in cross section, with medial and lateral areas between the tibial and femoral condyles connected only anteriorly behind the patellar mechanism. Anteriorly, the **synovial membrane** attaches to the edges of the articular surface of the patella and lines the deep surfaces of the quadriceps tendon, both patellar retinacula, and the patellar ligament. The synovium corresponds to the fibrous capsule on either side of the joint. Toward the central part of the joint posteriorly, the synovium separates from the fibrous capsule and follows the deep edges of the articular surfaces anteriorly. These two layers of synovium are continuous across the anterior aspect of the intercondylar area. The result is a central area that is within the fibrous capsule but is not part of the synovial cavity. This area, the intercondylar area, contains the cruciate ligaments and the central attachments of the menisci.

The synovial cavity is further subdivided anteriorly. That part of the cavity above the patella, between the quadriceps tendon and the distal anterior femur, is the **suprapatellar bursa.** In this area the posterior aspect of the synovial membrane is partially separated from the femur by the **articularis genu muscle** and a fat pad. The small articularis genu extends from the distal anterior femur to the synovial membrane and functions to elevate the membrane during extension at the knee, thus keeping the membrane from getting caught between the bones. Inferiorly, a rather large **infrapatellar fat pad** attaches to the posterior aspect of the patellar ligament just below the patella. That portion of the synovial cavity between the patellar ligament and the fat pad is the **deep infrapatellar bursa.** It is important to note that the suprapatellar and deep infrapatellar bursae are part of the joint cavity and not separate closed spaces.

In addition, there are several true bursae around the knee. Inflammation of these bursae can produce characteristic swellings that usually are not connected to the knee joint per se. However, certain of the bursae occasionally or frequently communicate with the synovial cavity of the knee. Both the **prepatellar** and **infrapatellar bursae** are subcutaneous bursae associated with the anterior aspect of the knee. Although the two may be continuous, the prepatellar bursa is usually anterior to the lower part of the patella and the patellar ligament while the infrapatellar bursa is between the skin and tibial tuberosity. Either of these bursae can become inflamed, the former giving rise to "housemaid's knee" and the latter to "clergyman's knee." Neither typically communicates with the knee joint. Posteriorly, there are bursae deep to the medial and lateral heads of the gastrocnemius muscle. The bursa between the medial head of the gastrocnemius and the medial femoral epicondyle may communicate with the joint cavity; inflammation of this bursa may produce a swelling in the popliteal fossa, which is called a popliteal or Baker's cyst.

Because of the large and expansive joint cavity, effusion of the knee joint can be detected at various points, especially anteriorly. Marked effusion is readily detected by palpation or visualization on either side of the quadriceps tendon, patella, or patellar ligament. More subtle effusion can be detected by depressing the patella with the leg extended; depression pushes the fluid into the suprapatellar bursa, and a bulge appears

around the superior aspect of the patella and the quadriceps tendon. Marked effusion can also be detected by the postion of the joint. The volume of the joint space is greatest when the knee is positioned in 15 to 20 degrees of flexion. A patient with marked effusion will hold the knee in that position because there is the least amount of pressure on the capsule, and therefore it is the most comfortable position.

The capsule of the knee joint is innervated by branches of the saphenous, obturator, tibial, and common peroneal nerves. Importantly, knee pain can be referred to the hip joint, and vice versa, although the referral of pain from hip to knee seems more common.

Motion at the Knee Joint

The motions that occur at the knee joint are flexion and extension as well as medial and lateral rotation. Since the femoral condyles are much longer (anteroposteriorly) than those of the tibia, the majority of the motion that occurs between the two sets of articular surfaces is the sliding of the tibial condyles across the femoral condyles. In full flexion the more curved portions of the femoral condyles are in contact with the tibial condyles and the menisci, and the point of contact is on the posterior aspects of the tibial condyles. As extension occurs, the points of contact on the tibial condyles move very slightly anteriorly; the points of contact on the femoral condyles, however, move anteriorly rapidly as the tibial condyles slide across the femoral condyles. The anteroposterior length of the lateral femoral condyle is somewhat shorter than that of the medial femoral condyle. As a result, the motion producing extension between the lateral femoral and tibial condyles ceases before the motion on the medial side of the joint. When this occurs, the point of contact between the lateral condyles becomes a pivot as the extension motion continues between the medial condyles. This results in a small amount of lateral tibial rotation during the final few degrees of extension. (If the foot is fixed, of course, the femur rotates medially.) This rotation can be called "locking of the knee joint" and should not be confused with the pathological locking that may accompany a torn meniscus.

It is also important to note that during the final degrees of extension there is a small amount of "rocking motion" (point-to-point contact) between the articular surfaces and also that the flatter portions of the femoral condyles are in contact with the tibia. Both of these factors add to the stability of the joint. Flexion between these two bones is essentially the reverse of the process described above. However, the knee must be actively "unlocked" before flexion can occur; that is, the femur must be rotated laterally (if the foot is fixed). This rotation is provided by the action of the popliteus muscle.

As the leg is flexed or extended, both menisci are deformed: posteriorly during flexion, and anteriorly during extension. The amount of movement of either meniscus is small, but the lateral meniscus is probably deformed somewhat more than the medial.

Because of the patella's attachment to the tibia via the patellar ligament, its position is essentially fixed and its relationship to the tibia does

not change. Its relationship to the femur, however, changes continuously during flexion and extension at the knee. During flexion the patella slides distally in the patellar groove of the femur; and during extension it glides proximally. Due to the valgus angle formed by the femur and tibia, there is a natural tendency for the patella to move laterally as it slides proximally during extension. This tendency is counteracted by the high lateral lip of the patellar groove and the oblique pull of the vastus medialis muscle through the medial patellar retinaculum.

Motors of the Knee

The anterior and posterior muscles of the thigh are the principal muscles of the knee. The quadriceps femoris extends the leg and prevents flexion at the knee during the weight-bearing phase of gait. With the foot fixed on the ground, the gluteus maximus can produce and maintain extension at the knee, especially through its attachment to the iliotibial tract. The hamstring muscles are the major flexors at the knee, although both the sartorius and the gracilis muscles in the thigh and the gastrocnemius in the leg can assist. External rotation of the leg is produced only by the biceps femoris, but internal rotation is a function of the semimembranosus, semitendinosus, gracilis, sartorius, and popliteus muscles.

Thigh

The muscles of the thigh are arranged in three groups (Fig. 4-1A): the anterior femoral muscles, the medial femoral or adductor group, and the posterior femoral or hamstring group. A single arterial trunk, the femoral artery, passes through the entire thigh and supplies its large muscle mass. The femoral artery is the continuation of the external iliac artery of the abdomen; it becomes the popliteal artery as it passes from the anterior to the posterior compartment in the distal thigh. Anteriorly, just distal to the inguinal ligament, the femoral triangle contains the major neurovascular structures of the thigh.

Anterior Compartment of the Thigh

Muscles of the anterior compartment.   The major muscle of the anterior thigh is the **quadriceps femoris** (Fig. 4-26), which in reality consists of four separate muscles that share a common insertion. This mass of muscle is positioned more anterolaterally than anteriorly (Fig. 4-1A), and the component muscles are the **rectus femoris, vastus intermedius, vastus lateralis,** and **vastus medialis.** The **rectus femoris muscle** (Figs. 4-7B, 4-19B, 4-26) is the only member of the quadriceps that crosses the hip joint and thus arises from the os coxae. This muscle has two heads of origin, one from the anterior inferior iliac spine and the other from the ilium just superior to the acetabulum. The two heads join and form a long muscle that parallels the shaft of the femur. The muscle inserts into the patella via the quadriceps tendon, which in turn is connected to the tibial

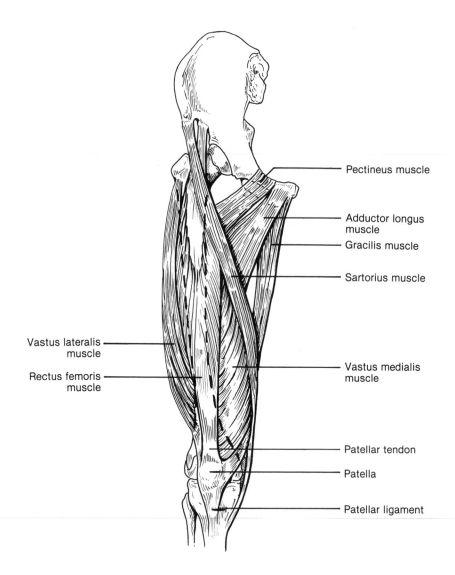

Pectineus muscle

Adductor longus muscle

Gracilis muscle

Sartorius muscle

Vastus lateralis muscle

Rectus femoris muscle

Vastus medialis muscle

Patellar tendon

Patella

Patellar ligament

Figure 4-26
Anterior view of the more superficial muscles in the anterior and
medial aspects of the thigh.

tuberosity by the patellar ligament. As with all components of the quadriceps, the true insertion is the tibial tuberosity.

The **vastus lateralis muscle** (Figs. 4-10B, 4-11B, 4-19B, 4-26) forms
most of the bulk of the anterolateral aspect of the thigh. It has a long,
thin origin from the femur that starts superiorly below the anterior aspect
of the greater trochanter and then wraps obliquely around the bone to
the linea aspera, where it attaches to its lateral aspect. In addition, it
arises from the lateral intermuscular septum. The muscle fibers pass
obliquely anteriorly and medially, the inferior being more oblique, and
insert into the quadriceps tendon (and the tendon of the rectus femoris)
and the patella. The most inferior fibers are continuous with portions of
the lateral patellar retinaculum.

The **vastus medialis muscle** (Figs. 4-10B, 4-11B, 4-19B, 4-26) is similar to the vastus lateralis but is on the medial aspect of the thigh, and it extends farther distally. Its origin begins superiorly just inferior to the intertrochanteric line, then curves medially around the femur, and continues inferiorly along the entire medial aspect of the linea aspera and onto the medial aspect of the supracondylar region. It also arises from the medial intermuscular septum. From this wide origin, its fibers pass obliquely laterally and inferiorly toward the quadriceps tendon and the patella. Importantly, the inferior fibers of the vastus medialis are more obliquely oriented than those of the vastus lateralis and extend more distally; these inferior fibers attach quite far distally on the patella and play an important role in stabilizing the patella against lateral dislocation. The most inferior fibers also are continuous with the medial patellar retinaculum.

The **vastus intermedius muscle** (Figs. 4-10B, 4-11B, 4-19B, 4-27) is the deepest of the quadriceps and is completely covered anteriorly, me-

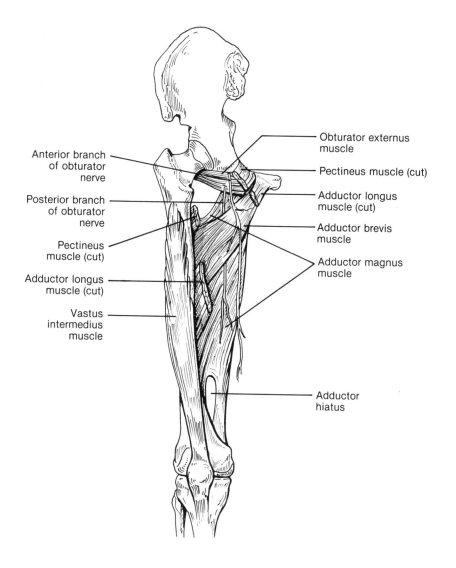

Anterior branch
of obturator
nerve

Posterior branch
of obturator
nerve

Pectineus
muscle (cut)

Adductor longus
muscle (cut)

Vastus
intermedius
muscle

Obturator externus
muscle

Pectineus muscle (cut)

Adductor longus
muscle (cut)

Adductor brevis
muscle

Adductor magnus
muscle

Adductor
hiatus

Figure 4-27
Anterior view of the deeper muscles in the anterior and medial aspects of the thigh.

dially, and laterally by the other muscles. It arises from the upper two-thirds of the anterior and lateral aspects of the shaft of the femur. Its fibers descend and insert into the deep surface of the quadriceps tendon and superior aspect of the patella.

The quadriceps femoris is the only extensor of the leg. The rectus femoris is also a flexor at the hip, but its role is limited to assisting the iliopsoas muscle. Loss of the quadriceps results in a complete loss of active extension at the knee. During gait a quadriceps deficit is apparent toward the end of the swing phase and through most of the stance phase. Since the limb cannot be prepared for heel strike with the knee slightly flexed, it must be fully extended and locked in that position prior to contact with the floor. This is accomplished by using momentum to swing the leg through and into full extension; the thigh is flexed during the early part of the swing phase and then abruptly stopped, and the momentum carries the leg forward into extension. As the leg moves into extension, the hip extensors contract to pull the thigh posteriorly and bring the heel into contact with the ground. The knee is held in extension by the contraction of the hip extensors, and flexion of the hip and vertebral column ensure the ground reaction is postioned well anterior to the knee joint. The knee is thus held in extension from heel strike through midstance. In addition, a patient may hold a hand on the anterior aspect of the thigh to ensure that the knee does not buckle. This gait is commonly called a vaulting type of gait because the weight-bearing limb is not shortened and the patient "vaults" over a rigidly extended limb. All four components of the quadriceps are innervated by the femoral nerve.

The **sartorius muscle** (Figs. 4-7B, 4-19B, 4-26), the longest muscle in the body, is positioned so it passes obliquely across the thigh. From its origin on the anterior superior iliac spine its fibers pass medially and inferiorly, cross the medial aspect of the knee, and insert on the anteromedial aspect of the tibial shaft just inferior to the tibial tuberosity. It shares that area of insertion with the gracilis and semitendinosus muscles; the common insertion for all three is the **pes anserinus.** Contraction of the sartorius results in flexion, abduction, and external rotation at the hip, and flexion and internal rotation at the knee. This combination of motions results in the limb being crossed over the other in the sitting position (the tailor's position) and hence the name the "tailor's muscle." All functions of this muscle are very much secondary to those of other muscles, so its loss results in virtually no active deficit, and its loss cannot be detected during gait. The sartorius is supplied by the femoral nerve.

Neurovascular structures of the anterior compartment. The **femoral triangle** (Fig. 4-28) is located in the proximal part of the anterior thigh. It contains several large neurovascular structures that are close to the surface and thus convenient for use in certain medical procedures. The triangle is defined superiorly by the inguinal ligament, laterally by the sartorius muscle, and medially by the medial border of the adductor longus muscle. The floor of the triangle is muscular and formed primarily by the pectineus and adductor longus muscles along with small portion of the iliopsoas laterally. The major neurovascular structures are positioned side by side as they pass deep to the inguinal ligament and include, from

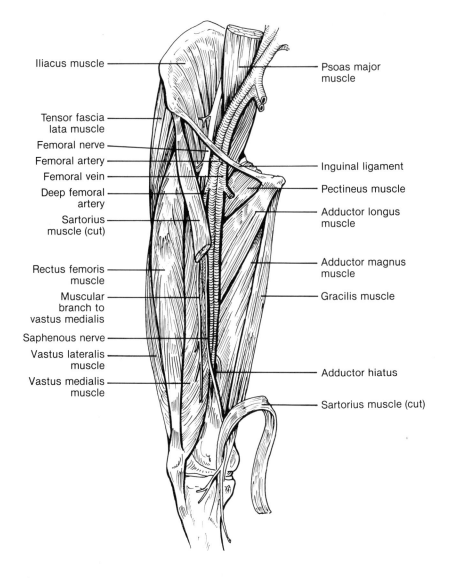

Iliacus muscle

Tensor fascia lata muscle

Femoral nerve

Femoral artery

Femoral vein

Deep femoral artery

Sartorius muscle (cut)

Rectus femoris muscle

Muscular branch to vastus medialis

Saphenous nerve

Vastus lateralis muscle

Vastus medialis muscle

Psoas major muscle

Inguinal ligament

Pectineus muscle

Adductor longus muscle

Adductor magnus muscle

Gracilis muscle

Adductor hiatus

Sartorius muscle (cut)

Figure 4-28
Anteromedial view of the thigh. The sartorius muscle is cut and reflected distally, exposing the contents of the adductor canal.

lateral to medial, the **femoral nerve,** the **femoral artery,** and the **femoral vein.** The femoral artery is easy to locate because its pulse can be palpated midway between the anterior superior iliac spine and the pubic tubercle.

The vein and artery are enclosed in a sleeve of fascia, the **femoral sheath,** that is derived from fascia in the abdomen. This sheath extends medial to the vein and presents an empty area, the **femoral canal,** which is the opening through which a **femoral hernia** can occur. The great saphenous vein joins the femoral vein in the triangle. A large number of lymph nodes, the **superficial** and **deep inguinal nodes,** are located, respectively, superficial and deep to the fascia lata in the region of the femoral triangle.

The inferior extension of the femoral canal is the **adductor** or **subsartorial canal** (Fig. 4-28). This canal is located deep to the sartorius muscle and transmits the femoral vessels, the nerve to the vastus medialis, and the saphenous nerve. This canal spirals medially and distally, deep to the sartorius muscle, and ends at a gap (the **adductor hiatus**) in the insertion of the adductor magnus muscle. This hiatus is found medial to the distal aspect of the femur, just proximal to the adductor tubercle of the femur, and serves as a communication between the adductor canal and the popliteal fossa (which is posterior to the knee). Both the femoral artery and vein pass through the adductor canal and into the popliteal fossa where they become the popliteal vessels.

The **femoral artery** (Figs. 4-28, 4-29) provides the blood supply to most of the lower limb. It is the direct continuation of the external iliac artery, entering the thigh by passing deep to the inguinal ligament and into the femoral triangle. It descends through the thigh by passing through first the femoral triangle and then the adductor canal; it becomes the popliteal artery where it enters the popliteal fossa after passing through the adductor hiatus. Most of the branches of the femoral artery occur in the femoral triangle. The most proximal branches arise just distal to the inguinal ligament. These small branches, the **superficial epigastric, superficial iliac circumflex,** and **external pudendal arteries,** enter the superficial fascia and supply superficial structures in the lower abdominal wall and proximal thigh. The **deep femoral artery** is the largest branch of the femoral and usually arises in the upper part of the femoral triangle. This branch arises from the posterolateral aspect of the femoral artery and then passes medially and deeply to descend just medial to the femur on the ventral aspect of the adductor muscles. The two most proximal branches of the deep femoral, the **medial** and **lateral femoral circumflex arteries,** pass medially and laterally around the femur and supply the large muscles of the thigh. The larger lateral femoral circumflex has ascending, transverse, and descending branches that are important in potential collateral arterial pathways around the proximal part of the femoral and external iliac arteries. Either or both of the circumflex arteries may arise from the femoral artery. The deep femoral artery has three or four **perforating branches,** each of which passes posteriorly to supply the medial and posterior structures of the thigh; the deep femoral ends as the lowest perforating artery. One of the arteries of the knee, the **descending genicular artery,** typically branches from the femoral just proximal to the adductor hiatus.

The **femoral nerve** (Figs. 4-9, 4-28) is formed within the psoas major muscle from fibers from spinal cord segments L2–L4; it emerges from the lateral aspect of that muscle in the iliac fossa of the abdomen, just proximal to the inguinal ligament. In its short abdominal course, the nerve is vulnerable to compression by abscess or hematoma within the psoas muscle. Also, it can be forced against the inguinal ligament in certain positions (for example, the lithotomy position if prolonged), and it can be injured during various surgical procedures (such as appendectomy or repair of an inguinal hernia). The nerve enters the thigh by passing deep to the inguinal ligament, where it is the most lateral structure in the femoral triangle. Very soon after entering the thigh (3–4 centimeters) the nerve branches into its terminal branches, which are muscular branches to the muscles in the anterior compartment of the thigh and cutaneous

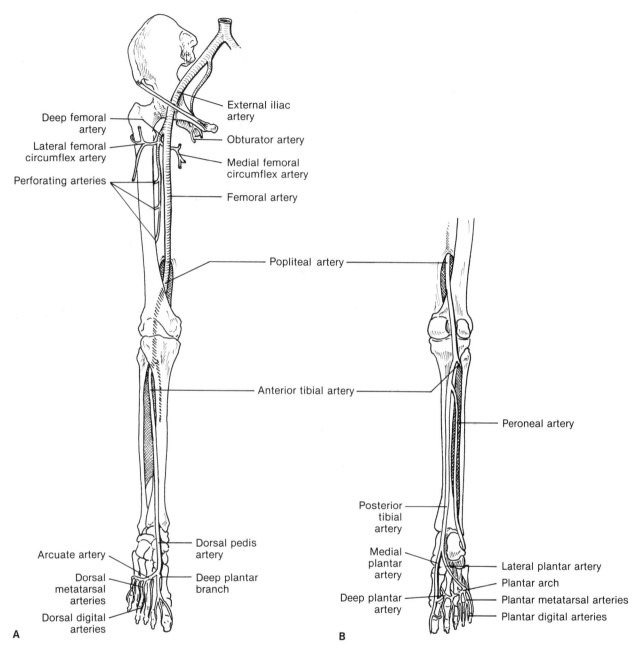

Figure 4-29
Anterior (A) and posterior (B) views of the major arteries of the lower limb.

branches to the anterior and medial aspect of the distal half of the thigh. One cutaneous branch, the **saphenous nerve,** descends through the adductor canal, and just proximal to the medial aspect of the knee, it enters the subcutaneous tissue by piercing the fascia lata. The nerve then descends through the medial aspect of the leg and foot along with the greater saphenous vein and supplies the skin of the medial aspects of the knee, leg, and foot. The main trunk of the femoral nerve can be injured by stretching during a prolonged period in the supine position with the hip and trunk fully extended. The nerve's position next to the femoral artery makes it vulnerable during procedures utilizing the artery. The saphenous nerve and its infrapatellar branch are vulnerable to entrapment as they pass respectively through the fascia lata and the sartorius muscle or tendon. The saphenous nerve is also vulnerable to surgical incisions on the medial aspect of the knee and during venous cutdown of the greater saphenous vein on the anteromedial aspect of the ankle.

Medial Thigh

Muscles of the medial thigh.   The structures that form the medial thigh are not within their own compartment but rather share the posterior compartment with the posterior femoral structures (Fig. 4-1A). The **medial femoral** or **adductor muscles** are positioned anteromedially in the thigh and are arranged in two layers with one muscle between the layers and one muscle oriented vertically and located medial to the rest. The anterior layer is composed of the **pectineus** and **adductor longus muscles;** the posterior layer, of the **adductor magnus** and **obturator externus;** the **adductor brevis** is between these two layers. The **gracilis muscle** is vertically oriented and the most medial of the group. Generally, this group of muscles interconnects the anteroinferior aspect of the os coxae—that is, the pubis and anterior aspect of the ischial ramus—with the femur. And, with the usual exception of the pectineus, the group is innervated by branches of the obturator nerve.

The **pectineus** (Figs. 4-7B, 4-11B, 4-26) is somewhat intermediate between the anterior and medial femoral muscles because of its position, variable innervation, and function. From an origin on the pecten of the pubis and adjacent part of the superior pubic ramus, the fibers of this muscle pass obliquely inferiorly and laterally to a vertical insertion on the pectineal line of the posteromedial aspect of the femur. This muscle is more of a flexor than adductor of the thigh, and it is more commonly innervated by the femoral than the obturator nerve.

The **adductor longus muscle** (Figs. 4-7B, 4-11B, 4-26) is the more medial and inferior of the muscles in the anterior layer. Its origin from the body of the pubis, just inferior to the pubic tubercle, is the most medial of the adductor muscles. From this rather restricted origin its fibers diverge as they pass inferolaterally toward a thin vertical insertion on approximately the middle third of the medial aspect of the linea aspera.

The **adductor magnus muscle** (Figs. 4-7B, 4-11B, 4-27) is the largest of the adductor muscles and forms virtually all of the posterior layer of these muscles. It is a two-part muscle in that it is dually innervated and it has two different functions. Although the separation of the two parts is not distinct, the anterior and posterior portions are functionally different. This muscle has an extensive origin from the inferior aspect of the os coxae that includes most of the lateral aspect of the inferior pubic ramus and all of the ischial ramus as far posteriorly as the ischial tuberosity. From this large origin its fibers diverge as they pass inferiorly and laterally to an even more extensive insertion on the posteromedial aspect of the femur. Its more anteriorly arising fibers insert into the upper portion of the medial aspect of the linea aspera; and the posterior fibers insert into the more distal aspect of the linea aspera and the medial supracondylar line as far distally as the adductor tubercle. There is a gap in this insertion, the **adductor hiatus,** just proximal to the adductor tubercle. The fibers arising more anteriorly constitute the more proximal portion of the muscle; this part functions as an adductor at the hip and is supplied by the obturator nerve. Fibers arising posteriorly (those from the ischium) are the posterior part of the muscle and function partially as a hamstring muscle. This part of the muscle produces extension at the hip and is innervated by the tibial portion of the nerve.

The **obturator externus muscle** (Figs. 4-11B, 4-27) is the deepest of the adductors and functionally belongs with the short external rotators of the thigh. It arises from the anterior, inferior, and posterior aspect of the obturator foramen and the obturator membrane (the fibrous membrane that partially closes the obturator foramen). Its fibers pass laterally and ascend somewhat as they pass posterior to the lower aspect of the hip joint and insert into the trochanteric fossa. This muscle is an external rotator of the thigh but a rather weak adductor.

The **adductor brevis muscle** (Figs. 4-7B, 4-11B, 4-27) is located between the two layers of adductors. Its fibers are more obliquely oriented than those of the muscles on either its superficial or deep aspects. It arises from the body and inferior ramus of the pubis and inserts on approximately the upper third of the linea aspera.

The **gracilis muscle** (Figs. 4-7B, 4-19B, 4-26) is the longest and most medial of the adductors. It arises from the body and inferior ramus of the pubis and inserts on the anteromedial aspect of the shaft of the proximal part of the tibia (pes anserinus). It has multiple functions at both the knee and hip, none of which is particularly strong. It can adduct and flex the thigh, and flex and medially rotate the leg.

In addition to their common action of adduction of the thigh, the adductor muscles also are capable of various combinations of flexion, extension, and rotation. During gait, the adductors are active at heel strike and during the initial stages of the swing phase. At heel strike the posterior portion of the adductor magnus is active, presumably assisting the hamstrings in preventing flexion at the hip. The more anteriorly arising muscles, such as the adductor longus, are active during the initial part of the swing phase, presumably functioning as flexors to propel the thigh forward. Loss of this muscle group logically results in a virtual loss of thigh adduction and a reduction in the strength of thigh flexion and medial rotation. The loss of these muscles can affect gait by causing circumduction of the lower limb during the swing phase. This change in gait, theoretically at least, supports the notion that the adductor muscles play a role in flexion of the thigh during ambulation.

Neurovascular structures of the medial thigh. The **obturator nerve** (Figs. 4-9, 4-27) arises from the lumbar plexus and is formed within the psoas major muscle by fibers from spinal cord segments L2–L4. This nerve emerges from the medial aspect of the psoas in the abdomen, crosses the pelvic brim to enter the pelvis, and descends along the lateral wall of the pelvis toward the obturator canal. The nerve passes through this foramen and into the medial thigh, where it splits into anterior and posterior divisions around the adductor brevis muscle. These divisions branch into muscular branches that supply the adductor muscles (with the usual exception of the pectineus and the constant exception of the posterior part of the adductor magnus), and cutaneous branches to the medial thigh and, on occasion, the medial proximal leg. The obturator nerve also has articular branches to the hip and knee joints, the former arising in the pelvis and the latter from the posterior division. The innervation of both joints is thought to be the means by which pain is referred from one joint to the other.

The obturator nerve has a rigidly fixed course through the abdomen and pelvis and therefore is vulnerable to entrapment-like syndromes more in those areas than in the thigh. It is vulnerable to psoas or other types of retroperitoneal abscess; it can be compressed against the pelvic brim during pregnancy; and it can be affected by space-occupying lesions in the pelvis or by pelvic abscesses. It can be compressed against the edge of the obturator canal by an obturator hernia or during extreme positioning of the hip for an extended period (lithotomy position).

Posterior Thigh

Muscles of the posterior thigh.   The **posterior femoral muscles** and related neurovascular structures occupy the lateral portion of the posterior compartment (Fig. 4-1A). Their location, however, is truly posterior in the thigh. The posterior femoral muscles, or **hamstrings** (Fig. 4-30), consist of the **semitendinosus, semimembranosus,** and **biceps femoris.** Most of these muscles cross both the hip and knee joints and do not attach to the femur. Generally these muscles arise from the most inferior aspect of the os coxae and cross either the posteromedial or posterolateral aspect of the knee.

The **semitendinosus muscle** (Figs. 4-7B, 4-19, 4-30) is the more superficial of the two medial hamstrings. From an origin on the ischial tuberosity, the fibers descend vertically and join the long tendon at about the midthigh level. The muscle and its tendon incline medially in the distal third of the thigh, pass posterior to the medial femoral condyle and cross the posteromedial aspect of the knee joint. The tendon curves anteriorly and inserts on the anteromedial aspect of the shaft of the proximal tibia (pes anserinus).

The **semimembranosus muscle** (Figs. 4-7B, 4-20, 4-30) is larger and deeper than the semitendinosus, and in the distal thigh it is considerably wider. It arises from the ischial tuberosity and inserts into the posteromedial aspect of the medial tibial condyle. In the distal thigh it is positioned between the medial femoral condyle and the tendon of the semitendinosus muscle.

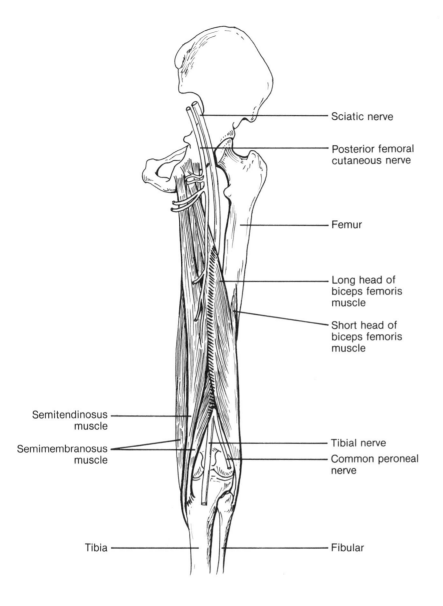

Sciatic nerve

Posterior femoral cutaneous nerve

Femur

Long head of biceps femoris muscle

Short head of biceps femoris muscle

Semitendinosus muscle

Semimembranosus muscle

Tibial nerve

Common peroneal nerve

Tibia

Fibular

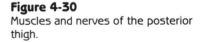

Figure 4-30
Muscles and nerves of the posterior thigh.

The **biceps femoris muscle** (Figs. 4-7B, 4-11B, 4-20, 4-30) is the only lateral hamstring and it has two heads of origin. Its long head arises from the ischial tuberosity, and its short head arises from approximately the lower half of the linea aspera and the lateral supracondylar line. The two heads join in the distal portion of the posterolateral thigh, just proximal to the formation of the muscle's strong tendon. This tendon crosses the posterolateral aspect of the knee joint and inserts on the head of the fibula.

Since all three hamstring muscles cross the posterior aspects of both the hip and knee joints, their actions include extension at the hip and flexion at the knee. However, their action is usually concentrated on one joint, that joint being the more movable of the two. The action of the short head of the biceps femoris, of course, is limited to flexion at the knee. In addition, both the semitendinosus and semimembranosus muscles medially rotate the flexed leg, and the biceps femoris rotates the flexed leg laterally.

Loss of the hamstring muscles results in a profound loss of flexion at the knee but only a weakening of extension at the hip. The hamstrings have a strong ally at the hip in the gluteus maximus; the other flexor of the leg, the gastrocnemius, is a strong muscle, but it also is a two-joint muscle and its action is limited primarily to the ankle. During gait the hamstrings are active during most of the swing phase and at heel strike. During the swing phase they produce flexion at the knee and thus shorten the limb. At heel strike they contract, along with the quadriceps, to provide a flexible yet rigid limb for landing. At heel strike the hamstrings and the gluteus maximus also prevent flexion of the pelvis on the thigh.

In quiet standing there is virtually no activity in the hamstrings because extension at the knee is limited by the posterior aspect of the joint capsule. However, surgical release of the hamstring muscles (including the short head of the biceps) in a child with spastic cerebral palsy frequently results in genu recurvatum. Whether this is sufficient reason to believe the hamstrings have a postural role in reinforcing the knee posteriorly is unclear.

Neurovascular structures of the posterior thigh. As the **sciatic nerve** (Figs. 4-17, 4-30) leaves the gluteal region, it emerges from beneath the gluteus maximus muscle where it is lateral to the ischial tuberosity and in a relatively superficial position. It then passes deep to the long head of the biceps femoris muscle and descends in a deep position that is posterior to the femur and generally between the medial and lateral hamstring muscles. In the distal thigh the sciatic nerve typically divides into its tibial and common peroneal portions as it enters the popliteal fossa. In the thigh, the tibial portion of the sciatic nerve has branches to all of the hamstring muscles except the short head of the biceps, which receives a branch from the common peroneal portion of the sciatic nerve. The sciatic nerve is somewhat vulnerable to injury just distal to the gluteus maximus muscle, where it is susceptible to laceration because of its relatively superficial position, and where it can be compressed if a person sits on a hard surface with a sharp edge. Throughout the majority of the thigh the nerve is deep and well protected, but it also can be injured by the ragged edge of a fractured femur.

There is no major arterial channel in the proximal portion of the posterior thigh. The majority of the blood supply is provided by the perforating branches of the deep femoral artery.

Popliteal Fossa

The **popliteal fossa** (Fig. 4-31) is the indented area posterior to the knee that is similar in several respects to the cubital fossa anterior to the elbow. This diamond-shaped depression is bounded superolaterally by the biceps femoris muscle and tendon, superomedially by the semitendinosus and

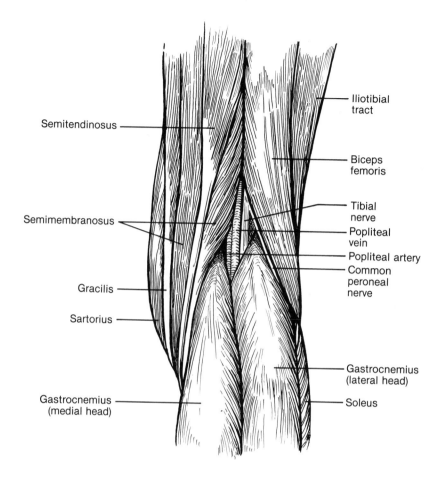

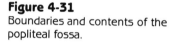

Semitendinosus

Semimembranosus

Gracilis

Sartorius

Gastrocnemius
(medial head)

Iliotibial
tract

Biceps
femoris

Tibial
nerve

Popliteal
vein

Popliteal artery

Common
peroneal
nerve

Gastrocnemius
(lateral head)

Soleus

Figure 4-31
Boundaries and contents of the
popliteal fossa.

semimembranosus, and inferomedially and inferolaterally by the two
heads of the gastrocnemius muscle. The fossa is deep, and its floor is
formed by the supracondylar portion of the femur, the posterior aspect of
the joint capsule of the knee, and the popliteus muscle. The fossa is covered by the investing fasciae of the thigh (fascia lata) and leg (sural);
when the leg is extended this fascial roof is quite taut, and thus structures
within the fossa are difficult to palpate.

The popliteal artery is the deepest structure in the fossa. It is the
continuation of the femoral artery, entering the fossa through the adductor hiatus and descending on the supracondylar surface of the femur. This
artery has multiple **genicular branches** that supply the knee and surrounding structures. The popliteal artery descends into the posterior compartment of the leg by passing between the two heads of the gastrocnemius muscle. The popliteal artery is vulnerable when the supracondylar
portion of the femur is fractured, because the gastrocnemius muscle typically pulls the distal fragment posteriorly. The **popliteal vein** is superficial
to the artery and accompanies it through the fossa. While in the fossa,
this vein is usually joined by the lesser saphenous vein.

The sciatic nerve typically splits into its component nerves, the **tibial** and **common peroneal nerves,** in the uppermost part of the fossa. The tibial nerve passes vertically through the fossa and enters the leg by passing deep to the gastrocnemius. This nerve is the most superficial structure passing through the central portion of the fossa and is thus vulnerable to laceration. In addition, it and the popliteal vessels are ensheathed by a connective tissue sleeve; therefore, the nerve can be compressed by an aneurysm within the sleeve. The common peroneal nerve follows the superolateral border of the fossa, descending along the medial border of the biceps femoris muscle and superficial to the posterior aspect of the lateral femoral condyle. It then crosses the lateral head of the gastrocnemius muscle as it passes toward the neck of the fibula. This nerve is particularly vulnerable to compression as it crosses the femoral condyle, where it can be compressed during prolonged periods of bed rest. Cutaneous branches of the tibial and common peroneal nerves, the **medial** and **lateral sural cutaneous nerves,** arise in the fossa and descend along the posterolateral leg. These two branches typically join to form the sural nerve, which supplies the posterolateral leg and the lateral aspect of the foot.

Surface Anatomy of the Thigh and Knee

Most of the contours of the thigh are formed by the underlying muscles. The anterior femoral muscles are positioned anterolaterally; the posterolateral vertical indentation marks the position of the **iliotibial tract** and the lateral extent of the anterior muscles. The medial extent of the anterior muscles generally corresponds to the position of the **sartorius;** this muscle may be visible and palpable if the motions of medial rotation and flexion of the leg, and flexion of the thigh, are resisted. Three components of the quadriceps femoris are usually visible and palpable. The **rectus femoris** presents a vertical bulge that parallels the femur and extends from the hip to the **quadriceps tendon** superior to the **patella.** The **vastus medialis** is usually more prominent than the **vastus lateralis;** both appear on their respective sides of the inferior half of the rectus femoris, quadriceps tendon, and patella. The vastus medialis extends somewhat more distally than the vastus lateralis. Although the muscle masses formed by both the adductors and hamstrings are easily defined in the thigh, the resolution of individual muscles other than the distal aspect of the hamstrings is difficult.

Many bony prominences and soft structures are palpable in the region of the knee. Anteriorly, the **quadriceps tendon, patella,** and **patellar ligament** are readily palpable, as is the **tibial tuberosity** at the inferior extent of the patellar ligament. On either side of the patellar ligament, with the leg flexed or extended but the muscles relaxed, the indentation between the edges of the **femoral** and **tibial condyles** marks the position of the **joint space.** As this space is palpated, so are the peripheral surfaces of the **medial** and **lateral menisci.** With the leg flexed, the anterior edges of the femoral condyles can be followed superiorly, where they form the edges of the patellar groove. As the medial joint space is followed medially, it is lost anteromedially, especially if the leg is extended, because the **medial collateral ligament** crosses the space in that area. Posteromedially, the muscular **semimembranosus** and the tendon of the **semitendinosus muscle** are readily palpable, as is the tendon of the **biceps femoris muscle** posterolaterally. The superior borders of the popliteal fossa are thus easily defined. The **popliteal pulse** can be felt in the depths of the fossa; however, the hamstring muscles must be relaxed to permit depression of the fascial roof. Laterally and slightly superior to the knee, a deep depression separates the biceps femoris tendon (posteriorly) from the **iliotibial tract** (anteriorly). Laterally, at the level of the joint space, the **fibular collateral ligament** can be felt as it stretches from the **head of the fibula** to the **lateral femoral epicondyle.** Medially, superior to the joint space, both the medial femoral epicondyle and the adductor tubercle are palpable.

Bones and Joints of the Foot and Ankle

Bones of the Foot

Although there are a number of similarities between the foot and hand, those between the bones are quite apparent. Yet it is also apparent that the bones of the hand are constructed and arranged for maneuverability, while those of the foot are adapted for weight bearing. Further, weight must be accommodated during quiet standing as well as during ambulation and a variety of other activities where the weight transmitted across the foot greatly exceeds that of the body. The foot must provide a forceful push-off and a soft landing (in walking and running), so it must be strong and flexible. Seven **tarsal bones** form the **tarsus,** the posterior or proximal portion, which is the junctional region with the ankle. Five **metatarsals** and fourteen **phalanges** form the **forefoot.**

The **tarsal bones** (Figs. 4-32 through 4-35) are commonly described as being arranged in two rows with one bone positioned between the rows. In the proximal, or posterior, row the **talus** is positioned on the superomedial aspect of the **calcaneus.** The distal (anterior) row, from medial to lateral, consists of the **medial, intermediate,** and **lateral cuneiforms,** and the **cuboid.** The **navicular** is positioned between the medial aspects of the two rows. In addition to the proximodistal positioning of these bones, there is a vertical arrangement resulting in only a few of these bones contacting the ground in the normal foot. The talus is the most superior and the only tarsal bone that articulates with the bones of the leg. The calcaneus is the most inferior bone and the only one that touches the ground. Of the remaining bones, the cuboid is the most inferior and the navicular is the most superior. The cuneiforms are between. The formation of the arches of the foot is described later in this chapter.

The **calcaneus** is the largest and most posterior of the tarsals, and it alone forms the heel of the foot. The **tuberosity of the calcaneus** is the posterior and inferior extension that contacts the ground. The medial, shelflike projection, the **sustenaculum tali,** supports and articulates with the superiorly positioned talus. The posterior and inferior aspect of the sustenaculum has a groove that houses the tendon of the flexor hallucis

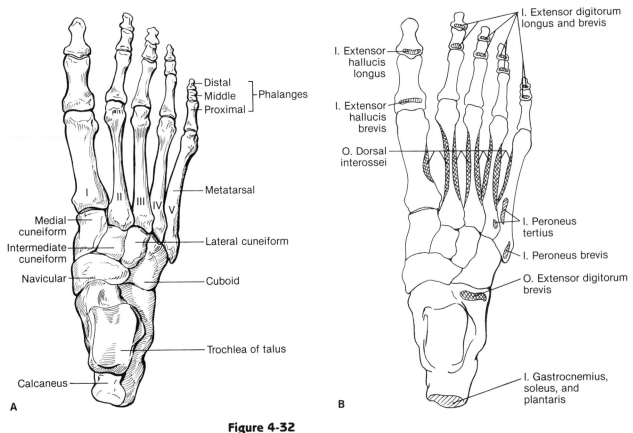

Figure 4-32
Superior views of the bones of the foot indicating their locations and bony prominences (*A*) and the locations of muscle attachments (*B*). The areas of origin are indicated by crosshatch, the insertions by parallel lines.

longus muscle. The calcaneus has three separate articular surfaces. Superiorly, there is a pair of articular surfaces that are separated by the nonarticular **calcaneal sinus.** These two surfaces articulate with the talus, and together they form an inclined plane that slopes anteriorly, medially, and inferiorly. The anterior aspect of the bone also presents an articular surface that articulates with the cuboid.

The **talus** consists of an anterior **head** and a posterior **body** that are separated by a constricted neck. The head is rounded and covered by an articular surface that articulates with the navicular and the plantar calcaneonavicular ligament. The most inferior portion of the head, which contacts the plantar calcaneonavicular ligament, is frequently flattened. The most prominent portion of the body is the superior **trochlea,** whose pulley shape is covered with articular surface on its superior, medial, and lateral aspects. These surfaces articulate with both the tibia and fibula to form the ankle joint. The posterior aspect of the bone is indented by a groove that accommodates the tendon of the flexor hallucis longus muscle. The inferior surface of the talus presents two articular surfaces that correspond to the surfaces on the superior aspect of the calcaneus; the

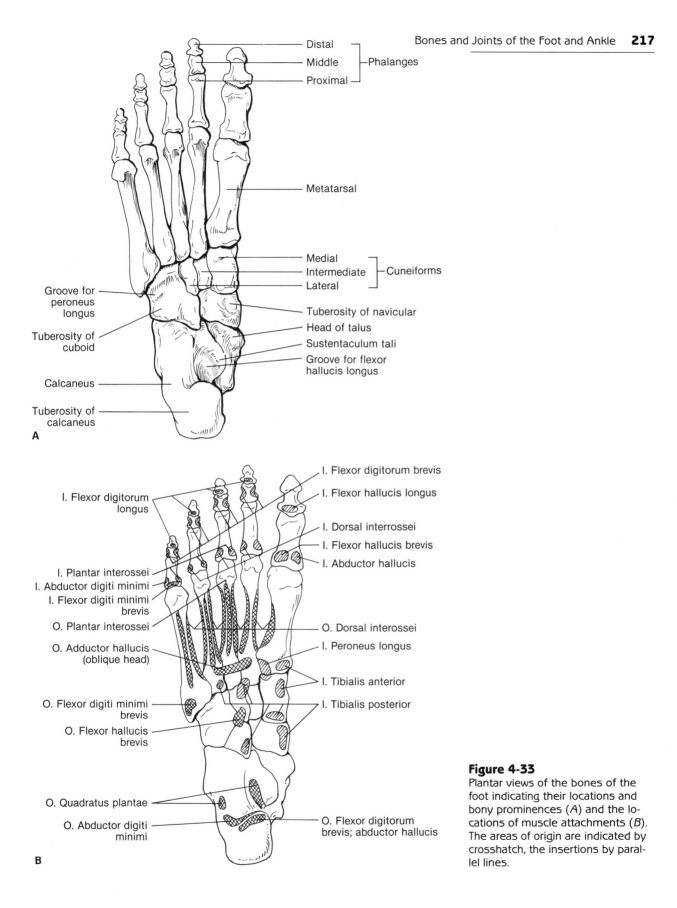

Distal
Middle — Phalanges
Proximal

Metatarsal

Medial
Intermediate — Cuneiforms
Lateral

Groove for
peroneus
longus

Tuberosity of navicular

Head of talus

Tuberosity of
cuboid

Sustentaculum tali

Groove for flexor
hallucis longus

Calcaneus

Tuberosity of
calcaneus

A

I. Flexor digitorum brevis

I. Flexor hallucis longus

I. Flexor digitorum
longus

I. Dorsal interrossei

I. Flexor hallucis brevis

I. Abductor hallucis

I. Plantar interossei
I. Abductor digiti minimi
I. Flexor digiti minimi
brevis

O. Plantar interossei

O. Dorsal interossei

O. Adductor hallucis
(oblique head)

I. Peroneus longus

I. Tibialis anterior

O. Flexor digiti minimi
brevis

I. Tibialis posterior

O. Flexor hallucis
brevis

O. Quadratus plantae

O. Abductor digiti
minimi

O. Flexor digitorum
brevis; abductor hallucis

B

Figure 4-33
Plantar views of the bones of the foot indicating their locations and bony prominences (A) and the locations of muscle attachments (B). The areas of origin are indicated by crosshatch, the insertions by parallel lines.

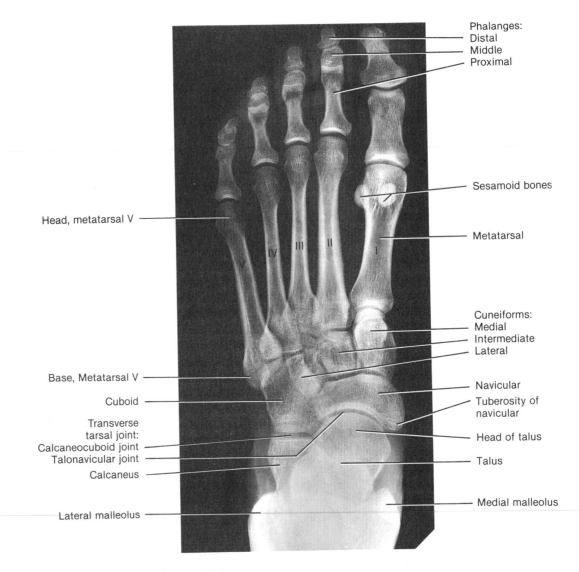

Figure 4-34
Anteroposterior (dorsoplantar) radiograph of the foot.

anterior surface is continuous with the articular surface of its head. These inferior articular surfaces of the talus are separated by the nonarticular oblique **talar sinus,** which together with the calcaneal sinus forms the **tarsal sinus.**

The **navicular** is concave posteriorly and convex anteriorly. Both of these surfaces are articular; the bone articulates with the head of the talus posteriorly and with the three cuneiforms anteriorly. Its prominent **tuberosity** projects from its inferomedial aspect.

The **medial, intermediate,** and **lateral cuneiform bones** fill the interval between the navicular and the medial three metatarsals; all three cuneiforms articulate with the navicular, and each articulates with one

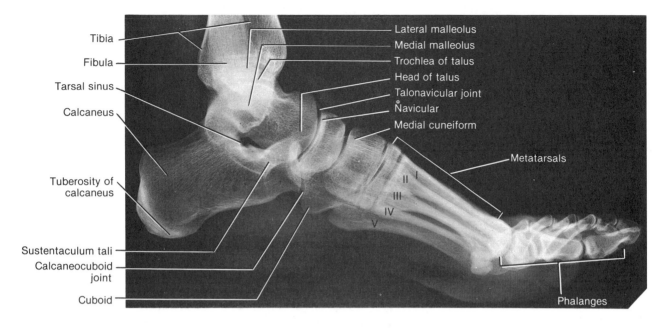

Tibia
Fibula
Tarsal sinus
Calcaneus

Tuberosity of calcaneus

Sustentaculum tali
Calcaneocuboid joint
Cuboid

Lateral malleolus
Medial malleolus
Trochlea of talus
Head of talus
Talonavicular joint
Navicular
Medial cuneiform
Metatarsals

II I
III
IV
V

Phalanges

Figure 4-35
Lateral radiograph of the foot and ankle.

or more of the metatarsals. The three bones also articulate with one another, and the lateral also articulates with the cuboid. All three of these bones are wedge-shaped, with the apex of the medial cuneiform directed superiorly, but the apices of the intermediate and lateral bones directed inferiorly. Viewed as a group, the three bones form a wedge, the apex of which is directed inferiorly.

The **cuboid** bridges the gap between the calcaneus and the two lateral metatarsals, articulating with each of those three bones as well as the lateral cuneiform. Its inferior surface is grooved to accommodate the tendon of the peroneus longus muscle; the posterior wall of this groove is formed by the large **tuberosity** of the cuboid.

The five **metatarsals** are quite similar to those of the hand, except they are larger and heavier. The first metatarsal is larger than the rest, an indication that it transmits more weight than any other. Each bone has a large **base** that articulates with the tarsal bones and a rounded **head** that articulates with its respective proximal phalanx. The base of the fifth metatarsal has a prominent inferolaterally projecting **tuberosity.** The shaft of each bone is slightly convex dorsally, whereas the ventral surface of the shaft is considerably concave. The head of each bone has a **tubercle** on either side for the attachment of the collateral ligament. The ventral aspect of each head, particularly that of the first metatarsal, is usually grooved to accommodate the flexor tendons.

The **phalanges** of the foot are arranged very much like those of the hand: Each toe has three phalanges except the great toe, which has two. The relative lengths of the phalanges and metatarsals, however, are quite different in the hand and foot. In each finger, the total lengths of its phalanges exceed that of the associated metacarpal. In the foot the reverse is true; the length of the metatarsal (with the frequent exception of the great toe) is usually greater than the sum of its associated phalanges. Each proximal phalanx has a concave base and a cylindrical head (side to side) that is grooved from superior to inferior. Each middle phalanx has a head similar to those of the proximal phalanges and a base that is concave from side to side and ridged from superior to inferior. The bases of the distal phalanges are similar to the bases of the middle, and their distal ends are expanded into blunted tuberosities.

Ankle Joint

The **ankle (talocrural) joint** (Fig. 4-36) is formed between the tibia and fibula proximally and the trochlea of the talus distally. The distal aspect of the tibia articulates with the superior surface of the trochlea; the deep aspect of the medial malleolus, with the medial surface of the trochlea; and the deep surface of the lateral malleolus, with the lateral aspect of the trochlea. The medial and lateral malleoli form a kind of mortise into which the trochlea fits. This mortise is strengthened by the interosseous membrane between the tibia and fibula and the **anterior** and **posterior tibiofibular ligaments** (Fig. 4-38).

The motion at the ankle joint consists essentially of the cylinder-shaped trochlea, and hence the rest of the foot, rotating around a horizontal axis that extends between the malleoli. Although some medial and lateral motion does occur, the major motion occurs in a sagittal plane around the horizontal axis. Movement of the foot superiorly, as in walk-

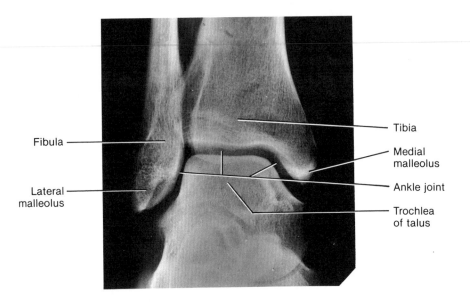

Fibula

Lateral malleolus

Tibia

Medial malleolus

Ankle joint

Trochlea of talus

Figure 4-36
Modified anteroposterior (mortise view) radiograph of the ankle joint.

ing on the heels, is **dorsiflexion.** Movement of the foot inferiorly, as in standing on the ball of the foot or the toes, is **plantar flexion.** No other significant motion occurs at this articulation. It is important to note that the stability of this joint, provided by the bones that form the joint, is not consistent throughout the range of motion. The distance between the malleoli is fixed, but the width of the trochlea is greater anteriorly than posteriorly. As a result, the wider portion of the trochlea is between the malleoli when the foot is dorsiflexed and the bony support is the greatest. Conversely, as the foot is plantar flexed the narrower portion of the trochlea passes between the malleoli and considerable medial-lateral play can occur; thus the ankle is more vulnerable to injury when the foot is plantar flexed.

A pair of **collateral ligaments** reinforce the ankle medially and laterally. The **medial (tibial, deltoid) collateral ligament** (Fig. 4-37) is a strong triangular ligament that extends from the medial malleolus to the talus, navicular, and calcaneus. Its components, the **anterior** and **posterior tibiotalar, tibiocalcaneal,** and **tibionavicular ligaments,** are fused together superiorly but diverge somewhat as they pass inferiorly. This ligament protects the ankle against eversion strains and provides some support to the medial longitudinal arch of the foot. The **lateral (fibular) collateral ligament** (Fig. 4-38) consists of three distinct bands that extend from the lateral malleolus to the talus and calcaneus. Both the **anterior** and **posterior talofibular ligaments** are horizontally oriented, passing, respectively, anteriorly and posteriorly from the lateral malleolus to the talus. The **calcaneofibular ligament** extends inferiorly from the talus. The vast majority of ankle sprains occur when the ankle "rolls over" laterally, as in stepping off a curb or on a stone. This is a plantar flexion-inversion sprain; the foot is plantar flexed, in a position with minimal bony support, and it is twisted medially. This motion places stress on the entire fibular collateral ligament, but most particularly on the anterior talofibular lig-

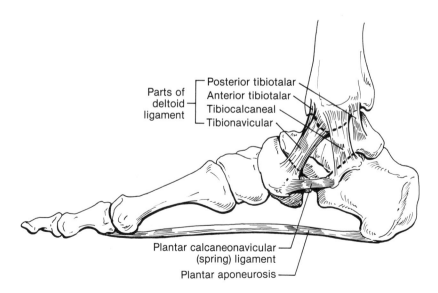

Parts of deltoid ligament
— Posterior tibiotalar
Anterior tibiotalar
Tibiocalcaneal
Tibionavicular

Plantar calcaneonavicular (spring) ligament
Plantar aponeurosis

Figure 4-37
Medial view of the ligaments of the ankle and foot. The components of the deltoid ligament actually are part of a single triangular sheet; they are pictured here separately.

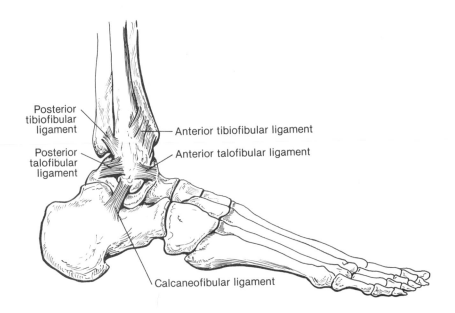

Posterior
tibiofibular
ligament

Anterior tibiofibular ligament

Posterior
talofibular
ligament

Anterior talofibular ligament

Calcaneofibular ligament

Figure 4-38
Lateral view of the ligaments of the ankle.

ament, which, perhaps, is the most commonly sprained ligament in the body.

The **joint capsule** of the ankle joint attaches to the edges of the articular surfaces of the three bones. This capsule is quite thin anteriorly and posteriorly but reinforced by the collateral ligaments medially and laterally. The ankle joint is controlled by the extrinsic muscles of the foot. The principal plantar flexors are the **gastrocnemius** and **soleus muscles;** they are assisted by the deep muscles (**tibialis posterior, flexor hallucis longus, flexor digitorum longus**) of the posterior leg and the peroneal muscles of the lateral leg. The major dorsiflexor is the **tibialis anterior muscle.** This muscle is assisted by the **extensor hallucis longus** and **extensor digitorum longus muscles.**

Articulations of the Foot

Motion within the foot occurs at the **intertarsal joints,** and motion of the toes occurs at the **metatarsophalangeal** and **interphalangeal joints.** There is a large number of intertarsal joints, and virtually all of them contribute to the movements of the foot. Even so, there are two articular areas where most of that motion occurs.

The **subtalar joint** (Fig. 4-35) is formed between the talus superiorly and the calcaneus inferiorly. Both the underside of the talus and the superior aspect of the calcaneus have a pair of articular surfaces that are separated, respectively, by the talar and calcaneal sinuses. The shapes of the opposing surfaces correspond quite well; and the two joints form a common plane that is inclined and sloped anteriorly, medially, and inferiorly. The posterior portion of the subtalar joint is enclosed by its own articular capsule. The anterior portion is part of a larger joint, the **talocalcaneonavicular joint,** and thus shares a joint cavity that extends beyond the articular surfaces of the talus and calcaneus. Ligamentous support of the subtalar joint is provided mainly by the **plantar calcaneonavicular** and **talocalcaneal interosseous** ligaments. The latter ligament is strong and interconnects the two bones within the tarsal sinus.

The **transverse tarsal (midtarsal) articulation** (Figs. 4-32A, 4-34) also consists of two sets of articular surfaces. It is appropriately named because it passes transversely across the foot. It is formed medially between the head of the talus and the navicular and laterally between the calcaneus and the cuboid. The calcaneocuboid joint is enclosed by its own articular capsule, but the talonavicular joint space is part of the larger talocalcaneonavicular joint. The major ligamentous support is provided by the spring ligament medially and the long plantar ligament laterally.

The articulation of the talus with the calcaneus, spring ligament, and navicular is the **talocalcaneonavicular joint.** This is a single anatomical joint (encased in a single joint capsule) that participates in the formation of both the subtalar and transverse tarsal joints. The spring ligament is its major support.

The motion that occurs within the tarsus, predominantly at the subtalar and midtarsal joints, is a combination of motions that results from the architecture of the tarsal bones that enables the foot to adapt to an uneven terrain. Traditionally, these motions are called **inversion** and **eversion.** Inversion is the elevation of the medial aspect of the foot (supination) combined with medial movement of the anterior part of the foot (adduction). Eversion is the reverse, a combination of elevation of the lateral aspects of the foot (pronation) combined with lateral movement of its anterior aspect (abduction). Clinically, however, the movements of the foot are described differently. **Supination** is the elevation of the medial aspect of the foot combined with medial movement of the anterior part of the foot. Since these movements are augmented by plantar flexion, supination is defined as a combination of inversion, adduction, and plantar flexion. **Pronation** is the reverse. Since elevation of the lateral aspect of the foot and lateral movement of its anterior part are amplified by dorsiflexion, pronation is defined as the combination of eversion, abduction, and dorsiflexion.

Even though the **tarsometatarsal** and **intermetatarsal** (between the bases of the metatarsals) **joints** (Fig. 4-34) are synovial articulations, very little motion occurs. The distal row of tarsal bones and the bases of the metatarsals are bound tightly together by a series of **interosseous, tarsometarsal,** and **metatarsal ligaments.**

The **metatarsophalangeal** and **interphalangeal joints** (Fig. 4-34) are all synovial joints and are quite similar to the metacarpophalangeal and interphalangeal joints of the hand. The **metatarsophalangeal joints** are formed between the concave bases of the proximal phalanges and the rounded heads of the metatarsals. The joint capsules are reinforced by collateral ligaments and strong **plantar ligaments** that are interconnected from toe to toe by the **deep transverse metatarsal ligament.** The plantar ligament of the great toe contains a pair of sesamoid bones that are important in the weight-bearing function of that toe. The **interphalangeal**

joints of all toes are similar: Each is formed by a cylindrically shaped phalangeal head and the concave base of the more distal phalanx. These joints also are reinforced by collateral and plantar ligaments. The metatarsophalangeal joints permit flexion and extension along with adduction and abduction; the interphalangeal joints allow only flexion and extension.

Arches of the Foot

Weight is transferred from the foot to the ground through the **tuberosity of the calcaneus** posteriorly and the **heads of the metatarsals** anteriorly. In quiet standing the weight is distributed fairly evenly between front and back; and approximately one-quarter to one-third of the anterior weight passes through the first metatarsal. Weight is distributed through a series of arches, two longitudinal and one transverse.

The **medial longitudinal arch** is the highest and the most important. The keystone of this arch is the talus; it is completed posteriorly by the calcaneus and anteriorly by the navicular, cuneiforms, and medial three metatarsals. The **lateral longitudinal arch** does not include the talus but does include the calcaneus, which is the common posterior pillar of both arches. This arch is completed by the cuboid and lateral two metatarsals.

The **transverse arch** is most obvious in the junctional region between the tarsus and the metacarpals. The cumulative shape of both the distal row of tarsal bones and the bases of the metatarsals is an arch that is oriented transversely with its concavity directed inferiorly. This arch is higher medially than laterally. Anteriorly, this arch flattens and all metatarsal heads are in contact with the ground.

The system of arches and the articulations between the component bones allow the foot to be a flexible and yet a rigid support. The foot can accommodate uneven surfaces, provide a soft landing during ambulation, and transmit force from one part to another and thus facilitate push-off. Each of the arches requires strong support. Loss of this support can lead to flattening of the arches, changes in the mechanics of the foot, and painful disabilities.

Three factors are important in the maintenance of the arches: the shapes of the bones, certain ligaments, and various muscles, particularly the intrinsic foot muscles. The shapes of certain of the tarsal bones, namely the wedge-shaped talus, cuneiforms, and metatarsal heads, are important to the shapes of the arches. A change in the shape of a bone, as the result of a fracture, for example, can lead to a change in the shape of an arch and subsequently a change in the mechanics of the foot.

Several ligaments are the most important supports of the arches of the foot. The **plantar calcaneonavicular (spring) ligament** (Figs. 4-37, 4-39) is clearly the most important ligament. This very strong ligament extends from the anteromedial aspect of the sustentaculum tali to the inferior and medial aspects of the navicular. It holds these two bones together and supports the head of the talus. This ligament also maintains the highest part of the arch and prevents the talus from sliding medially and inferiorly. The superior surface of the spring ligament is partially cov-

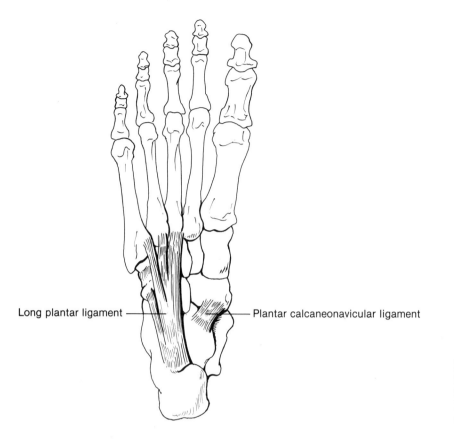

Long plantar ligament —————— Plantar calcaneonavicular ligament

Figure 4-39
Plantar view of the bones of the foot indicating the locations of the long plantar and plantar calcaneo-navicular ligaments.

ered by articular cartilage; the joint cavity between the inferior aspect of the head of the talus and the spring ligament is part of the **talocalcaneo-navicular joint.** The **long plantar ligament** (Fig. 4-39) extends from the calcaneus, anterior to its tuberosity, to the tuberosity of the cuboid and the lateral metatarsals. This ligament supports primarily the lateral longitudinal arch. The **plantar aponeurosis** (Fig. 4-37), a thickened portion of the investing fascia of the foot, interconnects the tuberosity of the calcaneus and the metatarsophalangeal joints anteriorly. This long fibrous band connects the anterior and posterior weight-bearing points of the foot and functions as a tie-rod—thus, it keeps the supporting columns of the longitudinal arches from spreading.

Although a number of muscles are considered to function as supports of the arches, the **intrinsic muscles of the foot** clearly are the more important. During quiet standing the ligaments provide most of the support of the arches. With any motion, the intrinsic muscles become active and provide added support. Several extrinsic muscles (muscles that have origins in the leg and insertions in the foot) also appear positioned to provide support to the arches. The amount of this support, however, is not yet fully determined. The **tibialis anterior** and **peroneus longus** insert, respectively, on the inferomedial and inferolateral aspects of the medial cuneiform and base of the first metatarsal. They thus form a sling that may support (elevate) the medial longitudinal arch. The tendon of the **tibialis posterior** enters the posteromedial aspect of the foot and passes inferior to the head of the talus and spring ligament before inserting into several of the anterior tarsal bones. This muscle also is in a position to support the medial arch.

Change in any of these supports may lead to a series of changes that can result in a flatfoot. The fracture of a tarsal bone, a connective tissue disease that weakens ligaments, a primary muscular disease or peripheral nerve injury that weakens or paralyzes muscles—any of these can contribute to the breakdown of the arches. Mechanical changes in weight transfer can also be caused by other factors, such as a sudden increase in body weight, a fracture more proximally in the lower limb, a change in the gait pattern due to joint pathology or muscle paralysis in the more proximal areas of the limb.

Flatfoot

The term **flatfoot** is relative because the "normal" height of the medial longitudinal arch varies considerably. In the pathologic sense a flatfoot occurs when the height of a person's normal longitudinal arch has been reduced or the arch has "fallen," and the ultimate flatfoot occurs when the head of the talus becomes weight bearing. The medial longitudinal arch is the focus of the discussion that follows because it is the highest part of the arch system, and the talus is the bone that usually moves the most.

The events involved in the breakdown of the supports of the arches and hence the formation of a flatfoot are described in a circular and progressive fashion. It is important to understand, however, that any part of this circle could be the problem that initiates the cycle. Once this sequence of events is established, it is virtually impossible to reverse and very difficult to arrest.

Several points are important in understanding this process. The talus receives all weight that is transferred from the leg to the foot; and because of its keystone position, the weight is transferred anteriorly and posteriorly from that single bone. The bony platform on which the talus rests, through the subtalar joint, is an inclined plane that slopes anteriorly, medially, and inferiorly. The position of the talus is maintained to a large extent by the spring ligament that directly supports the talar head. Finally, the point where the body weight is transferred from the tibia to the talus is medial to the point where the weight passes from the calcaneal tuberosity to the ground. As a result, there is a natural tendency for the calcaneus to roll medially or into eversion. Such movement of the calcaneus is restricted by the spring ligament.

The sequence of events that leads to the formation of a flatfoot can be initiated by a variety of events, such as a change in the mechanics of the foot, a weakened ligament, or a fractured tarsal bone. For purposes of this discussion the assumption is made that the precipitating event is a slight increase in the length of the spring ligament. The direct result is a reduction in the support that "holds up" the head of the talus so the talus slides ever so slightly down the inclined plane of the subtalar joint. Even a very small medial shift of the talus changes the path of weight transfer through the foot, because the weight enters the foot more medially and thus must pass farther laterally to the calcaneal tuberosity, the point where it enters the ground. This medial shift of the weight as it enters the foot places a greater rotational force on the calcaneus; and any eversion of the calcaneus increases the slope of the subtalar joint, which places greater stress on the spring ligament. The vicious cycle is complete. What is important is not the exact sequence of the events but rather the relationships and interdependence of the factors involved.

Leg

Lateral Compartment of the Leg

The lateral compartment of the leg (Fig. 4-1B) is small and located superficial to the fibula in the anterolateral aspect of the leg. In addition to the fibula, its boundaries are the anterior and posterior intermuscular septa and the investing fascia. This compartment contains only two muscles, the peroneus longus and brevis, and a single nerve, the superficial peroneal. There is no major artery in this compartment.

The **peroneus longus muscle** (Figs. 4-19B, 4-33B, 4-40, 4-41) is the more proximal and superficial of the two muscles. It arises from the proximal half to two-thirds of the lateral aspect of the fibula, adjacent portions of both intermuscular septa, and the investing fascia. Its attachment to the fibula is interrupted by a gap in the region of the fibular neck, through which the common peroneal nerve passes. The tendon of this muscle parallels the fibula as it passes superficial to the peroneus brevis and enters the foot by passing posterior to the lateral malleolus. It then crosses the lateral aspect of the calcaneus and then passes medially in a groove on the plantar aspect of the cuboid. Its insertion is on the plantar and lateral aspects of both the medial cuneiform and base of the first metatarsal. The major function of this muscle is eversion of the foot, although it does assist (weakly) in plantar flexion. The peroneus longus muscle is supplied by the superficial peroneal nerve.

The **peroneus brevis muscle** (Figs. 4-19B, 4-20B, 4-40) arises from the distal half to two-thirds of the lateral aspect of the fibula and adjacent portion of the intermuscular septa. Its tendon descends initially deep to and then anterior to that of the peroneus longus; it occupies a groove in the posterior aspect of the lateral malleolus before inserting on the superolateral surface of the base of the fifth metatarsal. This muscle everts the foot and weakly assists in plantar flexion, and is innervated by the superficial peroneal nerve.

Loss of the peroneus longus and brevis muscles results in both greatly weakened eversion of the foot and a static deformity in which the foot is somewhat inverted. The major problem is a loss of balance between inversion and eversion and a definite tendency to walk on the lateral aspect of the foot. At heel strike the tibialis anterior muscle contracts strongly to regulate the contact of the ball of the foot with the floor. Since this

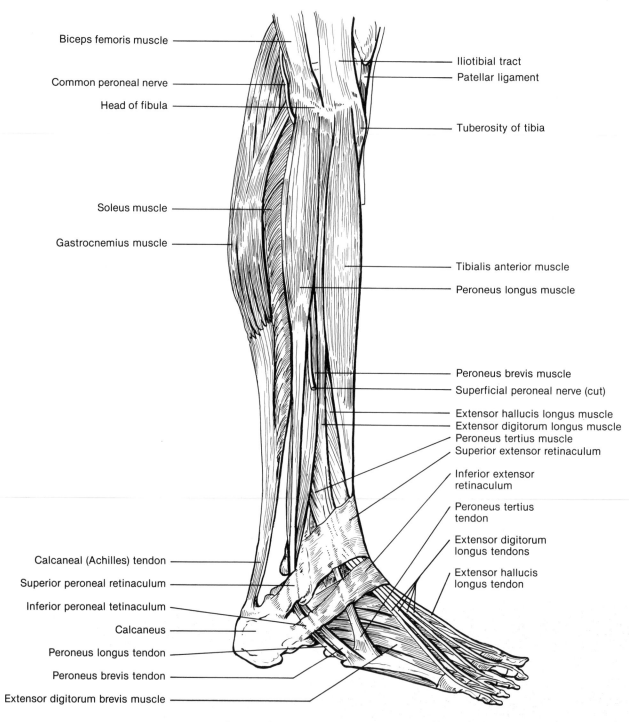

Biceps femoris muscle

Common peroneal nerve

Head of fibula

Soleus muscle

Gastrocnemius muscle

Iliotibial tract

Patellar ligament

Tuberosity of tibia

Tibialis anterior muscle

Peroneus longus muscle

Peroneus brevis muscle

Superficial peroneal nerve (cut)

Extensor hallucis longus muscle

Extensor digitorum longus muscle

Peroneus tertius muscle

Superior extensor retinaculum

Inferior extensor retinaculum

Peroneus tertius tendon

Extensor digitorum longus tendons

Extensor hallucis longus tendon

Calcaneal (Achilles) tendon

Superior peroneal retinaculum

Inferior peroneal tetinaculum

Calcaneus

Peroneus longus tendon

Peroneus brevis tendon

Extensor digitorum brevis muscle

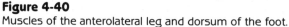

Figure 4-40
Muscles of the anterolateral leg and dorsum of the foot.

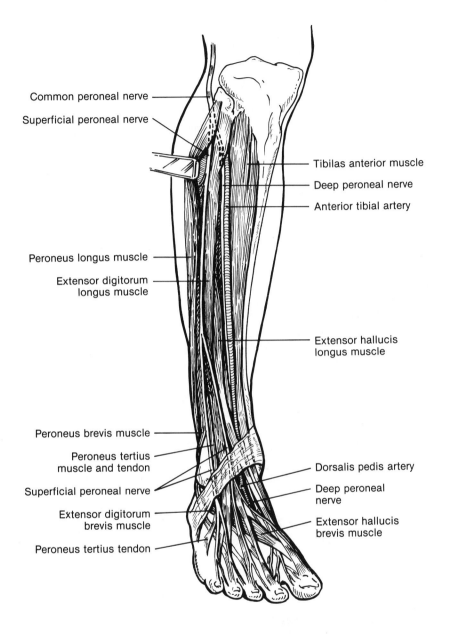

Common peroneal nerve

Superficial peroneal nerve

Tibilas anterior muscle

Deep peroneal nerve

Anterior tibial artery

Peroneus longus muscle

Extensor digitorum longus muscle

Extensor hallucis longus muscle

Peroneus brevis muscle

Peroneus tertius muscle and tendon

Dorsalis pedis artery

Superficial peroneal nerve

Deep peroneal nerve

Extensor digitorum brevis muscle

Extensor hallucis brevis muscle

Peroneus tertius tendon

Figure 4-41
Anterolateral view of the contents of the lateral and anterior compartments of the leg and the dorsum of the foot.

muscle is also a very strong invertor, the neutral position of the foot must be maintained by the evertors, which are principally the peroneus longus and brevis. When these muscles are lost, the weight is borne more laterally and the ankle is vulnerable to inversion sprains.

The **superficial peroneal nerve** (Figs. 4-40, 4-41) supplies the muscles in the lateral compartment of the leg and the skin of the distal anterior leg and most of the dorsum of the foot. The common peroneal nerve enters the lateral compartment by curving around the lateral aspect of the neck of the fibula and passing through the origin of the peroneus longus muscle (fibular tunnel). This is a potential entrapment point, particularly since the edges of the muscle tend to be fibrous. In addition to entrapment, the nerve is vulnerable to injury from fibular fracture and to compression against the bone by a variety of external forces, such as a short leg cast, tight boots, or pressure from a mattress during a prolonged illness. The common peroneal typically splits into its superficial and deep branches as it passes around the fibula, so entrapment at that point would likely involve both branches. The superficial peroneal nerve descends between the peroneus longus and brevis muscles, enters the subcutaneous tissue the distal third of the anterolateral leg, and then descends onto the dorsum of the foot. Entrapment may also occur as the nerve passes through the crural fascia into the superficial fascia; the resulting symptoms would be limited to changes in sensation on the dorsum of the foot.

Anterior Compartment of the Leg

The anterior compartment of the leg (Fig. 4-1B) is positioned lateral to the tibia and bounded additionally by the interosseous membrane posteromedially, the anterior intermuscular septum posterolaterally, and the crural fascia anterolaterally. The fascial layers that form this compartment are quite fibrous, strong, and relatively inelastic. Since the compartment is packed very tightly with muscles and other soft structures, there is little room for the addition of pus or blood as might occur in disease or injury. An **anterior compartment syndrome** can occur when such material accumulates, which necessitates prompt medical care to prevent compression of the structures within the compartment.

The **tibialis anterior muscle** (Figs. 4-19B, 4-33B, 4-40, 4-41) is the largest and strongest muscle in this compartment. Its pennate construction makes it one of the strongest muscles per unit volume in the body. The muscle has an extensive origin from the proximal two-thirds of the lateral aspect of the tibia, the adjacent portion of the interosseous membrane, and the deep surface of the investing fascia. Its strong tendon descends across the anteromedial aspect of the ankle, inclines medially across the tarsus, and then wraps around the medial aspect of the foot to insert on the inferomedial aspects of the medial cuneiform and the base of the first metatarsal. This muscle is both the major dorsiflexor and a strong invertor of the foot. The strength of the muscle belies its role in gait. It shortens the limb throughout the swing phase by dorsiflexing the foot; at heel strike its strong activity prevents forceful plantar flexion; the ball of the foot does not slap the ground, but rather is quietly positioned. Loss of the tibialis anterior results in a profound loss of dorsiflexion and a significant weakening of inversion. The change in gait pattern resulting from a weakened tibialis anterior is different from that produced by a totally paralyzed muscle. The weakened muscle results in a noticeable "foot slap" at heel strike; the muscle is strong enough to dorsiflex the foot during the swing phase, but it cannot counteract the forces that produce plantar flexion at the point of heel strike. As a result, immediately following heel strike, the ball of the foot hits the ground with a resounding slap. Paralysis of the tibialis anterior muscle results in a "steppage gait," one significantly altered in pattern and cadence. During the swing phase the limb cannot be shortened at the ankle, and therefore a high step must be taken to prevent the toes from dragging. Heel strike is replaced by the front of the foot hitting the ground before the heel. The end result is a labored gait that is greatly slowed. The tibialis anterior is innervated by the deep peroneal nerve.

Of the anterior muscles of the leg, the **extensor digitorum longus muscle** (Figs. 4-19B, 4-32B, 4-40, 4-41) arises the most laterally. It arises from the anterior aspect of the upper three-quarters of the fibula and adjacent portion of the interosseous membrane, the inferior aspect of the lateral tibial condyle, and the deep surface of the investing fascia. The muscle's tendon crosses the anterior aspect of the ankle laterally and then separates into four smaller tendons, one going to each of the four lateral toes. Each tendon then gives rise to an extensor aponeurosis that has a central band (which inserts on the dorsal base of the middle phalanx) and lateral bands (which insert on the dorsal base of the distal phalanx). The action of the extensor digitorum is limited for the most part to extension of the proximal phalanges. This is due to the balances of the toes, which favor flexion at both the PIP and DIP joints. This muscle is also a weak dorsiflexor and evertor of the foot. Loss of this muscle results in greatly weakened extension of the four lateral proximal phalanges, but no functional loss or change in gait. The extensor digitorum longus is innervated by the deep peroneal nerve.

The **peroneus tertius muscle** (Fig. 4-40) is more a portion of the extensor digitorum longus than a separate muscle, because they usually share a common muscle belly. The distal aspect of the common muscle mass gives rise to the tendon of the peroneus tertius, which usually appears deep to the inferior extensor retinaculum, where it is positioned lateral to the tendon of the extensor digitorum longus. The tendon inclines laterally toward its insertion on the dorsal aspect of the base of the fifth metatarsal. Even though this muscle is both a dorsiflexor and an evertor of the foot, both motions are weak and of very little functional value, and its loss results in no appreciable functional deficit. The peroneus tertius is innervated by the deep peroneal nerve.

The **extensor hallucis longus muscle** (Figs. 4-19B, 4-32B, 4-40, 4-41) is the deepest of the anterior muscles. Its fibers arise from the middle half of the anteromedial aspect of the fibula and adjacent aspect of the interosseous membrane and join its tendon in the distal leg. This tendon descends between those of the tibialis anterior and extensor digitorum longus and inserts on the dorsal aspect of the distal phalanx of the great toe. This muscle is the main extensor of the great toe and the only extensor at its interphalangeal joint; it also assists in both dorsiflexion and inversion. Its main function appears to be in contributing to the flexion-extension balance of the great toe; that is, the flexor hallucis longus muscle is quite strong and inserts on the plantar aspect of the distal phalanx. Loss of the extensor hallucis longus could result in a statically flexed IP joint of the great toe, which would interfere with the push-off function of that toe during gait. Loss of the extensor hallucis longus would not otherwise significantly affect the static position or movement of the foot. This muscle is innervated by the deep peroneal nerve.

Loss of all muscles in the anterior compartment, which is more common than loss of any one, results in an absolute loss of dorsiflexion, greatly weakened extension of the toes, and weakened inversion and eversion. Gait is affected much the same way as it is when only the tibialis anterior is lost, except the steppage gait may be more pronounced. Even with a paralyzed tibialis anterior, some dorsiflexion may be produced by the extensor hallucis longus and extensor digitorum longus muscles, and so a high step during the swing phase would not be required. With all muscles paralyzed, the step is very high and the change in gait is marked.

The **deep peroneal nerve** (Fig. 4-41) enters the proximal portion of the anterior compartment by piercing the anterior intermuscular septum, a point where the nerve is vulnerable to entrapment. The nerve joins the anterior tibial vessels and descends on the anterior aspect of the interosseous membrane, deep to the anterior compartment muscles. In the distal leg the nerve emerges from beneath the muscles, where it is positioned between the tendons of the tibialis anterior and extensor hallucis longus muscles. It then enters the foot by crossing the anterior aspect of the ankle deep to the inferior extensor retinaculum, which is another potential entrapment point (anterior tarsal tunnel syndrome). The deep peroneal nerve is vulnerable to either temporary or permanent injury from the compression that results from an anterior compartment syndrome. Since the pressure usually increases in the entire compartment, the nerve is vulnerable at any point along its course.

The **anterior tibial vessels** (Figs. 4-29, 4-41) accompany the deep peroneal nerve through the anterior compartment of the leg. The anterior tibial artery is one of the terminal branches of the popliteal artery; it enters the anterior compartment of the leg by passing above the proximal border of the interosseous membrane. This artery descends through the compartment on the ventral aspect of the interosseous membrane and deep to the muscles. In the distal leg it is between the tendons of the tibialis anterior and the extensor hallucis longus muscles. It enters the dorsal aspect of the foot by passing deep to the inferior extensor retinaculum with the deep peroneal nerve. Distal to this retinaculum, where it crosses the ankle, its name changes to the **dorsalis pedis artery.**

Posterior Compartment of the Leg

The posterior compartment of the leg (Fig. 4-1B) is the largest compartment in the leg; it contains the muscles that provide the forward propulsion necessary for gait and that are capable of lifting the entire body's weight. This compartment, commonly called the calf, is separated into superficial and deep portions by the **transverse intermuscular septum.** The superficial muscles function as strong plantar flexors; the deep muscles function more in inversion and eversion and in flexing the toes.

The **gastrocnemius, soleus,** and **plantaris muscles** are located within the superficial portion of the posterior compartment. The gastrocnemius and soleus, which share a common insertion but have three heads of origin, are referred to as the **triceps surae.** The plantaris is of clinical interest because it is commonly injured; however, it is of little functional value.

The **gastrocnemius muscle** (Figs. 4-11B, 4-32B, 4-42) forms the upper half of the contour of the calf. Its medial and lateral heads arise respectively from the medial and lateral aspects of the supracondylar surface of the femur, just superior to the femoral condyles. The two heads form the inferior borders of the popliteal fossa and converge as they descend. The muscle fibers join the **calcaneal (Achilles) tendon** in the middle of the calf and through this tendon insert into the posterior aspect of the calcaneus. Both heads of origin are typically separated from the posterior aspects of the femoral condyles by bursae; that on the medial side commonly communicates with the joint space and is thought to contribute to the formation of a **popliteal,** or **Baker's, cyst.** Although either head may contain a sesamoid bone, the presence of such a bone is more com-

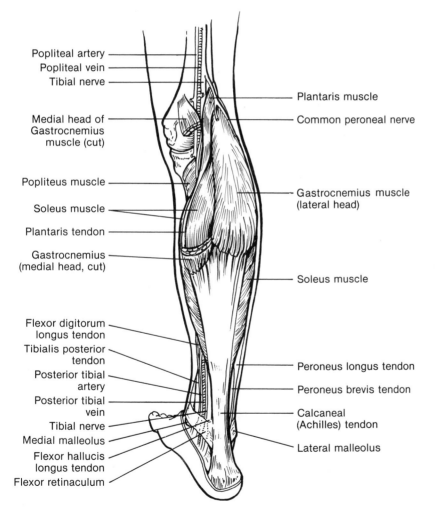

Figure 4-42
Superficial structures of the posterior compartment of the leg. A portion of the medial head of the gastrocnemius muscle is removed.

Popliteal artery
Popliteal vein
Tibial nerve

Plantaris muscle
Common peroneal nerve

Medial head of Gastrocnemius muscle (cut)

Popliteus muscle

Gastrocnemius muscle (lateral head)

Soleus muscle

Plantaris tendon

Gastrocnemius (medial head, cut)

Soleus muscle

Flexor digitorum longus tendon
Tibialis posterior tendon
Posterior tibial artery
Posterior tibial vein
Tibial nerve
Medial malleolus
Flexor hallucis longus tendon
Flexor retinaculum

Peroneus longus tendon
Peroneus brevis tendon
Calcaneal (Achilles) tendon
Lateral malleolus

mon in the lateral head, where it is known as a **fabella.** The gastrocnemius is supplied by the tibial nerve.

The **soleus** (Figs. 4-20B, 4-32B, 4-42, 4-43) does not cross the knee, but is positioned deep to the gastrocnemius and provides the contour of the distal half of the calf. A strong fibrous arch interconnects its points of origin from the posterior surfaces of both bones of the leg—that is, from the proximal quarter of the fibula and the soleal line of the tibia. From this rather extensive origin the fibers converge toward the strong, flat tendon that contributes to the formation of the calcaneal tendon and inserts on the posterior aspect of the calcaneus. The soleus is innervated by the tibial nerve.

The gastrocnemius and soleus muscles are the major plantar flexors of the foot. The function of the soleus is not affected by the position of the knee, but since the gastrocnemius crosses the knee it plantar flexes

Figure 4-43
Posterior compartment of the leg, deeper structures. The superficial muscles are removed.

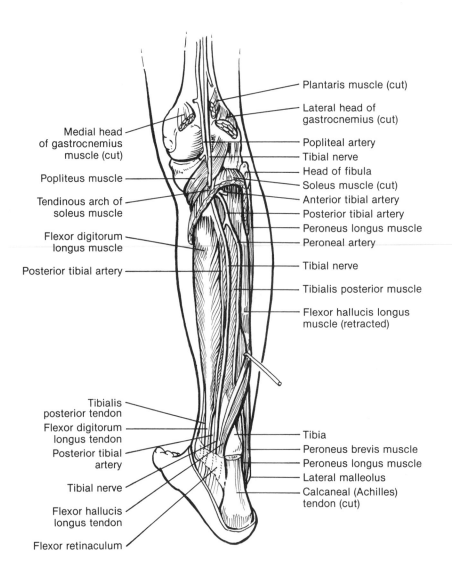

most strongly when the leg is extended. The gastrocnemius is also a flexor at the knee. Both muscles are extremely important during gait and contract strongly at the end of the stance phase when the push-off of the limb occurs and the body is propelled forward. Loss of these two muscles does not result in a complete loss of plantar flexion because the deeper muscles are also plantar flexors. However, functional plantar flexion against resistance is lost and gait is significantly affected. Also, useful push-off is lost. If the loss of muscles is unilateral, there is a significant lag in forward progress at the point where push-off of the involved side should occur. Walking is slowed and laborious, but possible. Running is virtually impossible.

The variably present **plantaris muscle** (Fig. 4-42) has a small muscle belly and a long, thin tendon. It arises from the posterior aspect of the femur just superior to the lateral head of the gastrocnemius. Its muscle belly is usually short and joins the tendon in the proximal part of the leg. However, the muscle belly may be found at any point along the tendon. The tendon descends first between the gastrocnemius and soleus muscles and then on the medial aspect of the calcaneal tendon, inserting medial to that tendon on the calcaneus. Although this muscle is potentially a plantar flexor and flexor at the knee, it is of virtually no functional value. Its tendon is vulnerable to rupture, which tends to occur most often in middle-aged "weekend athletes." The plantaris is supplied by the tibial nerve.

The muscles in the deep portion of the posterior compartment are the **flexor hallucis longus, flexor digitorum longus, tibialis posterior,** and **popliteus.** These muscles are positioned on the posterior aspects of the tibia, fibula, and interosseous membrane and have tendons that enter the foot by passing posterior to the medial malleolus to insert on the more anterior bones of the foot.

The **flexor hallucis longus muscle** (Figs. 4-20B, 4-33B, 4-43) is positioned posterior to the fibula and arises from approximately the distal half to two-thirds of the posterior aspect of that bone. The muscle's tendon of insertion is quite long and extends proximally into the muscle. The muscle fibers are arranged in a bipennate fashion and thus are short and obliquely oriented. The tendon enters the foot as the most posterior structure behind the medial malleolus and passes toward the great toe, where it inserts on the plantar surface of the base of its distal phalanx. The flexor hallucis longus is the strongest flexor of the great toe; its size and pennate construction reflect its function in providing the final push-off through flexion of the great toe during gait. Although this muscle is positioned to both plantar flex and invert the foot, it does so weakly because its contraction range is quite limited. Loss of this muscle results in a loss of flexion of the great toe and a slight lag in the final phase of push-off because the position of the great toe cannot be maintained. The flexor hallucis longus muscle is supplied by the tibial nerve.

The **flexor digitorum longus muscle** (Figs. 4-20B, 4-33B, 4-43) is located posterior to the tibia and arises from the middle half of the shaft of that bone. Its tendon descends posterior to the medial malleolus between the tendons of the tibialis posterior and flexor hallucis longus muscles and then passes anteriorly around the inferior aspect of the sustentaculum tali. At about the level of the distal row of tarsal bones, the tendon splits into four separate tendons, one passing to each of the four lateral toes where they insert on the plantar aspects of the bases of the distal phalanges. This muscle is the only flexor of the distal phalanges of those toes; it is also capable of producing weak plantar flexion and inversion of the foot. Loss of this muscle results in the loss of flexion of the distal phalanges of the toes, but there is no interference with gait. The flexor digitorum longus is innervated by the tibial nerve.

The **tibialis posterior muscle** (Figs. 4-20B, 4-33B, 4-43) occupies the interval between and deep to the flexor hallucis longus and flexor digitorum longus muscles. It arises from portions of the upper halves of both the tibia and fibula, along with the intervening interosseous membrane. The distal part of the muscle (and/or its tendon) is directed medially and passes deep to the tendon of the flexor digitorum longus. The tendon then occupies a groove in the posterior aspect of the medial malleolus, where it is the most anterior of the structures entering the foot in that area. The tendon continues distally inferior to the sustentaculum tali and the spring ligament, and separates into slips that insert on the tuberosity of the navicular and the plantar aspects of all three cuneiforms, the cuboid, and the bases of the middle three metatarsals. This muscle is a strong invertor as well as a plantar flexor of the foot. Its more important function, however, may be the support it provides for the medial longitudinal arch of the foot. Its loss would weaken inversion significantly but have little effect on gait. A prolonged paralysis of this muscle may contribute to the development of a flatfoot. The tibialis posterior is supplied by the tibial nerve.

The **popliteus** (Figs. 4-20B, 4-43) is a short muscle located proximally in the leg and crossing only the knee joint. The muscle is obliquely oriented, extending from an origin on the lateral aspect of the lateral femoral epicondyle to its insertion on the posterior surface of the proximal aspect of the tibia. The tendon of origin passes between the fibrous and synovial layers of the joint capsule of the knee, then attaches to the lateral meniscus. When the limb is not bearing weight, this muscle rotates the leg medially. When the foot is on the ground, the muscle rotates the femur laterally, which is the motion thought to "unlock" the knee before flexion occurs. The popliteus also is a weak flexor at the knee. It is supplied by the tibial nerve.

The **tibial nerve** (Fig. 4-43) enters the posterior compartment of the leg from the popliteal fossa by passing first between and then deep to the two heads of the gastrocnemius. It then passes deep to the fibrous arch that interconnects the two heads of origin of the soleus muscle, a point at which it is vulnerable to entrapment. Together with the posterior tibial vessels, it descends first on the posterior surface of the tibialis posterior muscle and then on the tibia in the distal aspect of the leg. The tibial nerve may be compressed by increased pressure that accompanies a deep posterior compartment syndrome; also it is vulnerable to injury when the distal portion of the tibia is fractured. The tibial nerve enters the foot by passing posterior and then inferior to the medial malleolus and deep to the flexor retinaculum. The area deep to the flexor retinaculum is the **tarsal tunnel.** From anterior to posterior this tunnel houses the tendons of the tibialis posterior and flexor digitorum longus muscles, the posterior tibial artery and vein, the tibial nerve, and the tendon of the flexor hallucis longus. The nerve typically bifurcates into its two terminal branches, the **medial** and **lateral plantar nerves,** in the tarsal tunnel. While in the tarsal tunnel, the tibial nerve (or either the medial or lateral plantar nerve) is vulnerable to entrapment (tarsal tunnel syndrome) from a variety of sources, such as irritation of the nerve by fibrous edges, tendinitis, and vascular engorgement.

The popliteal artery ends in the proximal portion of the posterior compartment by dividing into the anterior and posterior tibial arteries. The **posterior tibial artery** (Figs. 4-29, 4-43) accompanies the tibial nerve through the posterior compartment of the leg. At the ankle, this artery is positioned posterior to the medial malleolus between the tendon of the flexor digitorum longus muscle anteriorly and the tibial nerve posteriorly. Its largest branch, the **peroneal artery,** arises in the proximal portion of the leg and descends through the lateral aspect of the posterior compartment between the superficial and deep groups of muscles. In the region of the ankle, the peroneal artery typically has branches that anastomose with branches of the posterior and anterior tibial arteries. The **posterior tibial** and **peroneal veins** accompany their respectively named arteries.

Foot

The soft tissue structures of the foot are similar to those of the hand, but the functional demands of weight bearing and maintenance of the arches along with the lack of dexterity are reflected in their construction. Those muscles utilized for support are larger than their counterparts in the hand; those concerned with dexterity are usually smaller. The fibrous tissue bands and septa of the foot are larger, thicker, and usually more firmly anchored than those of the hand. As a result, most structures in the foot are more firmly held in place and interconnected, reflecting their functions in maintenance of the arches. Those structures in the foot that have homologs in the hand are so indicated.

The compartmentation of the foot (Fig. 4-1C) is similar to that of the hand, but it is less well defined. The muscles in the plantar aspect of the foot are arranged in layers and are discussed on that basis. Since the major function of the plantar intrinsic muscles is to support the arches of the foot and the loss of a single muscle is both uncommon and usually of little functional consequence, the individual functions of each muscle are discussed but not stressed, and only the losses of groups of muscles are described.

Plantar Foot

Muscles of the plantar foot.   The muscles in the plantar aspect of the foot are organized into three layers, with a fourth layer consisting of those muscles, the **interossei,** that are positioned between the metatarsals. The **first,** or **superficial, layer** consists of the **flexor digitorum brevis, abductor hallucis,** and **abductor digiti minimi muscles.** The **second,** or **intermediate layer,** includes the **tendon of the flexor digitorum longus** and those muscles associated with that tendon: the **quadratus plantae** and **lumbricals.** The **third** or **deep layer** consists of the **adductor hallucis, flexor hallucis brevis,** and the **flexor digiti minimi brevis muscles.**

The **flexor digitorum brevis muscle** (Figs. 4-33B, 4-44) is homologous to the flexor digitorum superficialis of the hand, but differs because it is an intrinsic muscle of the foot. It is positioned deep to the plantar aponeurosis in the central region of the foot and arises from the anterior aspect of the tuberosity of the calcaneus and the deep aspect of the plantar aponeurosis. Its four tendons extend to the four lateral toes, each splitting to allow passage of the tendon of the flexor digitorum longus, and then inserting on the plantar aspect of the middle phalanx. This muscle flexes the proximal interphalangeal joints of those toes. The flexor digitorum brevis is supplied by the medial plantar nerve.

The **abductor hallucis muscle** (Figs. 4-33B, 4-44) forms the majority of the medial portion of the plantar aspect of the foot and extends from its origin on the medial aspect of the tuberosity of the calcaneus and

Figure 4-44
Superficial muscles of the plantar foot. Major portions of the plantar aponeurosis and the flexor digitorum brevis muscle are removed.

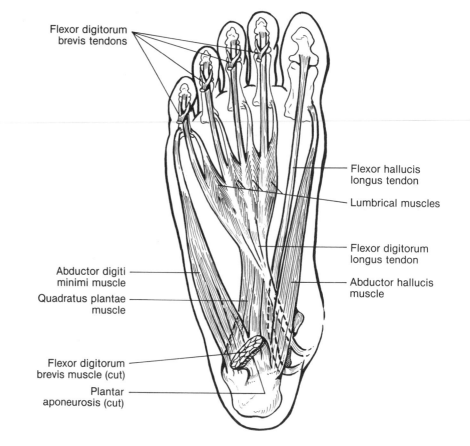

Flexor digitorum brevis tendons

Flexor hallucis longus tendon

Lumbrical muscles

Flexor digitorum longus tendon

Abductor hallucis muscle

Abductor digiti minimi muscle

Quadratus plantae muscle

Flexor digitorum brevis muscle (cut)

Plantar aponeurosis (cut)

adjacent connective tissue to its insertion on the medial aspect of the plantar base of the great toe. Unlike its homolog in the hand, the abductor pollicis brevis, this muscle is more of a flexor of the proximal phalanx of the great toe than an abductor. It is strong and supports the medial longitudinal arch. It is innervated by the medial plantar nerve.

The **abductor digiti minimi muscle** (Figs. 4-33B, 4-44) forms the lateral plantar border of the foot and extends from its origin on the calcaneal tuberosity and related connective tissue to its insertion on the lateral base of the proximal phalanx of the little toe. It functions to abduct the little toe. It is innervated by the lateral plantar nerve.

In the central region of the foot, the structures forming the second layer extend from the calcaneus to the toes. The **tendon of the flexor digitorum longus muscle** (Fig. 4-44) passes obliquely across the tarsus and branches into four smaller tendons that extend to the four lateral toes. Each of these tendons passes through the arch formed by the flexor digitorum brevis tendon and inserts on the plantar base of the distal phalanx.

The **quadratus plantae muscle** (Figs. 4-33B, 4-44) occupies the interval between the calcaneus and the tendon of the flexor digitorum longus. This muscle arises from the medial and lateral aspects of the plantar surface of the calcaneus and inserts into the flexor digitorum longus tendon, proximal to its division into its four tendons. The quadratus plantae clearly assists the long flexor in its action; and perhaps more importantly, it transforms the oblique pull of the long flexor into a force that is perpendicular to the flexon-extension axes of the toes. It is supplied by the lateral plantar nerve.

The **lumbrical muscles** (Fig. 4-44) are anatomically quite similar to those in the hand, arising from the tendons of the flexor digitorum longus and inserting into the extensor aponeuroses on the dorsal aspects of the toes. Although the potential actions of these muscles are the same as those of the hand, the muscles are typically small and the extensor aponeuroses is poorly defined. The three lateral lumbricals are usually supplied by the lateral plantar nerve, whereas the first is innervated by the medial plantar nerve.

The three muscles that form the deep, or third, layer are positioned on the plantar aspects of the metatarsals; and although they are associated with the great and little toes, they extend more or less across the foot. The **adductor hallucis muscle** (Figs. 4-33B, 4-46), like the adductor pollicis, has two heads of origin. Its oblique head arises from the plantar bases of metatarsals 2, 3, and 4; the transverse head arises from various connective tissue structures at the level of the metatarsal heads—the plantar and deep transverse metatarsal ligaments. The two heads converge toward their common insertion on the lateral aspect of the plantar base of the proximal phalanx of the great toe. This muscle obviously has the potential to adduct the great toe. It is supplied by the lateral plantar nerve.

The **flexor hallucis brevis muscle** (Figs. 4-33B, 4-46) is shorter than and positioned deep to the abductor hallucis muscle. From an origin on the adjacent aspects of the cuboid and the lateral cuneiform bones, the fibers of this muscle parallel the oblique head of the adductor hallucis muscle as they extend anteriorly and insert on the medial and lateral aspects of the plantar base of the proximal phalanx of the great toe. This muscle flexes the proximal phalanx of the great toe. It is supplied by the medial plantar nerve.

The **flexor digiti minimi brevis muscle** (Figs. 4-33B, 4-46) is deep to the abductor digiti minimi and extends between the plantar bases of the fifth metatarsal (origin) and the proximal phalanx of the little toe (insertion). It produces flexion at the metatarsophalangeal joint of that toe. It is innervated by the lateral plantar nerve.

The fourth layer of muscles is formed by the **dorsal** and **ventral interossei** (Figs. 4-33B, 4-46), which are positioned generally between the metatarsals. These muscles are similar to those of the hand in general position and function, but they differ in specific location because the reference for adduction and abduction is the second toe (rather than the middle finger). The three plantar interossei extend from the plantar shafts of the three lateral metatarsals to the medial aspects of the plantar bases of the corresponding proximal phalanges. These muscles adduct those toes at the metatarsophalangeal joints. Each of the dorsal interossei arises from the adjacent sides of two metatarsals. Two of these muscles insert on the base of the second proximal phalanx; muscles 3 and 4 insert on

Figure 4-45
Superficial neurovascular structures of the plantar foot.

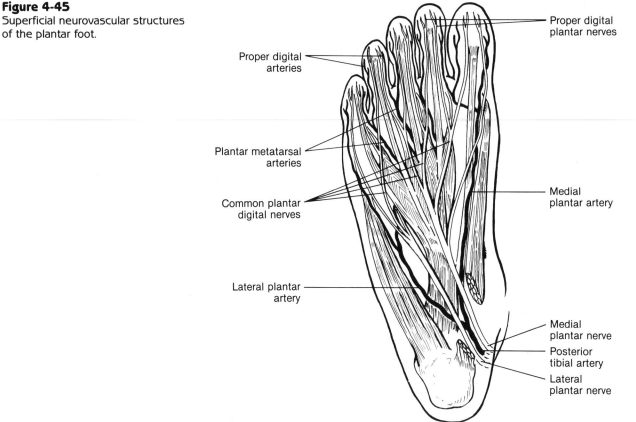

the lateral aspects of the plantar bases of the third and fourth proximal phalanges. The dorsal interossei abduct the third and fourth toes away from the second toe, and deviate the second toe either medially or laterally. Both sets of these muscles have potential insertions into the rudimentary extensor mechanism and thereby are potential flexors at the MP joints and extensors at the IP joints. As a rule, however, neither these attachments nor these actions are well developed. All interossei are supplied by the lateral plantar nerve.

Nerves of the plantar foot. The **medial** and **lateral plantar nerves** (Figs. 4-45, 4-46) are the terminal branches of the tibial nerve and typically begin in the tarsal tunnel. Together, these nerves pass deep to the abductor hallucis muscle into the central area of the foot, where their courses diverge. As they pass the abductor hallucis muscle, they are positioned between the spring ligament above and a fibrous band below; either or both nerves are vulnerable to entrapment at that point, especially as the foot is everted and the nerves are forced against the fibrous edges. The course of the **medial plantar nerve** is similar to that of the median nerve in the hand. It passes anteriorly between the abductor hallucis and flexor digitorum brevis muscles and divides into its digital (common and proper) nerves. This nerve supplies the flexor digitorum brevis,

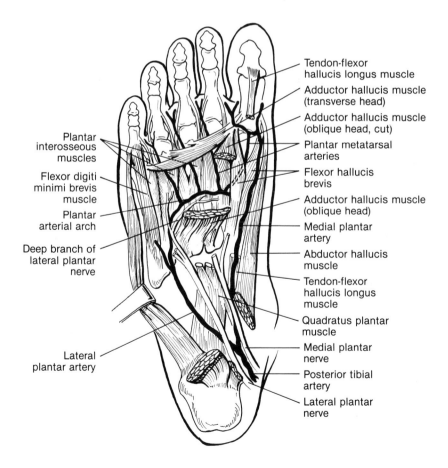

Figure 4-46
Deeper structures of the plantar foot.

Tendon-flexor hallucis longus muscle

Adductor hallucis muscle (transverse head)

Adductor hallucis muscle (oblique head, cut)

Plantar metatarsal arteries

Flexor hallucis brevis

Adductor hallucis muscle (oblique head)

Medial plantar artery

Abductor hallucis muscle

Tendon-flexor hallucis longus muscle

Quadratus plantar muscle

Medial plantar nerve

Posterior tibial artery

Lateral plantar nerve

Plantar interosseous muscles

Flexor digiti minimi brevis muscle

Plantar arterial arch

Deep branch of lateral plantar nerve

Lateral plantar artery

flexor hallucis brevis, and the first lumbrical. In addition, it supplies the plantar skin of the medial foot and the medial three and one-half toes. Similar in course and distribution to the ulnar nerve, the **lateral plantar nerve** passes laterally across the foot between the flexor digitorum brevis and quadratus plantae muscles. This part of the nerve supplies the quadratus plantae and abductor digiti muscles along with the skin of the lateral plantar foot. Near the base of the fifth metatarsal this nerve divides into superficial and deep branches. The superficial branch passes anteriorly and separates into both digital and muscular branches. The deep branch is entirely muscular and passes medially across the deep central region of the foot between the interossei and adductor hallucis muscles. It supplies the adductor hallucis, all the interossei, and a variable number of lumbricals. The superficial branch supplies the flexor digiti minimi, usually the lateral lumbrical, and the plantar skin of the lateral one and a half toes.

The **common digital branches** of both nerves pass inferior to the deep transverse metatarsal ligament and then incline somewhat superiorly into the toes. During weight bearing, especially as the toes are extended (push-off), these nerves are forced against the sharp edges of the ligament and are vulnerable to pressure. This is especially true for the common digital nerve between the third and fourth toes because it is usually formed by branches from both the medial and lateral plantar nerves and is therefore more firmly anchored proximally. As a result, this nerve is particularly vulnerable to friction where it crosses the ligament; it is more commonly irritated (**Morton's neuroma**) than any other of the common digital nerves.

Vessels of the plantar foot.   The **posterior tibial artery** (Figs. 4-39, 4-45, 4-46) enters the foot by passing deep to the abductor hallucis muscle along with the medial and lateral plantar nerves. This artery typically branches into the **medial** and **lateral plantar arteries** either deep to or proximal to that muscle. The **medial plantar artery** is the smaller of the two and passes anteriorly to supply the medial aspect of the foot. The **lateral plantar artery** (homologous to the ulnar artery of the hand) passes laterally across the foot with the lateral plantar nerve. At about the level of the base of the fifth metatarsal, the artery swings laterally and deeply and passes between the proximal aspects of the interossei and adductor hallucis muscles along with the deep branch of the lateral plantar nerve. This latter portion of the artery is the **plantar arterial arch** (Fig. 4-45), which is completed by the deep plantar branch of the dorsalis pedis artery. The plantar arch, which is similar to the deep arch of the hand, has plantar metatarsal branches, which in turn give rise to the digital arteries.

Dorsal Foot

The dorsum of the foot differs from that of the hand because it has intrinsic muscles; it is similar in that the superficial veins of the limb begin in the subcutaneous tissue of this surface. The **extensor digitorum brevis muscle** (Figs. 4-32B, 4-40, 4-41) is a small muscle that is positioned laterally and arises from the superior aspect of the distal calcaneus. The muscle belly gives rise to three tendons that pass anteriorly and join the lateral aspects of the extensor digitorum longus tendons to the second, third, and fourth toes. The **extensor hallucis brevis muscle** is positioned medial to the extensor digitorum brevis and frequently appears to be part of that muscle. The origin of the extensor hallucis brevis is also the superior aspect of the calcaneus, and its insertion is the dorsal base of the proximal phalanx of the great toe. Both of these muscles are supplied by the deep peroneal nerve, and they function to extend the proximal phalanges of their respective toes.

The **deep peroneal nerve** (Fig. 4-41) enters the foot by passing deep to the inferior extensor retinaculum in the anterior tarsal tunnel—where it can be entrapped—with the dorsalis pedis artery and between the tendons of the extensor hallucis longus and extensor digitorum longus muscles. The nerve has a lateral branch to the extensor hallucis brevis and extensor digitorum brevis muscle and also a medial branch that is cutaneous to a small area between the first and second toes. The **superficial peroneal nerve** (Fig. 4-40) enters the dorsum of the foot in the subcutaneous tissue. It supplies most of the skin of the dorsum of the foot and, since it is superficial throughout its course, is vulnerable to injury from laceration or external pressure.

The **dorsalis pedis artery** (Fig. 4-41) is the continuation of the anterior tibial artery; its course and distribution are similar to those of the radial artery of the hand. It enters the foot by passing deep to the inferior extensor retinaculum between the tendons of the extensor hallucis longus and extensor digitorum longus muscles. The artery continues distally toward the interval between the bases of the first and second metatarsals, through which its deep plantar branch passes to complete the plantar arterial arch. Proximal to the deep plantar branch, the arcuate branch arises and swings laterally, giving rise to the dorsal metatarsal arteries that extend toward the toes. The dorsal and plantar arteries are usually interconnected by perforating branches that pass between the metatarsals.

Surface Anatomy of the Ankle and Foot

The bony landmarks around the ankle are the medial and lateral malleoli, both of which are readily palpable. In the foot, a number of bony prominences also are easily palpable. The tuberosity of the calcaneus is posterior and inferior. The most inferior bony prominence below the medial malleolus is the medial aspect of the sustentaculum tali. Anterior to the sustentaculum is the head of the talus (and the spring ligament) and then the tuberosity of the navicular. The head of the talus is slightly superior to both the sustentaculum and the tuberosity of the navicular. Anterior and somewhat inferior to the navicular, the medial cuneiform and then the base of the first metatarsal are palpable. Laterally, the base of the fifth metatarsal is readily palpable as the obvious lateral bony protrusion just anterior to the tarsus. The lateral indentation posterior to the fifth metatarsal is the cuboid. The heads of all five metatarsals are palpable.

A number of the tendons of the extrinsic muscles of the foot and the arteries that cross the ankle are also palpable, and the positions of the major nerves can be related to these structures. A number of structures cross the anterior aspect of the ankle between the two malleoli. There are two tendons medially, a neurovascular bundle, and more laterally another tendon. The most medial tendon is that of the tibialis anterior muscle, and immediately lateral is the tendon of the extensor hallucis longus. Both of these tendons can be followed from the ankle to their insertions, and both are important in performing a segmental motor check. The tibialis anterior is the muscle used to check spinal cord segment L4; the extensor hallucis longus is used to check L5. Lateral to these tendons the deep peroneal nerve and dorsalis pedis artery enter the foot together. A dorsalis pedis pulse must be taken somewhat distally because at the level of the malleoli the artery (and the nerve) is in the anterior tarsal tunnel, where it is deep to the inferior extensor retinaculum and therefore not palpable. The most lateral tendon crossing the anterior ankle is that of the extensor digitorum longus muscle. This tendon is located just lateral to the neurovascular bundle. The greater saphenous vein also crosses the anterior aspect of the ankle. It is consistently positioned 1 to 2 cm lateral to the medial malleolus in the subcutaneous tissue, where it may or may not be visible.

Two tendons pass between the lateral malleolus and the calcaneus. These tendons are closely related to each other and occupy a groove on the posterior aspect of the lateral malleolus. The tendon of the peroneus longus muscle is superficial to that of the peroneus brevis; and although they are palpable just inferior to the malleolus, they may be somewhat difficult to differentiate.

A neurovascular bundle and three tendons enter the foot by passing posterior to the medial malleolus. All of these structures pass deep to the flexor retinaculum and thus through the posterior tarsal tunnel. As this tunnel is located more or less inferior to the medial malleolus, these structures are best palpated posterior to that part of the bone. The tendon of the tibialis posterior muscle is the most anterior structure and occupies a groove in the posterior aspect of the medial malleolus. The next posterior structure is the tendon of the flexor hallucis longus muscle. The neurovascular bundle containing the posterior tibial vessels and the tibial nerve is approximately 2 cm posterior to the malleolus; this bundle is positioned between the tendon of the flexor hallucis longus muscle anteriorly and that of the flexor digitorum longus posteriorly.

Most posteriorly, of course, is the common tendon of the gastrocnemius and soleus muscles. This calcaneal (Achilles) tendon is palpable just superior to the tuberosity of the calcaneus.

Nerve Injuries of the Lower Limb

The section begins with a comparison of peripheral and segmental patterns of innervation of the lower limb and is followed by a discussion of some of the more common injuries of lower limb nerves. The discussion of each nerve injury focuses primarily on the functional deficits that each produces, that is, changes in upright posture and gait. The descriptions of all injuries are based on a unilateral loss unless otherwise indicated.

The changes that occur in either standing or gait subsequent to muscle loss are compensatory. Such changes are usually positional and reflect the shifts in body weight that are necessary to maintain the upright position during standing and walking. In most instances there is a shift of the body toward the muscle loss above the joint that the paralyzed muscles control; for example, loss of the hip extensors results in a posterior shift of the trunk. Since most muscle activity is directed toward preventing rather than producing motion during either standing or walking (the muscles undergo lengthening rather than shortening contractions), loss of a muscle or muscle group allows gravity to produce an unwanted action. The only way such a loss can be counteracted is a shift in body weight that counteracts the loss.

Segmental Versus Peripheral Innervation of the Lower Limb

The basic differences between the segmental and peripheral patterns of innervation are discussed in the nerve injury section of the upper limb on page 147.

The dermatomes of the lower limb (Fig. 4-47) are as follows:

L1   proximal medial thigh
L2   proximal anterior thigh
L3   distal anteromedial thigh and knee
L4   anteromedial leg
L5   anterolateral leg, medial dorsal foot, plantar great toe
S1   heel, most of plantar foot, lateral dorsal foot
S2   posterior thigh and proximal leg

The cutaneous areas innervated by peripheral nerves of the lower limb (Fig. 4-47) are as follows:

Genitofemoral	proximal anterior thigh
Ilioinguinal	anteromedial proximal thigh, anterior perineum, skin over pubic symphysis
Femoral	most of anterior thigh; via its saphenous branch—medial knee, leg, and foot
Lateral femoral cutaneous	lateral thigh
Obturator	inferior medial thigh
Posterior femoral cutaneous	posterior thigh, posterior proximal calf
Sural	(formed by branches of common peroneal and tibial)—posterolateral leg and lateral foot
Tibial	via medial and lateral plantar branches—most of plantar foot
Superficial peroneal	distal anterior leg, most of the dorsum of the foot
Deep peroneal	dorsal web space between the first and second toes

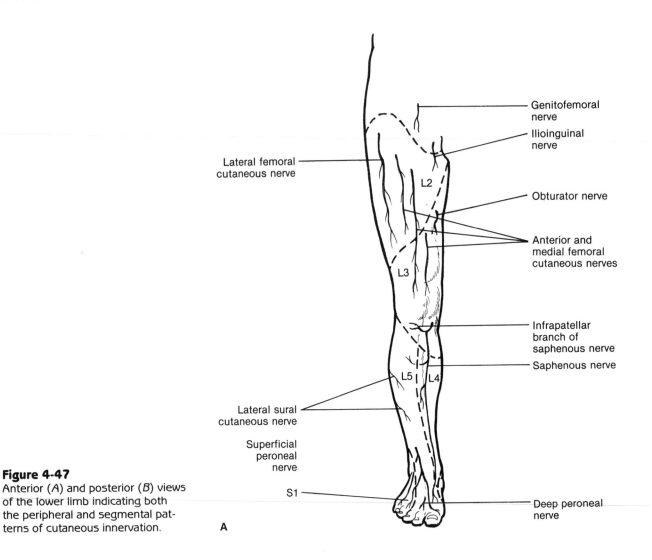

Genitofemoral
nerve

Ilioinguinal
nerve

Lateral femoral
cutaneous nerve

L2

Obturator nerve

Anterior and
medial femoral
cutaneous nerves

L3

Infrapatellar
branch of
saphenous nerve

Saphenous nerve

L5 L4

Lateral sural
cutaneous nerve

Superficial
peroneal
nerve

S1

Deep peroneal
nerve

A

Figure 4-47
Anterior (A) and posterior (B) views
of the lower limb indicating both
the peripheral and segmental patterns of cutaneous innervation.

The segmental muscular (motor) innervation of the lower limb is easy to
remember because it is consecutive from proximal to distal anteriorly and
then posteriorly: anterior hip, L2; anterior knee, L3; anterior ankle, L4;
anterior great toe, L5; all joints posteriorly, S1. The specifics and variability of this segmental motor innervation are as follows:

L2 (L1–3)   iliopsoas (flexion of the thigh)
L3 (L2–4)   anterior compartment of the thigh (extension of the
              leg), medial compartment of the thigh (adduction
              of the thigh)
L4 (L5)   tibialis anterior (dorsiflexion of the foot)
L5 (L4–S1)   extensor hallucis longus (extension of the great toe)
S1 (L5–S2)   gluteus maximus and hamstrings (extension at the hip
              and flexion at the knee), posterior compartment of
              the leg (plantar flexion of the foot and flexion of
              the toes)

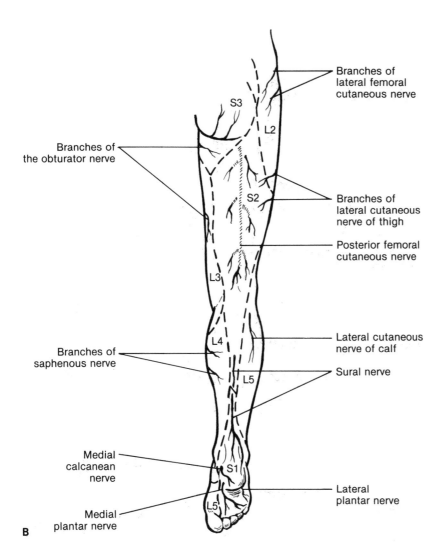

B

The peripheral pattern of muscular innervation of the lower limb is as follows:

Femoral	anterior compartment of the thigh (extension of the leg)
Obturator	medial compartment of the thigh (adduction at the hip)
Superior gluteal	gluteus medius and minimus (abduction at the hip)
Inferior gluteal	gluteus maximus (extension at the hip)
Tibial	hamstring muscles (extension at the hip and flexion at the knee), posterior compartment of the leg and intrinsic muscles in the plantar foot (plantar flexion of the foot and flexion of the toes)

| Superficial peroneal | lateral compartment of the leg (eversion of the foot) |
| Deep peroneal | anterior compartment of the leg (dorsiflexion and inversion of the foot, extension of the toes) |

Superior Gluteal Nerve

A lesion of the superior gluteal nerve results in total loss of the lateral gluteal muscles (the gluteus medius and minimus and the tensor fascia latae), but there is no cutaneous loss. The resulting changes in posture and gait are due predominantly to the loss of the two gluteal muscles, and the changes occur during weight bearing. A person with such a loss can easily stand on both feet, but must make dramatic changes to stand on one foot because the ability to prevent the pelvis from dropping on the uninvolved side is lost. To stand on one foot, the weight above the hip must be shifted well laterally (toward the involved side) so the line of gravity is positioned lateral to the hip joint. This position is neither stable nor comfortable. This same maneuver must occur during the stance phase of gait. As weight is shifted to the weight-bearing limb, the trunk shifts to that side. Since a limited time is spent in weight bearing during gait, the shift of the trunk may be less pronounced than that necessitated when standing.

Inferior Gluteal Nerve

Since this nerve supplies only the gluteus maximus muscle, there is a change in the gait pattern at heel strike and no cutaneous loss. At heel strike the gluteus maximus normally counteracts the tendency of the trunk to move forward—that is, it prevents flexion at the hip. To compensate for the loss, the trunk is shifted posteriorly so the ground reaction is positioned posterior to the hip joint. To add support to this maneuver, the patient may position his or her hand below the buttock and push the femur forward. Although there is little or no hip extensor activity necessary to maintain the upright position while standing, the line of gravity passes only slightly posterior to the hip joint so the patient may lean somewhat posteriorly to increase the feeling of stability.

Femoral Nerve

Loss of the femoral nerve results in denervation of the muscles in the anterior compartment of the thigh and the skin of most of the anterior thigh and the medial knee, leg, and foot. The anterior compartment muscles, essentially the quadriceps femoris, are active throughout the stance phase of gait and are solely responsible for preventing flexion at the knee. The major compensatory movement resulting from such a loss is the locking of the knee so the limb can support the body weight. The maneuvers involved in locking the knee are described on page 200. The rectus femoris muscle is also a flexor of the thigh, but its loss does not affect gait significantly because the iliopsoas is the main flexor at the hip.

Obturator Nerve

The obturator nerve supplies all of the muscles of the medial thigh, with the constant exception of the posterior portion of the adductor magnus. Loss of these muscles is discussed on page 209.

Tibial Nerve

The tibial nerve supplies all of the muscles in the posterior compartment of the leg and, through its medial and lateral plantar branches, all of the plantar intrinsic muscles of the foot. The major contribution to gait provided by all of these muscles occurs at push-off, when the plantar flexors push against the ground and propel the body forward. Loss of these muscles, specifically the gastrocnemius and the soleus, which are the strongest plantar flexors, virtually eliminates the push against the ground. There are no compensatory changes in position that are necessary to maintain the upright posture, nor is there any muscular substitution that can generate the push against the ground. The result of this loss is a definitive lag in forward progress at the point of heel-off. Loss of the flexor hallucis longus would appear to add to the loss of push-off since the great toe is the final part of the foot to leave the ground. Branches of the tibial nerve also supply most of the skin of the foot including the heel. The sensory information (proprioception and exteroception) transmitted through the tibial nerve provides valuable information relative to foot placement and position, and is an important part of the gait reflexes. Loss of this information may well cause an unsteady gait, particularly in the dark.

Deep Peroneal Nerve

A deep peroneal nerve injury results in loss of the muscles in the anterior compartment of the leg and on the dorsum of the foot, along with a small cutaneous area between the dorsal aspects of the great and second toes. The loss of both the cutaneous sensation and the dorsal intrinsic muscles of the foot is of little consequence. However, the loss of the anterior compartment muscles, primarily the tibialis anterior, results in a significant deviation in gait during both the stance and swing phases. The consequences of both a paralyzed and a weakened tibialis anterior muscle are described on page 232.

Superficial Peroneal Nerve

Loss of the superficial peroneal nerve results in paralysis of the muscles in the lateral compartment of the leg as well as loss of the cutaneous sensibility on the distal anterior leg and most of the dorsum of the foot. The cutaneous loss has little effect on gait. Loss of the peroneus longus and brevis muscles affects gait throughout the stance phase; the loss involves both positioning and stability of the foot. As the major evertors of the foot, the peroneal muscles balance the strong invertors and are necessary to maintain the neutral position of the foot. Loss of these muscles results in a chronically inverted foot, and weight is borne more laterally than normal. Additionally, important lateral stability of the ankle is lost making the ankle more vulnerable to inversion sprains.

Common Peroneal Nerve

Obviously, a common peroneal nerve injury is the same as injuries to both the deep and superficial peroneal nerves. There is little problem with quiet standing; however, gait is affected substantially. The most obvious loss and resulting changes in the gait pattern are due to loss of those muscles supplied by the deep peroneal nerve so that a pronounced steppage gait results. The balance between both inversion and eversion, and plantar and dorsiflexion, is lost, resulting in a foot that is statically plantar flexed (by all of the muscles in the posterior compartment of the leg) and inverted (by the deep muscles in the posterior compartment). The foot is thus positioned where the ankle has the least bony support (plantar flexion), and it is inverted so that it is especially vulnerable to inversion sprains.

Sciatic Nerve

An injury of the sciatic nerve in the gluteal region results in loss of all muscles below the knee as well as the posterior muscles of the thigh, in addition to denervation of the skin of the distal leg and foot except for their medial aspects. This loss is the same as a combined loss of the tibial and common peroneal nerves and all branches of the sciatic in the thigh. Since all hip musculature, except the hamstrings, and the extensors of the leg are intact, the limb can bear weight. However, in ambulating with no assistive devices, the limb can be used for little more than a rigid support that must be gingerly positioned on the ground. The leg must be fully extended to support and maintain weight, thus creating a vaulting gait. Loss of dorsiflexion produces a steppage gait; loss of the plantar flexors results in no push-off; loss of all muscles crossing the ankle produces an unstable ankle; and loss of both the intrinsic and extrinsic muscles of the foot results in poorly supported arches.

This chapter begins with a discussion of the structures found in the anterior cervical triangle and is followed by sections on the bones that form the skull, the various areas of the skull, and the contents of the cranial cavity. Thereafter, the majority of the discussion is centered around the cranial nerves. Both the anatomy and function of each nerve are considered. The discussion of each nerve includes its course, the types of fibers it contains, the structures it innervates and their functions, and, for most of the nerves, appropriate tests to evaluate the nerve. The discussion of each nerve also includes the head and neck anatomy that is relevant to the understanding of the nerve; for example, a description of the muscles of facial expression is included in the section on the facial nerve (CN VII).

Head and Neck

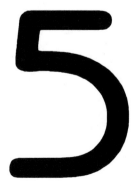

Anterior Cervical Triangle

The **anterior cervical triangle** (Fig. 5-1) is bounded medially by the midline, posteriorly by the anterior border of the sternocleidomastoid muscle, and superiorly by the inferior margin of the body of the mandible. Although a definitive floor limiting the depth of this triangle is not described, the structures encountered within this region extend posteriorly to the bodies of the cervical vertebrae. The contents include the thyroid and parathyroid glands, the inferior portion of the pharynx, the larynx and trachea, the esophagus, the infrahyoid muscles, and several major neurovascular structures. The skin of the anterior neck is supplied by branches of the transverse cervical nerve (C2, C3). The subcutaneous tissue in the area contains the large, flat platysma muscle, a muscle of facial expression. The investing layer of cervical fascia, covering the structures within the anterior triangle, is continuous posteriorly with the fascia of both the sternocleidomastoid and trapezius muscles.

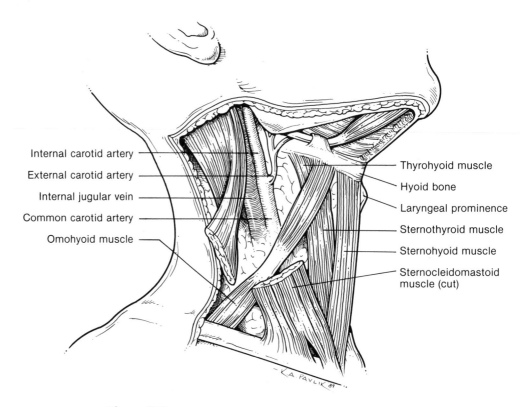

Internal carotid artery
External carotid artery
Internal jugular vein
Common carotid artery
Omohyoid muscle

Thyrohyoid muscle
Hyoid bone
Laryngeal prominence
Sternothyroid muscle
Sternohyoid muscle
Sternocleidomastoid muscle (cut)

Figure 5-1
Superficial view of the anterior cervical triangle.

Visceral Structures of the Neck

The **visceral structures** in the neck are a portion of the pharynx, the larynx and trachea, the esophagus, and the thyroid and parathyroid glands. The **pharynx** is a portion of both the respiratory and gastrointestinal systems; located posterior to the oral and nasal cavities, it is continuous with both. The most inferior portion of the pharynx, the laryngopharynx, extends into the upper part of the neck, where it separates into the esophagus and larynx. The **esophagus** (Fig. 5-2), collapsed except when transmitting food, descends through the neck just anterior to the cervical vertebrae. The **larynx** is anterior to the esophagus and extends from vertebral level C3 to C6, where it is continuous with the trachea. The larynx is composed of a system of cartilages and fibrous membranes that both maintain a patent airway and are responsible for the production and regulation of sound. A series of intrinsic laryngeal muscles, all supplied by branches of the vagus nerve (CN X), regulate the positions of the cartilages and vocal ligaments, thus determining the various parameters of the voice. The **trachea** (Fig. 5-2) passes inferiorly into the thorax.

The **thyroid** and **parathyroid** glands are endocrine glands that are closely related to the larynx. The thyroid gland is composed of large left and right lobes that are related to the lateral aspects of the larynx and upper part of the trachea and connected across the midline by the isth-

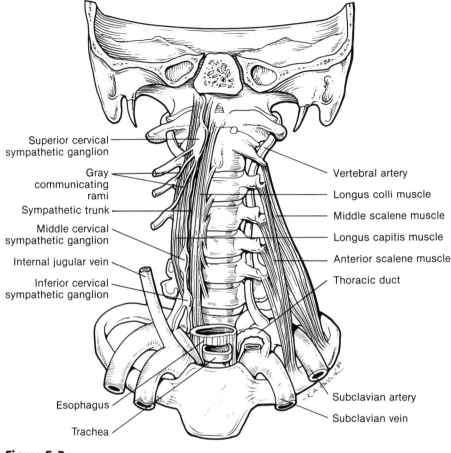

Superior cervical sympathetic ganglion

Gray communicating rami

Sympathetic trunk

Middle cervical sympathetic ganglion

Internal jugular vein

Inferior cervical sympathetic ganglion

Vertebral artery

Longus colli muscle

Middle scalene muscle

Longus capitis muscle

Anterior scalene muscle

Thoracic duct

Esophagus

Trachea

Subclavian artery

Subclavian vein

Figure 5-2
Deep structures of the anterior neck.

mus. The parathyroid glands, usually two pairs, are located on the posterior aspects of the thyroid gland.

Vascular Structures of the Neck

The **common carotid artery** (Fig. 5-1), along with the internal jugular vein and the vagus nerve, is encased in a tubular fascial sheath called the carotid sheath. The common carotid artery is deep to the sternocleidomastoid muscle and follows a line that interconnects the sternoclavicular joint and the midpoint between the mastoid process and the angle of the mandible. At the level of the interval between the hyoid bone (C3) and the laryngeal prominence (C4), the common carotid branches into the **internal** and **external carotid arteries.** The internal carotid artery has no branches in the neck and ascends through the carotid canal into the cranial cavity, supplying its contents as well as those of the orbit. The branches of the external carotid artery supply the structures of the anterior neck and face. Although the common carotid artery is readily palpable at any point, it should be palpated routinely *only inferior to the thyroid prominence.* Stimulation of the pressure-sensitive receptors within the carotid bifurcation can cause a pronounced drop in blood pressure, which can cause fainting.

The largest venous channel of the neck is the **internal jugular vein** (Fig. 5-1). This vessel begins at the base of the skull, at the jugular foramen, where it receives the venous blood from the cranial cavity. As it descends through the neck it receives multiple small veins that drain various structures of the neck and face. In a root of the neck the internal jugular vein joins the subclavian vein to form the brachiocephalic vein. The smaller **external jugular vein** drains more superficial structures; it usually begins in the region of the parotid gland and descends superficially across the sternocleidomastoid muscle before emptying into the subclavian vein.

Nerves of the Anterior Neck

The **vagus nerve** (CN X) descends through the neck with the common carotid artery and the internal jugular vein. Along its course in the neck it provides branches to the pharynx and larynx as well as to the heart. The vagus nerve then descends into the thorax.

The **phrenic nerve** contains fibers from spinal cord segments C3–C5. This nerve is formed on the anterior aspect of the anterior scalene muscle, crosses that muscle obliquely, and descends into the thorax.

The **cervical portion of the sympathetic trunk** (Fig. 5-2) is located on the anterior aspects of the longus capitis and colli muscles and usually consists of only three ganglia. The superior cervical ganglion is very large and positioned at the base of the skull; the smaller middle and inferior ganglia are found in the more inferior portion of the neck. All three ganglia provide gray communicating rami to cervical spinal nerves, and the superior ganglion has branches to cranial nerves and the periarterial plexuses through which most structures of the head receive sympathetic innervation.

Muscles of the Anterior Neck

The **infrahyoid muscles** (Fig. 5-1), commonly called the "strap muscles," cover the thyroid gland anteriorly. These small muscles are flat and extend from the hyoid bone to the thyroid cartilage of the larynx, the sternum, and the scapula. The muscles are arranged in two layers, and each muscle is named for its attachments. The superficial layer consists of the **sternohyoid** medially and the **omohyoid** laterally; the latter consists of two muscular bellies and extends from the hyoid bone to the superior aspect of the scapula (*omos* = shoulder). The deeper layer is composed of the **thyrohyoid** and the **sternothyroid.** These muscles depress the larynx and floor of the mouth during vocalization and swallowing.

The **longus capitis** and **colli muscles** (Fig. 5-2) are the deepest anterior muscles of the neck. These muscles are slightly oblique or vertical in orientation and interconnect the anterolateral aspects of the vertebral bodies and the transverse processes. The longus capitis extends from the occipital bone to lower cervical levels, the longus cervicis, from vertebra C1 to the upper thoracic levels. These two muscles, acting bilaterally, are the major flexors of the entire cervical spine. Functioning unilaterally, they produce rotation and side bending of the neck. Both muscles are innervated by branches of the ventral rami of the cervical nerves.

The **anterior, middle,** and **posterior scalene muscles** (Fig. 5-2) form most of the floor of the posterior cervical triangle and extend from the transverse processes of cervical vertebrae to the upper two ribs. Their role in thoracic outlet syndrome was discussed on page 60. Bilateral action produces flexion of the middle and lower portions of the cervical spine; unilateral activity results in rotation and side bending. These muscles also are supplied by branches of the cervical ventral rami.

Skull

The 29 bones of the skull (Fig. 5-3) can be grouped into those forming the calvaria, face, floor of the cranial cavity, orbit, nasal cavity, oral cavity, infratemporal fossa, and pterygopalatine fossa, and those occupying the middle ear cavity. However, a number of the bones participate in the formation of two or more of these areas. Most of the bones of the skull are constructed differently than many of the rest of the bones of the

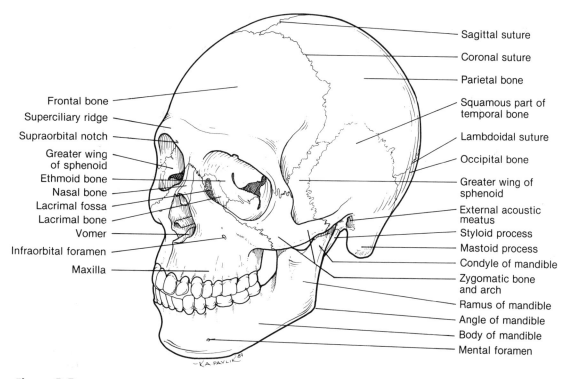

Figure 5-3
Anterolateral view of the bones of the skull.

body because they have no weight-bearing function and for the most part do not provide attachments for strong muscles. Although the mandible and the bones that encase the brain are strong and flat, many of the remaining bones are quite irregular in shape and delicate. In fact, portions of some of these bones are paper thin.

The **calvaria** (Fig. 5-3), or "skull cap," is formed primarily by the **frontal bone** anteriorly, the **occipital bone** posteriorly, with the paired **parietal bones** interposed between the two. The parietal bones are joined by the **sagittal suture,** which is continuous posteriorly between the occipital and both parietal bones as the **lambdoidal suture.** Anteriorly, the parietal bones are joined to the frontal bone through the **coronal suture.**

The Face

The **face** (Fig. 5-3) is formed superiorly by the **frontal bone** and inferiorly by the **mandible.** The two **maxillary bones** form the majority of the cheeks and meet in the midline inferior to the nose. Laterally, the maxillae (singular: *maxilla*) articulate with the **zygomatic bones,** which form the zygomatic portions of the face. Superiorly and medially, the two small **nasal bones** articulate with both the frontal bone and the maxillae and form the bridge of the nose. The mandible consists of an anterior body and posterosuperior ramus, which are joined at the angle of the mandible. The superior aspect of the ramus has two projections: the anterior coronoid process and the posterior condylar process, whose head articulates with the temporal bone to form the temporomandibular joint. Anteriorly, the bodies of the two mandibles are fused in the midline. Three large foramina open onto the face: the **supraorbital foramen** in the frontal bone, the **infraorbital foramen** in the maxilla, and the **mental foramen** in the mandible.

Cranial Cavity

The **floor of the cranial cavity** (Fig. 5-4) can be separated into the anterior, middle, and posterior cranial fossae. The **anterior cranial fossa** is formed predominantly by the **orbital plate of the frontal bone** as well as the **cribriform plate** and **crista galli of the ethmoid** medially and the **lesser wing** and **body of the sphenoid** posteriorly. These bones separate the anterior fossa from the more inferiorly positioned nasal cavity, ethmoid sinuses, and orbit. The multiple perforations in the cribriform plate of the ethmoid form a communication between the anterior fossa and the nasal cavity.

The **middle cranial fossa** (Fig. 5-4) has a median or central portion and two lateral areas. The central portion is formed by the **body of the sphenoid,** which consists of the **chiasmatic groove** anteriorly and the **sella turcica** posteriorly. The **optic canal** forms a communication between the orbit and the central part of the middle cranial fossa. The **lateral portion of the middle fossa** is formed primarily by the **greater wing of the sphenoid,** but also by the **squamous** and **petrous portions of the temporal bone.** This fossa is related inferiorly to the infratemporal fossa and the middle ear cavity, medially to the sphenoid sinus, and anteromedially to

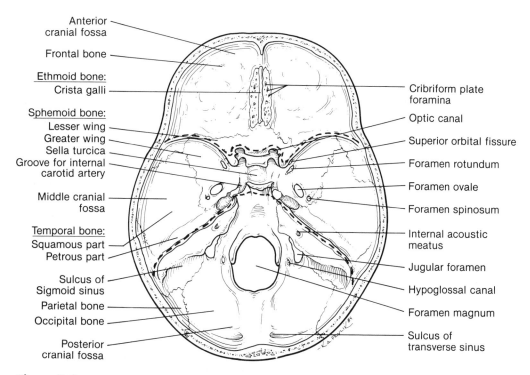

Anterior cranial fossa
Frontal bone
Ethmoid bone:
Crista galli
Sphemoid bone:
Lesser wing
Greater wing
Sella turcica
Groove for internal carotid artery
Middle cranial fossa
Temporal bone:
Squamous part
Petrous part
Sulcus of Sigmoid sinus
Parietal bone
Occipital bone
Posterior cranial fossa

Cribriform plate foramina
Optic canal
Superior orbital fissure
Foramen rotundum
Foramen ovale
Foramen spinosum
Internal acoustic meatus
Jugular foramen
Hypoglossal canal
Foramen magnum
Sulcus of transverse sinus

Figure 5-4
Superior view of the bones forming the floor of the cranial cavity. The anterior, middle, and posterior cranial fossae are delineated by broken lines.

the orbit. There are multiple openings between the lateral portion of the middle cranial fossa and adjacent areas of the skull: the **superior orbital fissure** with the orbit, the **foramen rotundum** with the pterygopalatine fossa, the **foramen ovale** and **foramen spinosum** with the infratemporal fossa, and the **hiatus of the facial canal** with the facial canal. The **foramen lacerum** is not an actual opening, its floor being filled by connective tissue.

The **posterior cranial fossa** (Fig. 5-4) is the largest of the fossae and is formed predominantly by the **occipital bone.** In addition, the **dorsum sellae of the sphenoid** is anterior and the **petrous and mastoid portions of the temporal bone** are lateral. Inferiorly, the large single **foramen magnum** is the communication between the cranial cavity and the vertebral canal. The other major openings in the posterior fossa are the **internal auditory meatus** (which is continuous with the facial canal), the **jugular foramen,** and the **hypoglossal canal.**

Orbit

The **orbit** (Fig. 5-3) is nearly pyramidal in shape, its base formed by the rim of the orbital opening and its apex directed posteromedially. Its walls are formed superiorly by the **orbital plate of the frontal bone,** laterally by the **greater wing of the sphenoid** and the **zygomatic bone,** inferiorly by the **maxilla,** and medially by the **maxilla, lacrimal, ethmoid,** and **palatine**

bones. The orbit is related superiorly to the anterior cranial fossa and the frontal sinus, laterally to the middle cranial fossa, medially to the ethmoid sinuses and inferiorly to the maxillary sinus.

Nasal Cavity

The **nasal cavity** is triangular in coronal section, its floor being considerably wider than its apex. The lateral wall is formed by the **maxillary, palatine, and ethmoid bones** and the **inferior nasal concha,** the floor by the **palatine process of the maxilla** and the **palatine bone,** and the roof by the **cribriform plate of the ethmoid.** The **nasal septum,** consisting of bony (**vomer** and the **perpendicular plate of the ethmoid**) and cartilaginous portions, separates the cavity into right and left portions. The nasal cavity is related inferiorly to the oral cavity, posteriorly to the pharynx, laterally to the maxillary and ethmoid sinuses, and superiorly to the anterior cranial fossa and the frontal sinus.

Oral Cavity

The walls of the **oral cavity** are only partially bony since both the floor and lateral walls are predominantly muscular. The roof of the oral cavity is the palate, which is formed anteriorly by the **maxilla** and **palatine bones (hard palate)** and posteriorly by muscular tissue **(soft palate).** Although both the maxillae and mandible would appear to form portions of the anterior and lateral walls, they form neither because a part of each bone extends into the cavity. The oral cavity is related superiorly to the nasal cavity and the maxillary sinuses and is continuous posteriorly with the pharynx.

Deeper Areas of the Skull

The **infratemporal fossa** is located inferior to the middle cranial fossa and medial to the ramus of the mandible, and is limited medially by the pterygoid portion of the sphenoid. Its major contents are structures related to mastication.

The **pterygopalatine fossa** is a small crevice located between the maxillary and sphenoid bones, and between the nasal cavity and the infratemporal fossa. It is mentioned here only because it contains the maxillary nerve and pterygopalatine ganglion.

The **middle ear (tympanic) cavity** is a cavitation within the petrous portion of the temporal bone. This cavity contains a series of three very small bones, the **malleus, incus,** and **stapes,** which transmit the motion of the tympanic membrane across the middle ear cavity to the internal ear.

Contents of the Cranial Cavity

The neural structures within the cranial vault are the brain, brain stem, and proximal portions of the cranial nerves (Fig. 5-5). The **frontal lobes**

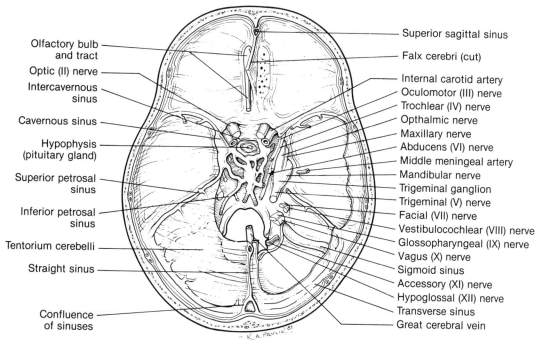

Olfactory bulb and tract
Optic (II) nerve
Intercavernous sinus
Cavernous sinus
Hypophysis (pituitary gland)
Superior petrosal sinus
Inferior petrosal sinus
Tentorium cerebelli
Straight sinus
Confluence of sinuses

Superior sagittal sinus
Falx cerebri (cut)
Internal carotid artery
Oculomotor (III) nerve
Trochlear (IV) nerve
Opthalmic nerve
Maxillary nerve
Abducens (VI) nerve
Middle meningeal artery
Mandibular nerve
Trigeminal ganglion
Trigeminal (V) nerve
Facial (VII) nerve
Vestibulocochlear (VIII) nerve
Glossopharyngeal (IX) nerve
Vagus (X) nerve
Sigmoid sinus
Accessory (XI) nerve
Hypoglossal (XII) nerve
Transverse sinus
Great cerebral vein

Figure 5-5
Superior view of the cranial cavity, showing the positions of the neurovascular structures and the dural septa.

of the brain occupy the anterior cranial fossa. The **temporal lobes** occupy the lateral portions of the middle cranial fossa. In the central portion of the middle cranial fossa, the **hypophysis (pituitary gland)** occupies the sella turcica and the **optic chiasm** the chiasmatic groove. The posterior fossa contains both the **cerebellum** and the majority of the **brain stem.** The two lobes of the cerebellum fill the fossa posterior and lateral to the foramen magnum, and the brain stem sits on the inclined plane that is found anteriorly. The junction of the brain stem and spinal cord is positioned at about the level of the foramen magnum; the midbrain is at the level of the dorsum sellae.

Meninges and Meningeal Specializations

The **meningeal coverings of the brain** are generally similar to those that surround the spinal cord. Both the **pia mater** and **arachnoid** are related to the brain much the same way as they are related to the spinal cord (see page 45). The **cranial dura mater,** however, differs substantially both in the way it is related to the bones of the skull and due to the presence of **dural septa** and **dural venous sinuses.** At the point where the cranial and spinal layers of dura mater are continuous, the foramen magnum, the cranial dura fuses with the periosteum on the deep surface of the bones of the skull. As a result, there is no actual epidural space in the cranial cavity as there is in the vertebral canal. Even though the attachment of the dura to the bone is rather firm, it can be separated from the bone by a collection of blood as in the case of an epidural hematoma. The two layers of the dura mater, even though fused, are named separately. The layer adjacent to the bone is the **periosteal layer of dura,** and the layer next to the arachnoid is the **meningeal layer.**

At various locations the meningeal layer separates from the periosteal layer and forms a septum (a **dural septum**) that extends centrally into the cranial cavity and thus separates parts of the brain. The major dural septa (Fig. 5-5) are the **falx cerebri,** which separates the hemispheres of the brain, the **tentorium cerebelli,** which separates the occipital lobes from the cerebellum, the **falx cerebelli,** which partially separates the right and left portions of the cerebellum, and the **diaphragm sellae,** which partially encloses the hypophysis.

The **dural venous sinuses** (Fig. 5-5) are a system of venous channels within the dura, most of which are formed between the two layers. These sinuses are valveless, enabling blood flow in either direction, and are connected to veins outside of the cranial cavity by a number of **emissary veins.** The blood in these sinuses usually drains toward the jugular foramen, where the sigmoid and inferior petrosal sinuses are continuous with the internal jugular vein. The **superior** and **inferior sagittal sinuses** are within the falx cerebri. These two sinuses are connected posteriorly by the straight sinus, which is located at the junction of the falx cerebri and the tentorium cerebelli. The **great cerebral vein,** a large vein conveying blood from the brain to the sinuses, joins the inferior sagittal sinus to form the straight sinus. The junction of the straight and superior sagittal sinuses is the **confluens of sinuses,** from which point the two **transverse sinuses** pass laterally in the fixed edge of the tentorium cerebelli. These sinuses turn inferiorly toward the jugular foramina as the **sigmoid sinuses.** The **cavernous sinuses** are large sinuses on either side of the sella turcica. These sinuses have emissary connections with the veins of the face via veins in the orbit, are connected to the transverse sinuses through the **superior petrosal sinuses,** and communicate with the sigmoid sinuses via the **inferior petrosal sinuses.**

The cranial dura mater is supplied by the **anterior, middle,** and **posterior meningeal arteries.** The middle meningeal artery (Fig. 5-5), a branch of the maxillary artery, is the largest of the three and supplies the dura of most of the cranial cavity. This artery is encased in dura and usually occupies a groove on the deep surface of the bones of the skull. Its position makes it vulnerable to fractures of the skull; fractures that cross the path of the artery may lacerate both the artery and the layer of dura separating it from the bone, resulting in an **epidural hematoma.** The anterior and posterior ethmoidal arteries are small and supply portions of the anterior and posterior cranial fossae, respectively.

Cranial Nerves and Related Structures

Most of the cranial nerves are similar to the spinal nerves in that they contain different types (functional components) of nerve fibers. They differ, however, in several respects. First, in addition to the fibers designated as "general," the cranial nerves contain the "special" components (see page 14) that innervate structures of the head and neck. Second, the cranial nerves contain varying numbers of fiber types; in fact, some contain only one. Third, certain types of fibers branch from one cranial nerve to branches of another as they pass toward their destinations. For example, parasympathetic fibers exit from the brain stem in cranial nerves III, VII, IX, and X, but many reach their target organs in branches of the fifth cranial nerve.

Cranial Nerve I

The fibers of the **olfactory nerve** are multiple and short. They are special visceral afferent neurons that innervate the olfactory epithelium in the superior aspect of the nasal cavity. The nerve fibers pass superiorly, through the openings in the cribriform plate of the ethmoid, into the anterior cranial fossa. There they synapse with neurons of the olfactory tract, whose cell bodies are located in the olfactory bulb (Fig. 5-5). The olfactory bulb and tract are positioned on the floor of the anterior cranial fossa, and both are part of the rhinencephalon, or "smell brain." Lesions of the olfactory system affect the perception of smell.

Cranial Nerve II

The **optic nerve** is a segment of the afferent system that connects the receptor cells of the retina with the visual cortex. This nerve, composed of special somatic afferent neurons, extends from the middle cranial fossa to the bulb of the eye. In the central part of the middle cranial fossa it is continuous with the optic chiasm and tract. It enters the orbit through the optic canal (Fig. 5-5) and extends to the eyeball through the center of the orbit. All three layers of meninges extend along the nerve to its junction with the eyeball, thus forming a sleeve of subarachnoid space and cerebrospinal fluid that surrounds the nerve. Since the central artery and vein of the retina are within the nerve, changes in cerebrospinal fluid pressure can affect the flow of blood in these vessels and can be detected by examination of the vessels within the eyeball. A lesion involving the optic nerve affects visual acuity. This nerve is the afferent limb of the pupillary light reflex.

Cranial Nerves III, IV, and VI

The **oculomotor (III), trochlear (IV),** and **abducens (VI) nerves** are discussed together because they innervate the extraocular muscles of the eye. Since these muscles work in concert to control the movements of the eyeball, it is helpful to consider these muscles and nerves together. The description of the muscles precedes the discussions of the three nerves.

Extraocular eye muscles. The mechanics of the movements of the eyeball and the actions of the extraocular muscles are complicated by the differences in the orientation of the **orbital** and **visual axes.** Each orbit is pyramidal in shape with its apex directed posteromedially and its base directed anterolaterally. As a result of this orientation, the axes of the orbits, which pass through the centers of both the apices and bases, diverge from each other as they are projected anteriorly. The visual axes correspond to the lines of vision of the eyes and thus are anteroposteriorly oriented and nearly parallel. Thus, the orbital and visual axes differ.

The eyeball can be deviated medially (**adduction**), laterally (**abduction**), superiorly (**elevation**), and inferiorly (**depression**), and it can be rotated. Rotation is described by the direction of the superior aspect of the eyeball (12 o'clock). If that point moves medially or toward the nose the movement is **intortion**; if that point moves laterally, the motion is **extortion**. Functionally, however, most motions of the eyeball are combinations of these movements.

The **extraocular muscles** consist of the **superior, inferior, medial, and lateral rectus muscles,** the **superior** and **inferior oblique muscles,** and the **levator palpebrae superiorus muscle.** The levator palpebrae superiorus elevates the upper eyelid, while the rest of the muscles position the eyeball. The specific actions of each muscle, acting independently, are listed in Table 5-1. The four rectus muscles extend from the apex of the orbit to the eyeball and are named by their positions. If the orbital and visual axes corresponded, each of these muscles would produce a single motion; the superior rectus would elevate the eyeball, the lateral would abduct, and so forth. Because the axes are not the same, only the medial and lateral rectus muscles produce single motions; the superior and inferior recti generate motions in addition to elevation and depression. Pure elevation and depression are possible because of the presence of the oblique muscles. These two muscles are positioned above (superior oblique) and below (inferior oblique) the eyeball. The lines of action of both muscles are toward the anteromedial aspect of the orbit.

Even though most of the extraocular muscles are capable of multiple actions, the eyeball can be positioned so each muscle is limited to a predominant motion and thus can be tested. To do this, the examiner asks the patient to follow his or her finger as it draws the letter "H." Adduction

Table 5-1   Extraocular Muscle Functions (Each Muscle Acting Independently)

Muscle	Elevation / Depression	Adduction / Abduction	Intorsion / Extorsion
Lateral rectus	—	Abduction	—
Medial rectus	—	Adduction	—
Superior rectus	Elevation	Adduction	Intorsion
Inferior rectus	Depression	Adduction	Extorsion
Superior oblique	Depression	Abduction	Intorsion
Inferior oblique	Elevation	Abduction	Extorsion

tests the medial rectus; elevation of the adducted eye tests the inferior oblique; and depression of the adducted eye tests the superior oblique. Abduction tests the lateral rectus; elevation of the abducted eye tests the superior rectus; and depression of the abducted eye tests the inferior rectus.

The **oculomotor nerve** (CN III) contains general somatic efferent fibers to most of the extraocular muscles and general visceral efferent fibers to certain of the smooth muscles of the eyeball. This nerve emerges from the interpeduncular fossa of the midbrain between the posterior cerebral and superior cerebellar arteries in the posterior cranial fossa. It crosses the free edge of the tentorium cerebelli, passes through the cavernous sinus (Fig. 5-5), and enters the orbit through the superior orbital fissure. It supplies the levator palpebrae superiorus, the inferior oblique, and the superior, medial, and inferior rectus muscles. In addition, it has a branch (containing preganglionic parasympathetic fibers) to the **ciliary ganglion.** In this ganglion, these fibers synapse with postganglionic parasympathetic neurons that pass to the eyeball and innervate the **ciliary muscle,** which controls the thickness of the lens, and the **sphincter pupillae muscle,** which reduces the size of the pupil. Loss of the oculomotor nerve results in diplopia (double vision), mydriasis (dilated pupil), ptosis (drooping eyelid), and lateral strabismus (statically laterally deviated eye). In addition, the patient is incapable of active movement of the eye medially or superiorly and the accommodation-convergence reaction is lost. The integrity of the third cranial nerve can be evaluated by testing the extraocular muscles it innervates (see above) and by the pupillary light and accommodation-convergence reflexes.

The **trochlear nerve** (CN IV) contains only the general somatic efferent fibers that supply the superior oblique muscle. This nerve emerges from the dorsal aspect of the midbrain and passes ventrally around the brain stem, just inferior to the tentorium cerebelli. It passes through the cavernous sinus (Fig. 5-5) along its lateral wall, enters the orbit through the superior orbital fissure, and then passes directly to the superior oblique muscle. Loss of this nerve results in diplopia and a statically deviated eye that is directed somewhat medially and superiorly and in an active inability to depress the adducted eye.

The **abducens nerve** (CN VI) also contains only general somatic efferent fibers and supplies only the lateral rectus muscle. This nerve arises from the ventral aspect of the brain stem, just lateral to the midline at the pons-medulla junction. It passes anteriorly and pierces the dura on the basilar portion of the occipital bone (Fig. 5-5); it then enters the cavernous sinus, where it is the most medial of the nerves in that sinus. The abducens nerve enters the orbit through the superior orbital fissure and then passes laterally toward the lateral rectus muscle. Loss of this nerve results in a medial strabismus and the loss of active abduction of the eye.

Cranial Nerve V

The **trigeminal nerve** (Fig. 5-6) contains both general somatic afferent and special visceral efferent fibers. This nerve provides all the general

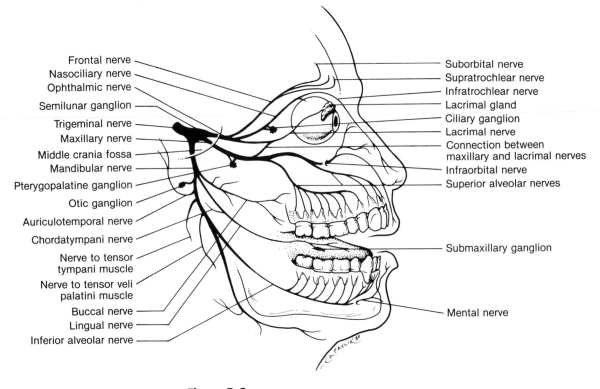

Figure 5-6
Trigeminal nerve (CN V) and its branches.

sensory innervation of the head anterior to vertical planes that parallel the petrous portions of the temporal bones, including the skin of the face and the cornea, the membranes that line the cavities of the head (sinuses, and nasal and oral cavities) and the deep receptors in the muscles, tendons, and ligaments. The special visceral efferent fibers supply the muscles of mastication.

The trigeminal nerve emerges from the anterolateral aspect of the pons at about the midpons level. It passes anterolaterally and pierces the dura of the posterior cranial fossa, just inferior to the tentorium cerebelli (Fig. 5-5). The main trunk of the nerve terminates in the middle cranial fossa, where it joins the **trigeminal (semilunar) ganglion,** which occupies a depression near the apex of the petrous portion of the temporal bone. This ganglion contains the cell bodies of the general somatic afferent neurons that form the majority of the nerve. Distal to the ganglion, the trigeminal nerve branches into its three divisions: the **ophthalmic, maxillary,** and **mandibular nerves.** An additional portion of the trigeminal nerve, the **motor root,** contains the special visceral efferent fibers. This root passes deep to the ganglion before becoming part of the mandibular nerve.

The **ophthalmic nerve** (Figs. 5-5, 5-6) contains only general somatic afferent fibers and is the most superior of the three terminal branches of the trigeminal nerve. It begins as the most medial extension of the trigeminal ganglion where it is positioned within the cavernous sinus. After passing through the sinus, the nerve enters the orbit via the superior orbital fissure, then separates into its terminal branches. These branches include the frontal nerve (which in turn branches into the supraorbital and supratrochlear nerves), the lacrimal nerve, and the nasociliary nerve (which provides branches to the nasal cavity, ethmoid air cells, and the bulb of the eye). These branches supply the skin of the forehead, bridge of the nose, upper eyelid, and the cornea of the eyeball, as well as the mucous membranes of the ethmoid sinuses and part of the nasal cavity. A lesion of this nerve results in loss of general sensation in those areas. This nerve can be tested via the corneal reflex because it provides the afferent limb.

The **maxillary nerve** (Figs. 5-5, 5-6) also contains only general somatic afferent fibers. It begins from the middle portion of the trigeminal ganglion where it is the most inferior nerve in the cavernous sinus. It exits from the middle cranial fossa by passing through the foramen rotundum into the pterygopalatine fossa. The nerve has multiple branches within the fossa and continues anteriorly into the orbit as the **infraorbital nerve.** The infraorbital nerve passes along the floor of the orbit and onto the face through the infraorbital foramen. The branches within the pterygopalatine fossa supply the nasopharynx (**pharyngeal**), palate (**greater** and **lesser palatine**), maxillary teeth (**posterior superior alveolar**), and nasal cavity (**nasopalatine, lateral nasal**). In addition, the maxillary nerve has branches (**pterygoid**) that interconnect it with the **pterygopalatine ganglion.** (The preganglionic input to this ganglion is discussed with the facial nerve.) This connection is the source of the postganglionic parasympathetic fibers (secretomotor) within those branches that supply the mucous membranes of the nasal cavity, palate, and nasopharynx, as well as the lacrimal gland. While in the orbit the infraorbital nerve has branches to the maxillary teeth (**middle** and **anterior superior alveolar**), and to the lacrimal gland and anterior temporal region (**zygomatic**). The zygomatic branch contains postganglionic parasympathetic fibers to the lacrimal gland (secretomotor). The cutaneous areas supplied by branches of the maxillary nerve include the cheek, upper lip, lateral nose, lower eyelid, and anterior temporal region. A lesion of this nerve at its beginning would result in a loss of general sensation in the cutaneous areas just described, but lacrimation and secretion of the mucous membranes would be unaffected (The parasympathetic fibers would be affected only if the lesion involved the branches distal to the ganglion or the facial nerve or certain of its branches.) The maxillary nerve can be evaluated only by testing general sensation in the appropriate areas.

The **mandibular nerve** (Figs. 5-5, 5-6) is the only division of the trigeminal nerve that contains both general somatic afferent and special visceral efferent fibers. It is formed by the motor root and fibers from the lateral portion of the semilunar ganglion. Its intracranial course is short because it passes into the infratemporal fossa (through the foramen ovale) soon after it begins. Its course in this fossa is also short because it divides into multiple branches high in the fossa. Several muscular branches supply the muscles of mastication (see below), the tensor tympani (a small muscle in the middle ear), and the tensor veli palatini (a muscle of the soft palate). Cutaneous branches are distributed to the lower lip and chin (**mental**), lower cheek and mandibular region (**buccal**), and posterior temporal region (**auriculotemporal**); other sensory branches supply the tongue (**lingual**) and mandibular teeth (**inferior alveolar**).

The **otic ganglion** (parasympathetic) (Fig. 5-6) is located deep to the main trunk of the mandibular nerve and near the roof of the infratemporal fossa. The mandibular nerve provides no preganglionic input to the ganglion (they are from the ninth cranial nerve), but the postganglionic fibers from the ganglion join the auriculotemporal nerve and are part of it until it passes through the parotid gland.

The **chorda tympani nerve** (Fig. 5-9), a branch of the facial nerve containing both preganglionic parasympathetic and taste (SVA) fibers, joins the lingual nerve in the infratemporal fossa. The taste fibers innervate the taste receptors on the anterior two-thirds of the tongue. The parasympathetic fibers pass to the **submandibular ganglion** (parasympathetic), which is located very close to the lingual nerve in the floor of the mouth. The postganglionic parasympathetic fibers beginning in this ganglion are the secretomotor fibers to the submandibular and sublingual salivary glands, and to the mucous membrane of the anterior two-thirds of the tongue.

A lesion involving the entire mandibular nerve as it branches from the trigeminal ganglion would result in both muscular and general sensory losses, but neither taste nor parasympathetic fibers would be affected. The loss of general sensation would involve the cutaneous areas described above as well as the lower teeth and anterior two-thirds of the tongue. All muscles of mastication (unilaterally) would be lost, resulting in an obvious asymmetry during chewing. The motor fibers of this nerve can be tested by depressing the mandible (opening the mouth) against resistance. If the muscles are paralyzed, particularly the lateral pterygoid, the mandible deviates toward the side of the lesion (see Muscles of Mastication, below). Loss of the tensor veli palatini usually causes some difficulty swallowing along with nasal speech because the palate cannot be fully elevated. The uvula deviates away from the side of the lesion. This deviation increases significantly when the patient says "ah." Loss of the tensor tympani muscle results in hypersensitivity to loud sounds (hyperacousis) because the muscle presumably functions to dampen the vibration of the ossicles in the middle ear.

Temporomandibular joint.   The temporomandibular joints (Fig. 5-7) are unique in both construction and function. Structurally, each joint contains an intra-articular disk that separates the articulation into two definitive parts. Each of these parts is constructed to permit different motions. Functionally, since the mandible is a single bone, motion always occurs at the two joints simultaneously.

The articular surfaces forming this joint are considerably different in shape. The **mandibular fossa** and **articular tubercle** of the temporal bone consist of a horizontally oriented depression positioned just posterior to an elevated (projecting inferiorly) tubercle. The mandibular **head (con-**

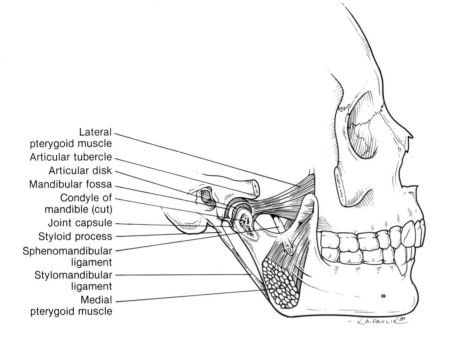

Lateral pterygoid muscle
Articular tubercle
Articular disk
Mandibular fossa
Condyle of mandible (cut)
Joint capsule
Styloid process
Sphenomandibular ligament
Stylomandibular ligament
Medial pterygoid muscle

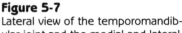

Figure 5-7
Lateral view of the temporomandibular joint and the medial and lateral pterygoid muscles.

dyle) is generally cylindrical and oriented horizontally. The articular surfaces of both bones are covered with fibrocartilage.

The **intra-articular disk** is thick and variably shaped. It is usually complete and thus separates two distinct joint cavities. The entire periphery of the disk is attached to the joint capsule; that part of the capsule between the temporal bone and the disk is quite loose, while the portion between the disk and the mandible is both thicker and tighter. Additionally, the entire lateral aspect of the capsule is reinforced by the **lateral temporomandibular ligament.** The looseness of the upper half of the capsule permits considerable excursion between the articular disk and the temporal bone. The tightness of the lower half of the capsule restricts that same type of motion between the mandibular condyle and the disk.

Both the **sphenomandibular** and **stylomandibular ligaments** (Fig. 5-7) suspend the mandible from the base of the skull. Although neither appears to have a major role in the support of the joint, both limit excursion of the mandible. The sphenomandibular ligament, particularly, plays an important role in determining mandibular movement. This ligament extends from the sphenoid bone to the lingula on the medial aspect of the mandibular ramus. Motion between the articular disk and the temporal bone occurs around a transverse axis that passes through the lingulae of the two mandibular rami. This motion involves anterior and posterior sliding of the disk and condylar process as a single unit. Such motion is produced as a result of the sling formed by the sphenomandibular ligaments. As this motion occurs anteriorly, the disk and condylar process slide "down" onto the articular tubercle.

The motion between the mandibular condyle and the disk takes place around a transverse axis through the mandibular head and consists of rotation of the condyle on the disk so that the anterior aspect of the mandible is elevated and depressed. Total motion of the mandible, therefore, is a combination of motion at two points: between the disk and temporal bone and between the disk and mandible.

When the mouth is opened the mandible is both **protracted** and **depressed.** Protraction occurs as the disk and mandible slide forward; depression occurs as the disk slides "down" onto the tubercle and as rotation occurs between the disk and mandibular head. Closing the mouth is the reverse motions and consists of **elevation** and **retraction.** The mandible can also be **deviated** to the right and left, enabling the grinding component of chewing. This oblique motion occurs predominantly between the articular disk and the temporal bone.

Muscles of mastication.   The muscles of mastication are innervated by the mandibular division of the trigeminal nerve. The **temporalis** and **masseter muscles** are located superficially; the **medial** and **lateral pterygoid muscles** are deep to the ramus of the mandible in the infratemporal fossa.

The **masseter muscle** (Fig. 5-8) virtually covers the superficial aspect of the ramus of the mandible. From an origin on the zygomatic arch, its fibers descend and insert into most of the lateral surface of the mandibular ramus. This muscle is a strong elevator of the mandible.

The **temporalis** (Fig. 5-8) is the largest of the masticatory muscles, arising from the entire temporal fossa. Its fibers converge as they descend toward an insertion on the coronoid process of the mandible. This muscle

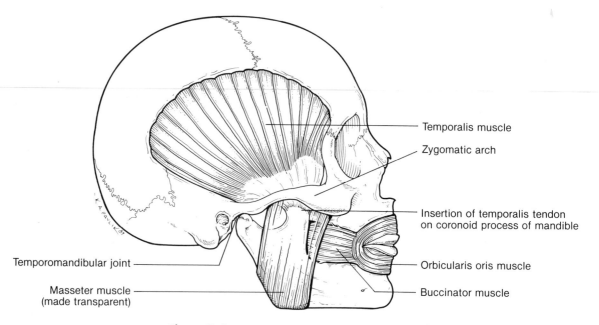

Temporalis muscle

Zygomatic arch

Insertion of temporalis tendon on coronoid process of mandible

Orbicularis oris muscle

Buccinator muscle

Temporomandibular joint

Masseter muscle
(made transparent)

Figure 5-8
Lateral view of the temporalis, masseter, buccinator, and orbicularis oris muscles.

also is a strong elevator, and its most posterior fibers are nearly horizontal and thus are oriented ideally to retract the mandible.

The **medial pterygoid muscle** (Fig. 5-7) extends from the sphenoid bone (origin) to the medial surface of the inferior aspect of the ramus of the mandible (insertion). Its vertical orientation is similar to that of the masseter, so it is an elevator of the mandible. Its insertion, however, is considerably lateral to its origin, so it can deviate the mandible to the opposite or contralateral side.

The fibers of the **lateral pterygoid muscle** (Fig. 5-7) are very nearly horizontal in orientation, and its origin is both anterior and medial to its insertion. From its origin on the sphenoid bone its fibers converge as they pass posterolaterally toward insertions on the neck of the mandible and the articular disk. Contraction of this muscle moves both the disk and mandible anteriorly (protrusion). Since the mandible slides inferiorly onto the tubercle during protrusion, the muscle is also a depressor. Like the medial pterygoid, it moves the mandible strongly to the opposite side.

Cranial Nerve VII

The **facial nerve** contains special visceral efferent fibers to the muscles of facial expression (as well as several other muscles), general visceral efferent fibers (parasympathetic) to the submandibular and pterygopalatine ganglia, special visceral afferent (taste) fibers from the anterior two-thirds of the tongue, and general somatic afferent fibers from the skin of a small portion of the external auditory meatus. The facial nerve begins in the posterior cranial fossa, where it arises from the brain stem at the lateral aspect of the pons-medulla junction (cerebellopontine angle). It then passes laterally into the internal auditory meatus of the temporal bone.

The facial nerve (Fig. 5-5) passes through the temporal bone in both the internal auditory meatus and the facial canal (which are continuous). The nerve passes first laterally, then posteriorly, and finally descends to exit from the bone through the stylomastoid foramen. In the temporal bone the nerve has several branches (Fig. 5-9). The **greater petrosal nerve** branches from the facial nerve at the **geniculate ganglion,** a sensory ganglion (taste) of the facial nerve. The preganglionic parasympathetic fibers in this branch are destined for the pterygopalatine ganglion, where they synapse with postganglionic fibers that supply the lacrimal gland and mucosa of the nasal cavity and paranasal sinuses along with the palate. The **chorda tympani nerve** branches just proximal to the stylomastoid foramen, then passes through the middle ear cavity and into the infratemporal fossa where it joins the lingual nerve. It contains preganglionic parasympathetic fibers to the submandibular ganglion and taste fibers to the anterior two thirds of the tongue.

After emerging from the stylomastoid foramen, the facial nerve passes anteriorly through the substance of the parotid gland (Fig. 5-10). Within this gland the nerve separates into multiple branches that fan out over the entire face. The branches are named regionally on the basis of the areas supplied: **temporal, zygomatic, buccal, marginal mandibular,** and

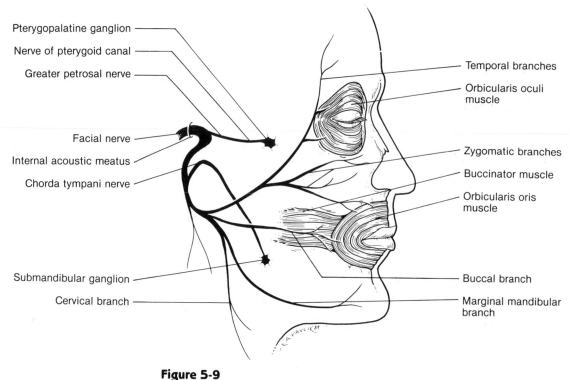

Pterygopalatine ganglion

Nerve of pterygoid canal

Greater petrosal nerve

Facial nerve

Internal acoustic meatus

Chorda tympani nerve

Submandibular ganglion

Cervical branch

Temporal branches

Orbicularis oculi muscle

Zygomatic branches

Buccinator muscle

Orbicularis oris muscle

Buccal branch

Marginal mandibular branch

Figure 5-9
Facial nerve (CN VII) and its branches.

cervical. Each of these branches contains only special visceral efferent fibers and supplies the muscles in the area to which it is distributed.

For the most part the **muscles of facial expression** (Figs. 5-9, 5-10) function to control the openings on the face—the eyes, mouth, and external nares. These skeletal muscles are different from other skeletal muscles because they attach primarily to the skin and thus move skin rather than bones. Certain muscles, the **orbicularis oris** (mouth) and **orbicularis oculi** (eye), are arranged as sphincters and thus can close the openings. Most of the remaining muscles are offshoots of these muscles and function to modify the shapes of the openings. Of particular importance is the **buccinator muscle,** which interconnects the lateral aspects of the mandible and maxilla. This is the only muscle in the interval between these bones and, thus, it alone is responsible for controlling the cheek. The buccinator plays an important role in chewing because it (along with the tongue) keeps food between the teeth. In addition, the buccinator regulates the tautness of the cheek and thus prevents it from slipping between teeth.

The other muscles innervated by the facial nerve are the **stapedius,** the **stylohyoid,** and the **posterior belly** of the **digastric.** The stapedius is a very small muscle within the middle ear that attaches to the stapes and presumably functions to dampen the vibration of the ossicles. Both the stylohyoid and posterior belly of the digastric extend from the base of the

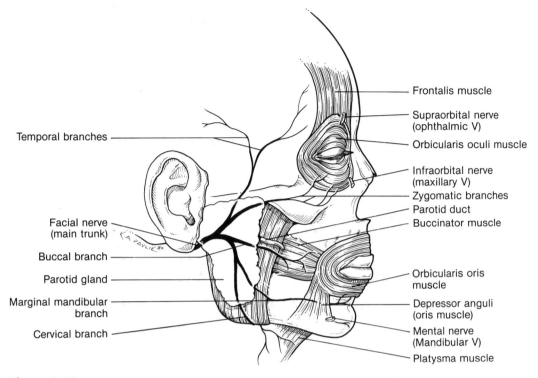

Figure 5-10
Facial nerve, parotid gland, masseter muscle, and the major muscles of facial expression.

skull to the hyoid bond and thus support the floor of the mouth, which they are capable of elevating.

A lesion affecting the facial nerve at its beginning results in a myriad of symptoms. There is a unilateral paralysis of all muscles of facial expression as well as the two muscles in the floor of the mouth and the stapedius. The face on the affected side is flat and expressionless and may be shifted (pulled) to the uninvolved side, expecially in the region of the mouth. There is an inability to wrinkle the forehead, close the eye, purse the lips, and tightly close the mouth. Fluid may leak out of the corner of the mouth, and the cheek may be lacerated internally because it gets caught between the teeth. Chewing also may be difficult because food collects laterally between the gum and cheek. Loss of the stapedius may produce a hypersensitivity to loud sounds (hyperacousis). Taste on the anterior two-thirds of the tongue also is lost. Autonomic symptoms include loss of salivary secretion of the submandibular and sublingual glands as well as part of the mucous membrane of the oral cavity, loss of secretion of the mucous membranes of the nasal cavity and paranasal sinuses, and loss of lacrimation ("dry eye"). Lesions of this nerve at various points along its course, depending on the location, produce partial losses. For example, involvement of the nerve as it passes through the parotid gland results in loss of the facial muscles, but taste and autonomic function are unaffected. **Bell's palsy** is the eponym most commonly used to describe a facial nerve paralysis. Although this term usually is used in conjunction with a unilateral paralysis of the facial muscles, the nerve may be affected at any point along its course resulting in additional symptoms.

Of the various structures innervated by the facial nerve, the muscles of facial expression are the easiest to test. Inspection and active performance of the various facial maneuvers are usually adequate for an accurate evaluation. In addition, the facial nerve is the motor limb of the corneal reflex. Taste on the anterior two-thirds of the tongue can be tested, but sometimes the results are inconclusive. Of the parasympathetic functions, lacrimation is the easiest to evaluate and certainly a major problem for a patient, particularly with a complete lesion of the facial nerve because the eye cannot be closed.

Cranial Nerve VIII

The **vestibulocochlear nerve** contains special somatic afferent fibers from the organs of both hearing (cochlea) and equilibrium (semicircular canals, utricle, saccule) that are located within the temporal bone in the internal ear. This nerve begins in the posterior cranial fossa, where it joins the brain stem as the most lateral nerve at the pons-medulla junction (cerebellopontine angle). It has a very short course in the posterior fossa, passing laterally into the internal auditory meatus (Fig. 5-5). Its course in that canal is also short. After only a few millimeters, the nerve separates into its vestibular and cochlear portions, and each passes to the nearby organs it supplies. Interference in the function of the vestibular fibers affects balance and postural reflexes; interference with the function of cochlear fibers affects hearing.

Cranial Nerve IX

The **glossopharyngeal nerve** contains general visceral afferent fibers from the middle ear, pharynx, posterior tongue, and carotid sinus, special visceral afferent fibers (taste) from the posterior tongue, and general visceral efferent (parasympathetic) fibers to the parotid gland. In addition, it contains a small number of general somatic afferent fibers from the external ear and special visceral efferent fibers to the small stylopharyngeus muscle in the pharynx. It arises in the posterior cranial fossa, as the most superior nerve in the postolivary sulcus, and then passes laterally and exits from the cranial cavity through the jugular foramen (Fig. 5-5).

The glossopharyngeal nerve descends along the stylopharyngeus muscle, has branches to the pharyngeal plexus and carotid sinus, and finally passes across the tonsilar fossa. While in the jugular foramen, the nerve has the small **tympanic branch,** which passes through a bony canal into the middle ear cavity. This branch contains both general visceral efferent (GVE) and general visceral afferent (GVA) fibers, which supply the middle ear cavity and participate in the formation of the **tympanic plexus** within the cavity. The small **lesser petrosal nerve** (containing GVE fibers) is resolved from the plexus. This nerve enters the middle cranial fossa and then the infratemporal fossa, where it joins the parasympathetic **otic ganglion,** which is located medial to the main trunk of the mandibular division of the trigeminal nerve. The postganglionic parasympathetic fibers from the otic ganglion join the **auriculotemporal branch** of the mandibular nerve and pass to the parotid gland.

Although a lesion of the glossopharyngeal nerve results in loss of parotid secretion, taste on the posterior aspect of the tongue, some cutaneous sensation of the external ear, and paralysis of the stylopharyngeus muscle, the loss of sensory innervation of the pharynx and the carotid sinus are the easiest to evaluate. Both the gag and carotid sinus reflexes consist of the ninth (sensory limbs) and tenth (motor limbs) nerves.

Cranial Nerve X

The **vagus nerve** contains fibers of five different functional types. The large number of general visceral efferent and afferent fibers supply the same structures—the viscera of the thorax and the abdomen—and are the afferent and efferent limbs of most of the cardiovascular, pulmonary, and gastrointestinal reflexes. The special visceral efferent fibers innervate the skeletal muscles of the larynx, pharynx (except the stylopharyngeus), palate (except the tensor veli palatine), and upper esophagus. The special visceral afferent fibers supply taste receptors in the region of the epiglottis, and the general somatic afferent neurons innervate a small patch of skin in the area of the posterior external ear.

This nerve, as the meaning of its name (vagrant) implies, has an extensive course as it "wanders" a considerable distance. It begins in the posterior cranial fossa, arising from the lateral aspect of the medulla just inferior to the ninth nerve in the postolivary sulcus. It then passes laterally to exit from the cranial cavity through the jugular foramen (Fig. 5-5). It descends through the neck within the **carotid sheath,** along with the carotid artery and the internal jugular vein. Its branches in the neck are multiple. The most superior is typically the **pharyngeal branch,** which supplies the muscles of the pharynx. The **carotid branch** innervates the carotid sinus. The **superior laryngeal nerve** also arises superiorly but passes anteriorly to supply most of the mucous membrane of the larynx and the cricothyroid muscle. **Cardiac branches** arise in the middle to lower neck and descend into the thorax, where they enter the **cardiac plexus,** the autonomic plexus of the heart. The **recurrent (inferior) laryngeal nerve** branches at the base of the neck. This nerve wraps around a large artery (the aortic arch on the left and the subclavian artery on the right) and passes superiorly in the groove between the esophagus and the trachea. It enters the larynx and supplies all of its muscles (except the cricothyroid) and the mucous membrane inferior to the vocal ligaments.

The vagus nerves accompany the esophagus through the upper portion of the thorax, providing multiple branches to both the cardiac and pulmonary plexuses. In the lower thorax the nerves become enmeshed in the **esophageal plexuses,** and just before entering the abdomen they are resolved into **anterior** and **posterior vagal trunks.** Upon entering the abdomen these trunks are continuous with the **aortic plexus,** the autonomic plexus that supplies the viscera of the abdominal cavity. The vagal fibers supply the gut as far distally as the splenic flexure.

A lesion of the vagus nerve results in a variety of symptoms. A patient's main complaints would probably involve swallowing (pharynx and palate) and talking (palate and larynx). Examination would reveal deviation of both the pharynx and palate away from the side of the lesion. This deviation would be more pronounced upon vocalization. Inspection of the vocal cords would reveal the involved cord to be fixed in a paramedian position.

Cranial Nerve XI

The **accessory nerve** contains only general somatic efferent fibers that innervate the sternocleidomastoid and trapezius muscles. Unlike the rest of the cranial nerves, this nerve arises from the lateral aspect of the upper portion of the cervical spinal cord. It ascends through the foramen magnum into the posterior cranial fossa and then exits from the cranial cavity through the jugular foramen (Fig. 5-5). It initially descends deep to the sternocleidomastoid muscle and enters the posterior cervical triangle. It then passes laterally across the triangle and then deep to the superior border of the trapezius approximately 2 cm from its clavicular attachment.

Loss of the accessory nerve results in paralysis of both the trapezius and sternocleidomastoid muscles. Inspection should reveal a statically "dropped shoulder" on the involved side. The trapezius can be tested by elevation (hunching) of the shoulder; the sternocleidomastoid muscle is tested by turning the head to the contralateral side.

Cranial Nerve XII

The **hypoglossal nerve** contains only general somatic efferent fibers and innervates all muscles of the tongue, both intrinsic and extrinsic, except the palatoglossus. This nerve arises from the preolivary sulcus of the medulla and passes anterolaterally toward the hypoglossal canal, through which it exits from the cranial cavity (Fig. 5-5). It proceeds anteriorly toward the floor of the mouth, passing between the internal jugular vein and the internal carotid artery. In the floor of the mouth it is positioned between the mylohyoid and hyoglossus muscles.

The usual complaint resulting from loss of the hypoglossal nerve is difficulty with talking and eating. These problems are purely mechanical in that the muscles of one-half of the tongue are lost and the tongue simply does not work properly. The muscles of the tongue and hence the hypoglossal nerve can be definitively tested by protrusion of the tongue. If there is a lesion of the nerve, the tongue will deviate toward the side of the lesion (see genioglossus, below).

The **muscles of the tongue** consist of intrinsic and extrinsic muscles. The intrinsic muscles are situated completely within the tongue and are involved in shaping the tongue. The extrinsic muscles interconnect the tongue to adjacent structures and thus regulate the position of the tongue.

The tongue can be retracted (styloglossus, hyoglossus), protruded (genioglossus), elevated (styloglossus, palatoglossus), and deviated from side to side (genioglossus). Of importance in testing the muscles (and the hypoglossal nerve) is the genioglossus. This muscle arises from a small area of the mandible, just lateral to the midline. The muscle fibers diverge considerably laterally as they pass into the tongue. As a result, the genioglossus muscle deviates the tongue to the opposite side as it is protruded. The ability to protrude the tongue in the midline requires both genioglossus muscles; loss of one results in deviation of the tongue toward the loss as it is protruded.

The thorax is the portion of the trunk between the neck and abdomen. It contains the heart and lungs as well as a number of large vessels and structures that pass from the head and neck to the abdomen. The musculoskeletal walls, which form the "thoracic cage," not only protect the viscera of the thorax but also are capable of a series of complex motions that can change the volume of the thoracic cavity. The thoracic cavity contains the lungs and pleural cavities laterally and the heart and other structures centrally, in an area called the mediastinum.

Thoracic Wall

The bones forming the thoracic wall are the thoracic vertebrae, ribs, and sternum (Fig. 6-1). The 12 pairs of ribs are similar in that each articulates with the vertebral column. They differ, however, in the ways in which they end anteriorly (Fig. 6-1). The upper seven ribs articulate directly with the sternum through the costal cartilages and are thus called true ribs. The remaining five are false ribs because they do not articulate directly with the sternum. Ribs 8, 9, and 10 articulate indirectly with the sternum since their costal cartilages join the cartilages of the ribs above. The anterior ends of ribs 11 and 12 do not join the sternum and therefore are called "floating ribs."

Each **typical rib,** ribs 3–9, consists of a head, neck, tubercle, and shaft. The head contains two facets that articulate with facets on adjacent vertebral bodies. The short neck extends laterally to the tubercle, which contains a single facet that articulates with a facet on the transverse process of a vertebrae. From the tubercle, the shaft is directed laterally and then anteriorly and inferiorly. The junction between the lateral and anterior portions of the shaft is angular. This junction, the angle of the rib,

Thorax

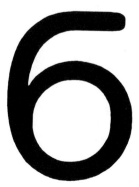

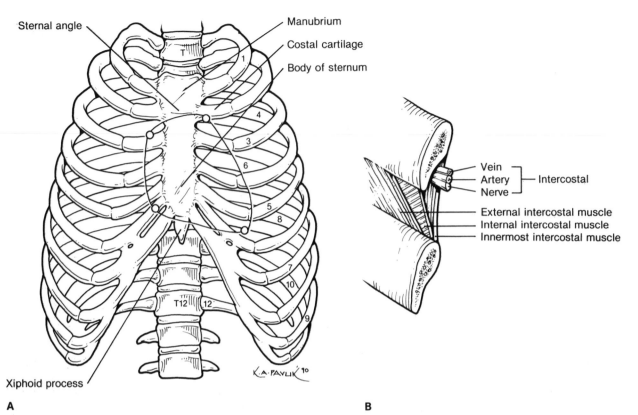

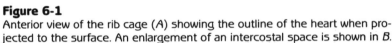

Figure 6-1
Anterior view of the rib cage (A) showing the outline of the heart when projected to the surface. An enlargement of an intercostal space is shown in B.

is the weakest portion of the rib, and therefore, the area most commonly fractured. The shaft is flattened and has a grooved inferior border, the costal groove.

The **first rib** is short, highly curved, and flattened superoinferiorly. It articulates only with the first thoracic vertebra and presents the subclavian groove superiorly. The **second rib** is longer than the first but shaped similarly. **Ribs 10–12** typically articulate with only one vertebra; ribs 11 and 12 have neither tubercles nor angles and do not articulate with the transverse processes. Since ribs 11 and 12 do not extend very far anteriorly, they are relatively short compared to typical ribs.

The articulations between the heads of the ribs and the vertebral bodies (**costovertebral joints**) and between the tubercles of the ribs and the transverse processes (**costotransverse joints**) are all synovial joints. These joints permit small amounts of sliding between the articular surfaces, enabling elevation and depression of both the anterior and lateral aspects of the ribs. Such motions permit changes in both the anteroposterior and lateral dimensions of the thoracic cage.

The **intercostal spaces** (Fig. 6-1B) are the areas between adjacent ribs; the first intercostal space is between ribs 1 and 2, the second between ribs 2 and 3, and so on. These spaces are filled by layers of muscles and fascia and contain the intercostal vessels and nerves. Each muscle is oriented differently from the others and extends from the inferior border or the rib above to the superior border of the rib below. The fibers of the most superficial muscle, the **external intercostal muscle,** are obliquely oriented and pass medially from above downward. The fibers of the next deeper layer, the **internal intercostal muscle,** are oriented at an angle of approximately 90 degrees to those of the external intercostal, so they pass laterally as they descend. The deepest layer, the **innermost intercostal muscle,** is incomplete and composed of fibers that parallel those of the internal intercostal muscle. These muscles are supplied by the intercostal nerves and are active in respiration.

The **intercostal neurovascular bundle** (Fig. 6-1B) occupies the subcostal groove on the inferior border of the shaft of the rib and is positioned deep to the internal intercostal muscle. The **intercostal nerves** are the continuations of the ventral rami of the thoracic spinal nerves. Each supplies a strip of the entire body wall, both laterally and anteriorly, including the skin and muscle as well as the parietal pleura. The lower intercostal nerves (nerves 7–11) continue beyond the subcostal margin onto the abdominal wall where they supply strips of skin, muscle, and the parietal peritoneum. There are two intercostal arteries and veins in each space: The **posterior intercostal artery** is a branch of the thoracic aorta, and the **anterior intercostal artery** is a branch of the internal thoracic artery. These two vessels form a potential anastomosis and thus a potential collateral route around portions of the aorta and the proximal portions of the subclavian arteries. The two **intercostal veins** are tributaries to the azygos (posterior intercostal) and internal thoracic (anterior intercostal) veins.

Lungs and Pleurae

Lungs

The shapes of the lungs reflect the contours of their adjacent structures: the thoracic walls along with the various individual structures within the mediastinum and the abdomen that are adjacent to the lungs. Each lung is somewhat conical with a rounded apex and a concave base (**diaphragmatic surface**). The anterior, lateral, and posterior surfaces (**costal surface**) are rounded, while the medial, or **mediastinal, surface** is irregular due to indentations by various organs. Anteriorly, the lungs overlap the mediastinum. Inferiorly, the lungs overlap various abdominal organs and are separated from these organs by the thin, muscular respiratory diaphragm.

All structures entering or leaving the lungs pass through the medially positioned **hilus** of the lung. These structures consist of the main bronchus, pulmonary and bronchial vessels, pulmonary nerve plexuses, and lymphatics. Collectively, these structures form the **root** of the lung.

Each lung has large subdivisions called **lobes,** and each lobe has subdivisions referred to as **bronchopulmonary segments.** Both the lobes and segments are functionally independent because each is completely separate anatomically and supplied by single bronchials and vessels. The lobes are separated by deep fissures, and the segments are separated by connective tissue septa. The right lung has three lobes, the **superior, middle, and inferior,** which are separated by the **oblique** and **horizontal fissures.** The left lung has only **superior** and **inferior lobes,** which are separated by the **oblique fissure.**

The outline of the lungs and positions of the fissures separating the lobes can be projected to the surface of the thoracic wall (Fig. 6-2). The apex of the lung is approximately 2.5 cm superior to the medial third of the clavicle. The medial border passes posterior to the sternoclavicular joint and descends to the sixth costal cartilage, where it inclines laterally. The left lung, though, inclines laterally a bit higher than the right (forming the cardiac notch) because of the position of the heart. The inferior border of the lung crosses the sixth rib in the midclavicular line, the eighth rib in the midaxillary line, and the tenth rib in the scapular line (medial border of the scapula). The **oblique fissure** follows a line that crosses the fourth rib posteriorly at the base of the spine of the scapula, the fifth rib in the midaxillary line, and the sixth rib in the midclavicular line. On the right, the **horizontal fissure** begins at the level of the fourth

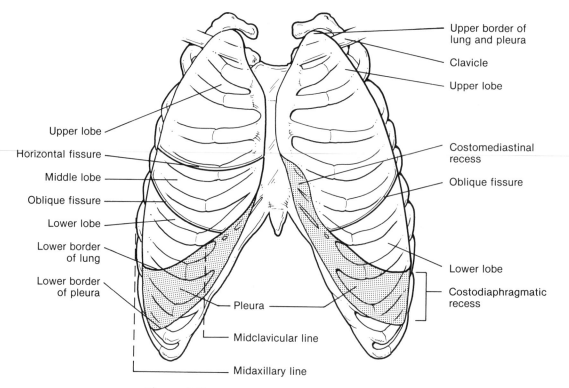

Figure 6-2
Anterior view of the rib cage showing the surface projections of both the lungs and pleural cavities.

costal cartilage anteriorly, then extends to the fifth rib in the midaxillary line, where it joins the oblique fissure.

Pleural Cavities

Each lung is nearly surrounded by a **pleural cavity** or **pleura** (Fig. 6-3), which is a closed space and formed by a double membrane. One layer of this membrane, the **visceral layer,** is firmly attached to the surface of the lung. The other layer, the **parietal layer,** is anchored to the deep surface of the thoracic wall as well as the diaphragm and structures of the mediastinum. These two layers are continuous around the root of the lung and thus form a closed cavity that nearly surrounds the lung. The air pressure within the lung is equal to that of the atmosphere, but within the pleura the pressure is less. This negative pressure holds the visceral layer (and the lung) firmly against the parietal layer (and thoracic wall). Consequently, the pleural cavity is only a potential space that contains a small amount of lubricating fluid. During quiet respiration, there are areas

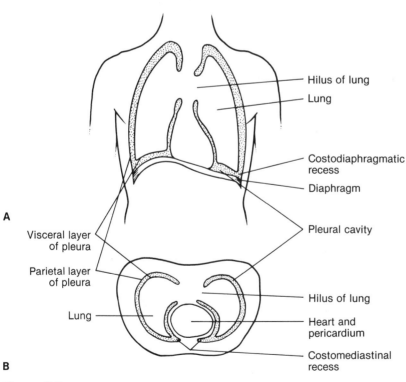

A

B

Figure 6-3
Coronal (*A*) and transverse (*B*) sections through the pleural cavities.

where two layers of parietal pleura are adjacent—for example, where the parietal pleura passes from the rib cage to the diaphragm. These areas are referred to as recesses and named according to location—for example, the **costodiaphragmatic** and **costomediastinal recesses.** These recesses can be entered with a needle without fear of hitting the lung. During deep inspiration, these recesses are obliterated as the lungs expand.

The outline of the pleural cavities, also known as the lines of pleural reflection, can also be projected to the surface of the thoracic wall (Fig. 6-2). Superiorly, the cupula of the pleura corresponds to the apex of the lung, approximately 2.5 cm above the medial third of the clavicle. The medial borders cross the sternoclavicular joints, meet in the midline posterior to the level of the second costal cartilages (sternal angle), and incline laterally at the level of the seventh costal cartilages. The inferior border crosses the eighth rib in the midclavicular line; the tenth rib in the midaxillary line; and the twelfth rib in the scapular line.

Respiratory Diaphragm and Respiration

The **respiratory diaphragm** (Figs. 6-6, 7-3) is a dome-shaped, thin, musculotendinous sheet that separates the thoracic and abdominal cavities. Its muscle fibers arise from the subcostal margin and upper lumbar vertebrae; the attachments to the lumbar vertebra are the **crura** of the diaphragm. From their origins, the muscle fibers arch superiorly and centrally as they converge to attach to the flat **central tendon** of the diaphragm, which is positioned just inferior to the heart. There are three openings in the diaphragm. The most superior is the opening for the inferior vena cava (vertebral level T8). The esophageal hiatus is at the level of vertebra T10, and the aorta and thoracic duct pass between the crura of the diaphragm at vertebral level T12. The esophageal hiatus is vulnerable to enlargement and may permit a portion of the stomach or abdominal esophagus to herniate superiorly into the thoracic cavity (hiatal hernia). The diaphragm is innervated by the right and left phrenic nerves, which contain fibers from spinal cord segments C3–C5. Injury of the spinal cord above the fourth cervical segment usually paralyzes the diaphragm, consequently precluding diaphragmatic breathing.

Normal **mechanics of respiration** involve two basic principles. First, the volume of the thoracic cavity must be both increased and decreased by motion of the ribs and diaphragm. Second, the lungs and thoracic wall must be held together by the negative pressure within the pleural cavities. Inspiration is largely an active process, because muscular activity increases the volume of the thoracic cavity, which, in turn, enlarges the volume of the lungs. The pressure within the lungs drops below that of the atmosphere and, therefore, air rushes into the lungs. Expiration is essentially passive, because the force needed to expel air from the lungs is provided by the elasticity of the lungs themselves. When the muscles of inspiration relax, the lungs recoil, and since their volumes are reduced, the air is forced from them. The thoracic wall follows the lungs and returns to its resting position. Loss of the lungs' elasticity is apparent in pathology such as emphysema, where the resting volume of the thoracic cavity is enlarged because the lungs cannot recoil their normal amount.

The major muscle of respiration is the respiratory diaphragm. As it contracts, it flattens, and the vertical dimension of the thoracic cavity increases. The diaphragm accounts for most of the change in volume during quiet respiration, but it is active during all respiration. The rest of the respiratory muscles regulate the positions of the ribs. The intercostal muscles are important because they maintain the sizes of the intercostal spaces as well as the rigidity of the soft tissues forming those spaces. Elevation of the ribs increases both the lateral and anteroposterior dimensions of the thoracic cavity, and becomes increasingly necessary as the depth of inspiration increases. This elevation is produced by the external intercostal and scalene muscles. The sternocleidomastoid muscle, considered as accessory breathing muscle, usually functions only during the deepest inspirations and in pathologic conditions such as emphysema.

Mediastinum

The mediastinum is the portion of the thorax between the two lungs and pleural cavities. It is bounded anteriorly by the sternum and posteriorly by the thoracic vertebrae. The mediastinum is separated into **superior** and **inferior** portions by a horizontal line that passes through the junction of the manubrium and body of the sternum anteriorly, and the intervertebral disk between thoracic vertebrae T4 and T5 posteriorly. The inferior mediastinum is further subdivided into three parts: The **middle mediastinum** is formed by the heart and pericardium; the **anterior mediastinum** is between the pericardium and the sternum; and the **posterior mediastinum** is between the pericardium and the lower eight thoracic vertebrae.

Heart

The **heart** and its enclosure, the **pericardium,** occupy the middle mediastinum and are positioned largely posterior to the sternum. However, they extend somewhat to the left of the sternum. The pericardial cavity, much like the pleural cavity, is a closed space containing only a small amount of lubricating fluid; it virtually surrounds the heart. The pericardium differs in that it has three layers. The outer, **fibrous pericardium** is a tough layer of fibrous tissue that blends with the adventitia of the great vessels and the central tendon of the diaphragm. A double layer of **serous pericardium** lines the fibrous pericardium and is firmly attached to the surface of the heart. These two layers are continuous around the great vessels and thus form a closed space. The layer lining the fibrous pericardium is the **parietal layer** of serous pericardium; the layer covering the heart is the **visceral layer** of serous pericardium, which also is considered the outer layer of the heart, or **epicardium.**

The heart (Figs. 6-4, 6-5) is bluntly conical in shape with its apex directed somewhat inferiorly and to the left. The **anterior surface** of the heart (Fig. 6-4) is related to the sternum and costal cartilages and formed

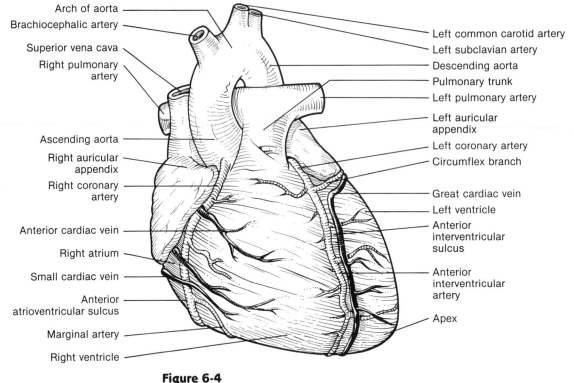

Arch of aorta
Brachiocephalic artery
Superior vena cava
Right pulmonary artery
Ascending aorta
Right auricular appendix
Right coronary artery
Anterior cardiac vein
Right atrium
Small cardiac vein
Anterior atrioventricular sulcus
Marginal artery
Right ventricle

Left common carotid artery
Left subclavian artery
Descending aorta
Pulmonary trunk
Left pulmonary artery
Left auricular appendix
Left coronary artery
Circumflex branch
Great cardiac vein
Left ventricle
Anterior interventricular sulcus
Anterior interventricular artery
Apex

Figure 6-4
Anterior view of the heart.

by portions of both ventricles, the right atrium, and both the left and right auricular appendages. The **inferior,** or **diaphragmatic, surface** (Fig. 6-5) rests on the central tendon of the diaphragm and is formed by portions of both ventricles and the inferior aspect of the right atrium into which the inferior vena cava empties. The **base** of the heart, its **posterior surface** (Fig. 6-5), is related to the esophagus and formed predominantly by the left atrium. The **apex** is directed inferiorly and to the left and is formed by the tip of the left ventricle.

The outline of the heart can be traced on the surface of the thoracic wall by interconnecting four points (Fig. 6-1). These points are (1) the left second costal cartilage, approximately 1 cm lateral to the sternum; (2) the right third costal cartilage, about 1 cm lateral to the sternum; (3) the right sixth costal cartilage, about 1 cm lateral to the sternum; and (4) the left fifth intercostal space, approximately 8 cm lateral to the sternum.

The septa that separate the chambers of the heart are indicated by grooves, or sulci, on its surface. These sulci contain the major vessels that supply the heart. The **coronary,** or **atrioventricular, sulcus** rings the heart and indicates the separation between the atria and the ventricles. Since the atria form the right and posterior aspects of the heart and the ventricles the left, anterior, and inferior aspects, this sulcus is oriented nearly vertically and passes obliquely downward to the right from above.

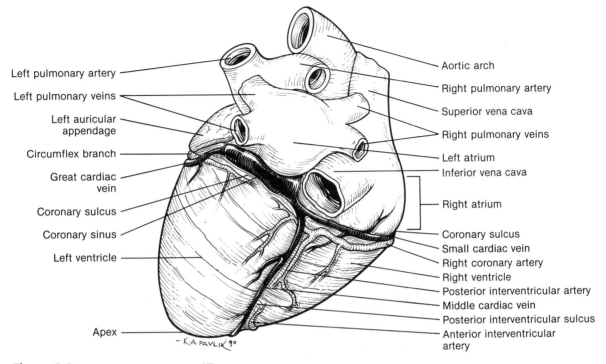

Left pulmonary artery

Left pulmonary veins

Left auricular appendage

Circumflex branch

Great cardiac vein

Coronary sulcus

Coronary sinus

Left ventricle

Apex

Aortic arch

Right pulmonary artery

Superior vena cava

Right pulmonary veins

Left atrium

Inferior vena cava

Right atrium

Coronary sulcus

Small cardiac vein

Right coronary artery

Right ventricle

Posterior interventricular artery

Middle cardiac vein

Posterior interventricular sulcus

Anterior interventricular artery

— K.A. PAVLIK '90

Figure 6-5
Posterior view of the heart, showing its posterior and diaphragmatic surfaces.

The **interventricular sulcus** is approximately perpendicular to the coronary sulcus, so it descends and passes inferiorly from right to left. That part of the sulcus on the anterior surface of the heart is the **anterior interventricular sulcus**; that portion on the inferior surface is the **posterior interventricular sulcus.**

Atria. Each **atrium** has two portions. The larger portions are composed of smooth, thin muscular walls, while the smaller portions, including the **auricular appendages,** are ridged internally by the presence of the **pectinate muscles.** The **right atrium** forms most of the right side of the heart. It receives the superior vena cava superiorly and the inferior vena cava and the coronary sinus inferiorly. It opens into the right ventricle anteriorly and to the left, via the **right atrioventricular ostium.** The **interatrial septum,** separating the atria, is almost coronal in orientation, so the left atrium is both posterior and to the left of the right atrium. The **left atrium** receives the four pulmonary veins posterolaterally, two on either side. Anteriorly and inferiorly, the left atrium communicates with the left ventricle via the **left atrioventricular ostium.**

Ventricles. While the walls of both **ventricles** are considerably thicker than those of the atria, the walls of the left ventricle are even thicker than those of the right. The walls of both chambers, internally, are roughened by muscular ridges called **trabeculae carnae.** The **right ventricle** occupies a large portion of the anterior surface of the heart and extends almost to the apex. Its cavity is crescent-shaped in cross section because of the thicker bulging wall of the left ventricle. Superiorly and anteriorly, this cavity communicates with the pulmonary trunk via the **ostium of the pulmonary trunk.** The **interventricular septum** consists of a small superior **membranous portion** and the large **muscular portion.** The thickness of the muscular portion is similar to that of the rest of the left ventricular wall. The **left ventricle** forms both the apex and most of the left surface of the heart and is positioned partially anterior to the left atrium. Superiorly and anteriorly, the chamber of the left ventricle narrows to its communication with the aorta through the **aortic ostium.**

Skeleton of the heart.   The **skeleton of the heart** consists of four strong, fibrous rings that surround the aortic, pulmonary, and atrioventricular ostia. These rings are firmly bound together and provide the structure for the openings as well as the base to which the muscle of the heart (**myocardium**) is attached. Since this fibrous skeleton is the firm attachment of the muscle, contraction produces movement of a chamber toward that skeleton. This is particularly apparent with the ventricles; when the ventricles contract, the apex of the heart moves toward its base.

Valves of the heart.   Anatomically and functionally, the **valves of the heart** are of two types. The **right (tricuspid)** and **left (mitral) atrioventricular valves** close the openings between the atria and ventricles when the ventricles contract. These valves are "active" because they are supported by the **papillary muscles.** These muscles are cylindrical extensions of the ventricular walls that are connected to the valve cusps through the tendinous **chorda tendinae.** These muscles are important in maintaining the closed positions of the valves.

Contraction of the ventricles is accompanied by shortening of their longitudinal dimensions; contraction of the papillary muscles compensates for this change in ventricular size and ensures proper positioning of the valve cusps. The **aortic** and **pulmonary valves** prevent flow of blood from the aorta and pulmonary trunk into the left and right ventricles. Each of these valves is composed of three cusps; each cusp consists of a thin core with a thickened free border; and each is constructed so it can collapse distally into its respective vessel. These valves are passive because they are not supported by muscles, and the positions of their cusps are dependent on pressure differences between the ventricles and large arteries. Ventricular contraction forces the blood into the pulmonary trunk and aorta, opening the valves by flattening the valve cusps against the vessel walls. When the pressure in the vessels exceeds that in the ventricles, the cusps are pushed toward the ventricles and the valves close.

Blood vessels of the heart.   The **blood supply to the heart** (Figs. 6-4, 6-5) is provided by a pair of **coronary arteries** that branch from the most proximal aspect of the aorta. These arteries arise from two of the **aortic sinuses,** pouchlike areas behind the cusps of the aortic valve, and are located in the sulci on the surface of the heart. The openings of these vessels are partially closed by the valve cusps during ventricular contraction. When the pressure in the aorta exceeds that in the left ventricle and the backflow of blood closes the valve, blood flows into the coronary arteries.

The larger **left coronary artery** (Figs. 6-4, 6-5) has a short main trunk that passes posterior to, and then to the left of, the pulmonary trunk. Upon reaching the atrioventricular sulcus, it branches into the **anterior interventricular** and **circumflex arteries.** The anterior interventricular artery descends toward the apex of the heart in the anterior interventricular sulcus and continues onto the diaphragmatic surface of the heart in the posterior interventricular sulcus, where it usually ends. This large branch is very important because it supplies a major portion of the left ventricle and the interventricular septum. The circumflex artery follows the atrioventricular sulcus to the left, passing onto the posterior aspect of the heart, where it usually ends.

The **right coronary artery** (Figs. 6-4, 6-5) also occupies the atrioventricular sulcus, passing first to the right on the anterior surface and then onto the posterior aspect of the heart. At the junction of the atrioventricular and posterior interventricular sulci, the artery branches into the larger **posterior interventricular artery,** which follows the posterior interventricular sulcus toward the apex of the heart and the smaller continuation of the right coronary in the atrioventricular sulcus. The **marginal artery** branches from the right coronary, as it passes around the right border of the heart, then passes along the inferior margin of the heart.

The terminal branches of the coronary arteries form two potential anastomoses. The first is between the anterior and posterior interventricular arteries in the posterior interventricular sulcus. The second, between the circumflex artery and termination of the right coronary, is in the posterior atrioventricular sulcus.

Most of the **venous blood from the myocardium** (Figs. 6-4, 6-5) empties into the **coronary sinus** prior to its opening into the right atrium. This sinus occupies the posterior atrioventricular sulcus and is the direct continuation of the **great cardiac vein,** which occupies the anterior interventricular sulcus. The other tributaries are the **middle cardiac vein** from the posterior interventricular sulcus and the **small cardiac vein** from the coronary sulcus. A variable number of **anterior cardiac veins** drain the anterior aspect of the right ventricle and empty directly into the right atrium.

Regulation of heart contraction. The **regulation of the contraction of the heart** involves both the **cardiac conduction system** and the autonomic nervous system. The cardiac conduction system, composed of specialized cardiac muscle cells, is located completely within the walls of the heart and functions to ensure the appropriate synchrony of contraction among the chambers of the heart. This system consists of two concentrations of cells called nodes and several bands of specialized muscle cells that pass along the walls of the heart. The **sinoatrial (SA) node,** commonly called the "pacemaker" of the heart, is located in the wall of the right atrium at the entrance of the superior vena cava. The contraction impulse begins in the SA node and spreads through the atrial myocardium to the **antrioventricular (AV) node,** which is positioned within the interatrial septum. The impulse then crosses the membranous part of the interventricular septum via the **atrioventricular (AV) bundle** (also called the **bundle of His**). This bundle then branches into right and left bundle branches, which spread through the walls of the ventricles. The AV bundle, as well as the bundle branches and their extensions, are composed of specialized cardiac cells called **Purkinje fibers.** Interruption of conduction across the AV bundle (AV block) disrupts the contraction sequence between the atria and ventricles and can cause an arrhythmic heart beat (arrhythmia). The **cardiac plexuses** are the autonomic plexuses through which sympathetic and parasympathetic stimuli modify, not initiate, cardiac contraction. Sympathetic stimulation, via cardiac branches of the sympathetic trunk, increases both the rate and force of cardiac contraction; parasympathetic stimulation, via the vagus nerve, produces the reverse effects.

Great Vessels

The proximal portions of the large blood vessels that are connected directly to the heart are referred to collectively as the **great vessels** (Figs. 6-4 through 6-6). These vessels are found in the superior and/or posterior

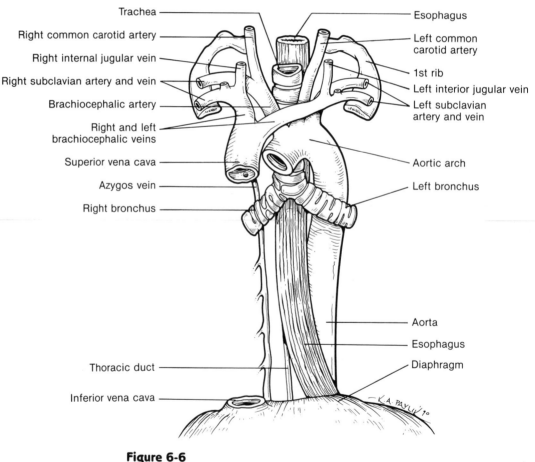

Figure 6-6
Anterior view of the great vessels, trachea, and contents of the posterior mediastinum.

portions of the mediastinum and consist of the **ascending aorta, vena cavae, pulmonary trunk,** and **pulmonary veins.**

The **thoracic portion of the aorta** (Fig. 6-6) consists of ascending and descending portions, which are united by an arch. The short **ascending aorta** is located within the superior mediastinum and is continuous with the most superior aspect of the left ventricle. It ascends very near the midline, slightly to the right and posterior to the pulmonary trunk, and has no branches other than the coronary arteries. The **arch of the aorta** continues posteriorly and to the left, passing lateral to both the trachea and esophagus. The arch is contained totally within the superior mediastinum and provides the large branches that supply the head as well as the upper limbs. In order of appearance, these branches are the **right brachiocephalic trunk, left common carotid,** and **left subclavian arteries.** The arch also passes superior to the left pulmonary artery, to which it is connected by the **ligamentum arteriosum,** which is the remnant of the **ductus arteriosus.** The **descending portion of the thoracic aorta,** in the posterior mediastinum, descends posterior to the root of the left lung, and is positioned anterolateral to the bodies of the thoracic vertebra. The aorta enters the abdomen at the level of the twelfth thoracic vertebra by passing between the crura of the diaphragm. The descending aorta provides bronchial and esophageal branches as well as the multiple posterior intercostal and the subcostal arteries to the body wall.

The **venae cavae** (Fig. 6-6) return systemic blood from the entire body to the right atrium. The **superior vena cava** is the most lateral structure (to the right) in the superior mediastinum. It is formed by the union of the two brachiocephalic veins and drains the head, both upper limbs, the body wall of the thorax, and upper part of the abdomen. The blood from the body walls of the thorax and upper part of the abdomen passes through the **azygos vein,** which joins the superior vena cava just before it enters the superior aspect of the right atrium. The **inferior vena cava** has an extremely short course in the thorax. It passes through the **esophageal hiatus** of the diaphragm at vertebral level T10 and immediately enters the most inferior aspect of the right atrium.

The **pulmonary trunk** (Fig. 6-4) conveys venous blood from the right ventricle to the lungs. This vessel is very short. It arises from the most superior aspect of the right ventricle anterior and to the left of the ascending aorta. Then, just inferior to the arch of the aorta, it bifurcates into the **right** and **left pulmonary arteries.** The longer right pulmonary artery passes horizontally to the right, posterior to the ascending aorta. The left pulmonary artery almost immediately enters the left lung.

The four **pulmonary veins** (Fig. 6-5), two from each lung, transmit arterial blood from the lungs to the left atrium. Since the left atrium forms most of the posterior aspect of the heart, these veins are all very short. Each enters the left atrium soon after exiting from the roots of the lung.

The **trachea** (Fig. 6-6) is the portion of the airway that extends from the larynx in the neck into the superior mediastinum, where it ends by branching into the **right** and **left primary bronchi.** The trachea is positioned in the midline, posterior to the left brachiocephalic vein and arch of the aorta and anterior to the esophagus. Its patent lumen is maintained by the presence of horseshoe-shaped cartilages within its wall. The right primary bronchus, which is shorter and more vertical than the left, passes posterior to the superior vena cava on its way to the right lung. The left primary bronchus passes inferior to the arch of the aorta as it passes toward the hilum of the left lung.

Esophagus

The **esophagus** (Fig. 6-6) begins in the neck, where it is continuous with the pharynx. It descends through the neck and then through both the superior and posterior portions of the mediastinum before passing through the esophageal hiatus (vertebral level T10) of the diaphragm. The esophagus is anterior to the bodies of the thoracic vertebrae; it is posterior to the trachea in the superior mediastinum and posterior to the left atrium in the posterior mediastinum. This tubular structure is collapsed except when food is transmitted.

Thoracic Duct

The **thoracic duct** (Figs. 5-2, 6-6) enters the thorax through the aortic opening of the diaphragm and then ascends through the thorax on the ventral aspects of the vertebral bodies. It enters the neck and empties into the junction of the left subclavian and internal jugular veins. This lymphatic vessel, the largest in the body, conveys lymphatic fluid from the entire body below the respiratory diaphragm and from the left half of the body above the diaphragm. Since the inferior deep cervical (scalene) lymph nodes filter this fluid just before it passes into the venous circulation, malignancy of these nodes can signify metastatic disease in one of the areas drained by the thoracic duct.

Phrenic and Vagus Nerves

Both the **phrenic** and the **vagus nerves** are found in the thoracic cavity. The phrenic nerves (C3–C5) descend through the superior mediastinum and pass anterior to the roots of the lungs. They end upon reaching the diaphragm, which they supply. The vagus nerves (CN X) also descend through the superior mediastinum, where they provide branches to both the cardiac and pulmonary autonomic plexuses. They then pass posterior to the roots of the lung before becoming entwined within the esophageal plexus. Just above the diaphragm the vagal fibers form anterior and posterior vagal trunks, which pass through the diaphragm into the abdomen.

Abdomen

The abdomen is the portion of the trunk between the thorax and the pelvis. The large abdominal cavity, separated from the thoracic cavity superiorly by the respiratory diaphragm, is continuous with the pelvic cavity inferiorly. Although it is a single cavity, there are a number of ways the abdominal cavity can be separated into regions. The simplest and clinically most commonly used system separates the abdomen into quadrants (Fig. 7-1). The **upper** and **lower left,** and **upper** and **lower right quandrants** are defined by vertical and horizontal lines that pass through the umbilicus. Another more extensive system separates the abdomen into nine regions (Fig. 7-1). These regional designations are commonly used to indicate areas of pain. The area surrounding the umbilicus is the **umbilical region;** above is the **epigastrium** and below the **hypogastrium.** The **left** and **right lumbar regions** are lateral to the umbilical region. The **left** and **right inguinal regions** are inferior and lateral, and the **left** and **right hypochondriac regions** are superior and lateral.

Abdominal Wall

Anterolateral Abdominal Wall

The abdominal wall is a muscular sheet filling the interval between the subcostal margin and the superior aspect of the pelvis. Four muscles form the anterior, lateral, and posterolateral portions of the abdominal wall (Fig. 7-2). Only the rectus abdominis forms the wall just lateral to the midline. Lateral to this muscle, the wall is composed of three layers, which are the external and internal abdominal oblique and the transversus abdominis muscles. Posteriorly and medially, the wall is considerably

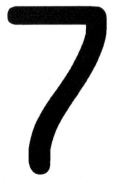

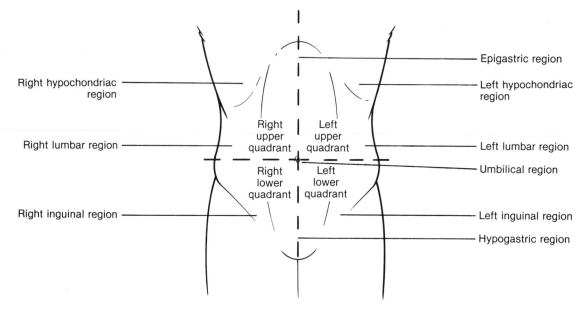

Figure 7-1
Anterior view of the abdomen showing its regions.

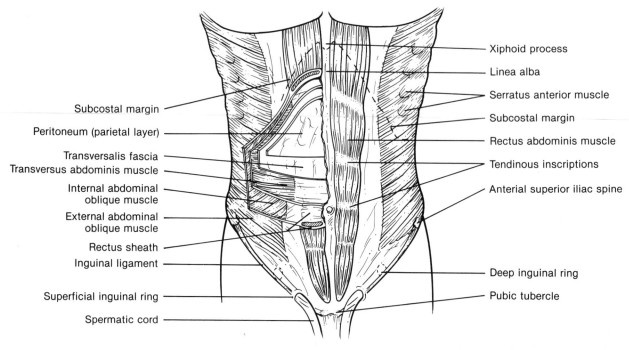

Figure 7-2
Anterior view of the muscles of the anterolateral abdominal wall. On the left, a section of each muscle is removed to reveal the deeper muscles.

thicker and formed by the quadratus lumborum and psoas major muscles (Fig. 7-3).

The **rectus abdominis muscle** (Fig. 7-2) consists of vertically oriented fibers that extend from the medial aspect of the subcostal margin and the xiphoid process to the body and superior ramus of the pubis. This muscle has three or four **transverse intersections,** which are transverse tendinous bands that separate the muscle into variably distinct segments. The sheath of the rectus abdominis is formed by the aponeuroses of the lateral abdominal wall muscles. These aponeuroses fuse lateral to the rectus abdominis, separate to enclose the muscle, and then fuse in the midline with similar layers from the opposite side. The fusion in the midline forms the vertically oriented **linea alba;** the fusion lateral to the rectus abdominis forms the slightly curved **semilunar line.**

The **external abdominal oblique muscle** (Fig. 7-2) is the most superficial of the anterolateral muscles. Its obliquely oriented fibers attach superiorly to the lower six or seven ribs and pass inferiorly and medially. The most posterior fibers attach inferiorly to the iliac crest. The rest of the fibers join the **aponeurosis of the external oblique,** the flat tendon of this muscle, in the region of the semilunar line. The lower portion of this aponeurosis attaches both to the anterior superior iliac spine and to the pubic tubercle. Through these attachments the lower border of the external oblique aponeurosis bridges the interval between the two bony points and forms the **inguinal ligament.** A split in the aponeurosis just superior to the most medial aspect of the inguinal ligament forms the **superficial inguinal ring.**

The fibers of the **internal abdominal oblique muscle** (Fig. 7-2) are oriented at an angle of approximately 90 degrees to those of the external oblique. From their attachments to the iliac crest and lateral half of the inguinal ligament, the fibers pass superomedially and attach to the lower two or three ribs and the **aponeurosis of the internal oblique** in the region of the semilunar line. The most inferior fibers of this muscle, those attaching to the inguinal ligament, arch medially above the spermatic cord and contribute to the **conjoined tendon.**

The **transversus abdominis muscle** (Fig. 7-2) is the deepest of the anterolateral muscles. Its fibers are oriented horizontally and extend from the subcostal margin, thoracolumbar fascia, iliac crest, and lateral half of the inguinal ligament to the **transversus abdominis aponeurosis,** which blends with the other aponeuroses at the semilunar line. The most inferior fibers of this muscle, together with those of the internal oblique, arch over the spermatic cord and form the conjoined tendon.

The muscles of the anterolateral abdominal wall support the viscera of the abdominal cavity, move the vertebral column, and assist in respiration. With the exception of the transversus abdominis, each of the other muscles, acting bilaterally, flexes the vertebral column. The rectus abdominis is the strongest flexor and is capable of effecting the greatest range of motion; in fact, it is the major flexor of the lumbar spine. Unilateral activity of either the internal or external abdominal oblique muscles produces rotation of the vertebral column; the external oblique rotates to the opposite side, the internal oblique, to the same side. Both oblique muscles laterally bend the lumbar spine to the same side. These muscles facilitate both inspiration and expiration. Simultaneous contraction of all of the muscles increases the intra-abdominal pressure. This action, coupled with relaxation of the diaphragm, aids expiration because compression of the contents of the abdominal cavity forces the diaphragm superiorly and thereby reduces the volume of the thoracic cavity. On the other hand, the abdominal muscles also stabilize the subcostal margin and provide a solid base against which the diaphragm can contract during inspiration. And, these muscles play a role in stabilizing the vertebral column. Simultaneous contraction of the extensors of the vertebral column and the abdominal muscles, particularly the rectus abdominis, forms a "splint" that protects the vertebral column. The muscles of the anterolateral abdominal wall are innervated by the lower seven intercostal nerves and the subcostal nerve (L1).

The **inguinal canal** (Fig. 7-2), a flattened tunnel through the inferior aspect of the abdominal wall, transmits the spermatic cord (ductus deferens and associated vessels and nerves) in the male and the round ligament in the female. This canal is immediately above and parallels the inguinal ligament. It extends from approximately the midpoint between the anterior superior iliac spine and the pubic tubercle to a point just lateral and slightly superior to the pubic tubercle. The ends of this tunnel are the **deep** and **superficial inguinal rings.** The deep inguinal ring is lateral and formed by an outpouching of the transversalis fascia. (The transversalis fascia is part of a fascial layer that lines the entire abdominopelvic cavity.) The structures that traverse the canal are covered by a sleeve of transversalis fascia that is called the **internal spermatic fascia.** The superficial inguinal ring consists of a split in the aponeurosis of the external oblique. As the spermatic cord passes through this canal, it acquires coverings in addition to the internal spermatic fascia. The **cremasteric fascia** and **muscle** are derived from the external oblique aponeurosis and muscle, and the **external spermatic fascia** is derived from the external oblique aponeurosis. The cremaster muscle is innervated by the genitofemoral nerve (L1); the cremasteric reflex, elicited by stroking the skin of the medial thigh, can be used to evaluate spinal cord segment L1.

The inguinal region is an area of potential weakness, particularly in males. **Inguinal herniae** are common and involve herniation of abdominal viscera, usually the small intestine, through the abdominal wall in the region of the inguinal canal. The most common type of inguinal hernia, the **indirect inguinal hernia,** follows the path of the testis during development. The hernia passes through the internal ring, through the canal, and then emerges through the superficial ring. The **direct inguinal hernia** passes directly through the abdominal wall, typically near the superficial ring. Either type of hernia is manifest by a bulge just superolateral to the pubic tubercle. This bulge enlarges with an increase in intra-abdominal pressure, as in lifting. Whether the hernia is direct or indirect, surgical intervention is usually required.

Posterior Abdominal Wall

The posteromedial aspect of the abdominal wall is formed by the **quadratus lumborum** and **psoas major muscles.** The psoas major is described on page 188. The quadratus lumborum (Fig. 7-3), alias the "hip-hiker muscle," is rectangular in shape and located lateral to the psoas major, where it fills the interval between the twelfth rib and the posterior aspect of the iliac crest. It also fills the gap between the muscles of the anterolateral wall and the vertebral column. The quadratus lumborum functions during respiration as well as in movement of the spine. Unilateral activity produces lateral bending of the lumbar spine; bilateral contraction extends the lumbar spine, thus increasing the lumbar curve. Although this muscle does elevate the pelvis on the same side, it does so only in concert with other muscles; for example, the deep muscles of the back. During

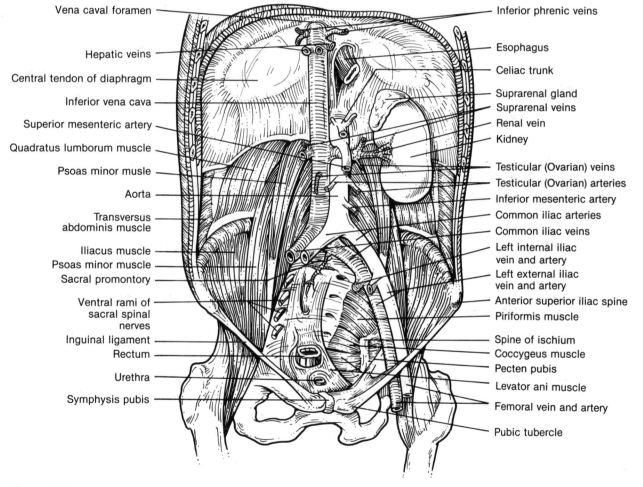

Figure 7-3
Anterior view of the posterior abdominal wall, respiratory diaphragm, and pelvic floor.

inspiration the quadratus lumborum stabilizes the twelfth rib, thereby providing a solid base against which the diaphragm can contract.

Abdominal Cavity

Abdominal and Peritoneal Cavities

The **abdominal cavity** extends both above and below the attachments of the abdominal wall muscles. Because of the arched shape of the diaphragm, this cavity extends superiorly to approximately the fifth intercostal space. Inferiorly, the abdominal cavity is continuous with the area within the pelvic ring, a single space containing portions of both the abdominal and pelvic cavities. The plane of separation between abdomen and pelvis is the pelvic inlet, which is formed by the sacral promontory, iliopectineal line, and superior aspect of the pubis. The area above the pelvic inlet and below the borders of the iliac crests is the most inferior portion of the abdominal cavity; it is also called the "false pelvis." The area inferior to the pelvic inlet is the pelvic cavity, hence the term "true pelvis." The abdominal and pelvic cavities are continuous, hence the term **abdominopelvic cavity.**

The **peritoneal cavity** or **peritoneum** should not be confused with either the abdominal cavity or the perineum. The peritoneal cavity is similar to the pleural cavities in its construction and contents; the peritoneum consists of parietal and visceral layers, and the cavity contains only a small amount of lubricating fluid. The peritoneal and pleural cavities differ, though, in the number of organs to which each is related. Each pleural cavity nearly surrounds only one lung, but the peritoneal cavity is related to a number of organs, almost surrounding some while only partially covering others.

The **parietal layer** of peritoneum lines the entire abdominopelvic cavity. It is firmly attached to the deep surface of the abdominal walls, the inferior surface of the diaphragm, and the superior aspect of the pelvic floor. The **visceral layer** of peritoneum is continuous with the parietal layer and attached to the surfaces of a number of the organs within the abdomen. The amount of an organ's surface covered by visceral peritoneum varies considerably among organs. Certain organs—the jejunum and ileum, for example—are almost completely encased in visceral peritoneum and are suspended from the posterior body wall by a double layer of peritoneum called a **mesentery.** These organs are considered to be **completely peritonealized** or **peritonealized.** The mesenteries are "life lines" because they convey the vessels and nerves that supply the organs. Other organs—the kidneys, for example—are firmly fixed to the posterior body wall and covered by peritoneum on only their anterior surfaces. These organs are outside or posterior to the peritoneum and called **retroperitoneal.** The amount of surface covered in other organs is between these two extremes. For example, the ascending and descending portions of the large intestine typically are covered on three sides and there is no mesentery; such organs are **partially peritonealized.**

The large number of organs, the variety of ways in which they are related to the peritoneum, and the positional changes of certain organs during development make the peritoneal cavity a morass of complex folds, nooks, and crannies that is very complex. There are, however, two major subdivisions. The smaller **omental bursa,** or **lesser sac,** is in the upper part of the abdomen posterior to the stomach. The rest of the peritoneal cavity is the **greater sac** and represents most of the cavity. These two parts of the peritoneum communicate at only one point, the **epiploic foramen (of Winslow),** which is located posterior to the free edge of the lesser omentum. The relationship of the peritoneum to each of the abdominal organs is covered with the discussion of the individual organs.

Organs of the Abdominal Cavity

Gastrointestinal tract. The components of the **gastrointestinal (GI) tract** occupy the majority of the abdominal cavity. This continuous system is composed of the terminal portion of the esophagus, the stomach, the small intestine, and the large intestine. Although the entire system is tubular, there is variation in shape and size, external and internal characteristics, and position and mobility. The parts of the GI tract are discussed from proximal to distal.

The abdominal portion of the **esophagus** (Fig. 7-4) is very short, joining the superomedial aspect of the stomach very high in the abdomen

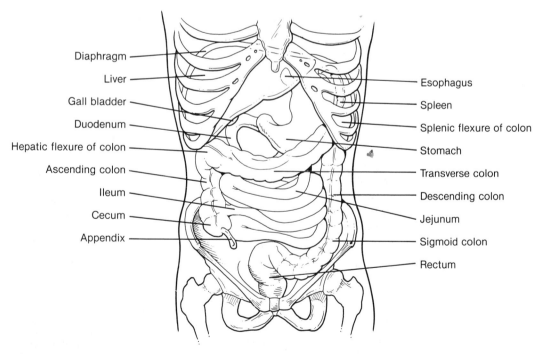

Figure 7-4
Anterior view of the organs of the abdominal cavity.

and just to the left of the midline. The part of the stomach surrounding the junction of the esophagus is the **cardiac portion** of the stomach.

The **stomach** (Fig. 7-4) is the most dilated portion of the GI tract and occupies a large percentage of the left upper quadrant. Although it is usually shaped like a reversed letter **C** with its convexity directed to the left and posteriorly, its shape is quite variable. And even though its proximal and distal aspects are fixed, it is variable in both size and position—sometimes extending into the lower abdomen. The dilated proximal portion the stomach consists of the **fundus,** above the entrance of the esophagus, and the main part, or **body,** below. Distally, the **pyloric portion** narrows to the **pyloric sphincter,** which marks its junction with the small intestine. The borders of the stomach are the concave **lesser curvature,** which is directed to the right, and the convex **greater curvature,** directed to the left. Its major relationships are the pancreas posteriorly and the liver and diaphragm anteriorly. Its peritoneal relationships include the **lesser omentum,** a peritoneal membrane connecting the lesser curvature to the liver, and the **greater omentum,** which hangs as an apron from its greater curvature.

The junction between the pylorus and the **duodenum** (Fig. 7-4), the most proximal portion of the small intestine, occurs just to the right of the body of vertebra L1. This junction is fixed because most of the duodenum is retroperitoneal. The duodenum is **C**-shaped but is divided into four parts. The **first,** or **superior, part** passes posteriorly and superiorly around the first lumbar body and then turns sharply inferiorly becoming the **second,** or **descending, part,** which descends to the level of the third lumbar vertebra. The second part receives both the common bile and pancreatic ducts. The duodenum then turns sharply to the left becoming the **third,** or **transverse, part,** passing in front of the inferior vena cava, aorta, and body of vertebra L3. The **fourth,** or **ascending, part** is very short and bends superiorly and anteriorly to the duodenojejunal junction. The head of the pancreas fits snugly within the curve formed by the duodenum.

The largest portion of the small intestine, averaging approximately 25 feet in length, is formed by the proximal **jejunum** and distal **ileum** (Fig. 7-4). This convoluted tube is attached to the posterior body wall by a **mesentery.** The body wall attachment of the mesentery is only 6 or 7 inches long and extends from the duodenojejunal junction inferiorly and to the right into the right iliac fossa. From this limited attachment the mesentery fans out to the entire jejunoileum, permitting considerable mobility of the jejunum and ileum. Even so, the jejunum is usually located in the umbilical region and the ileum, in the hypogastrium and pelvis. Although the jejunum and ileum have different characteristics, the junction between them is gradual. The jejunum is greater in diameter and has thicker walls because of the larger number of circular folds formed by its inner wall.

The **large intestine** (Fig. 7-4) differs from the small intestine in several ways: It is shorter (averaging approximately 4 to 5 feet in length), has a greater diameter, is characterized by sacculations (bulges), or **haustra,** along part of its length, has small fat-filled **epiploic appendages** hanging from its surface, and is more fixed in position. From proximal to distal the components of the large intestine are the **cecum, ascending colon, transverse colon, descending colon, sigmoid colon, rectum,** and **anal canal.** The small intestine joins the large intestine in the right iliac fossa at the **ileocecal junction.** The **cecum** is the short and dilated proximal portion of the large intestine, which is anchored in the right iliac fossa. The wormlike **vermiform appendix** attaches to its posteromedial aspect and most commonly is positioned posterior to the cecum. The appendix is very small in diameter but variable in length, sometimes reaching 7 or 8 inches. The **ascending colon** ascends along the right aspect of the posterior body wall where it is usually fixed because it has no mesentery; that is, it is partially peritonealized. It makes a bend to the left where it contacts the liver, forming the **hepatic,** or **right colic, flexure,** and becomes the transverse colon. The **transverse colon** traverses the upper part of the abdominal cavity toward the spleen where it makes a sharp inferior bend, the **splenic,** or **left colic, flexure,** and becomes the descending colon. The transverse colon is suspended from the posterior body wall by the **transverse mesocolon** and therefore is more mobile than either the ascending or descending portions of the colon. Since the length of the mesocolon varies, the transverse colon may extend inferiorly into the lower abdomen. The **descending colon,** usually partially peritonealized and therefore fixed in position, passes inferiorly along the posterior body wall on the left. It ends in the left iliac fossa, where the colon acquires a mesentery and becomes the sigmoid colon. The **sigmoid colon,** named for its configuration, varies in length but almost always folds on itself. It crosses the pelvic inlet and descends into the pelvis, where it joins the rectum. The **rectum** follows the curve of the sacrum through the pelvis and after passing through the pelvic floor, is continuous with the **anal canal.**

Liver and biliary system.   The **liver** (Fig. 7-4) is the largest organ in the abdomen, occupying the majority of the right upper quadrant and extending into the left. Its superior, or diaphragmatic, surface is rounded and corresponds to the shape of the diaphragm. Its inferior, or visceral, surface is generally flat and faces posteriorly and inferiorly. This surface presents an H-shaped group of fossae, the center bar of which is the **porta hepatis,** or hilum of the liver. The common hepatic duct, portal vein, and hepatic artery as well as autonomic nerve fibers and lymphatic vessels pass through the porta hepatis. The peritoneal coverings of the liver are complex because part is peritonealized and part is not.

The **gall bladder** (Fig. 7-4) occupies a fossa on the visceral surface of the liver. This organ is a dilated sac that narrows precipitously to the **cystic duct,** which joins the **common hepatic duct** from the liver. The junction of the cystic and common hepatic ducts forms the **common bile duct,** which descends posterior to the first part of the duodenum, joins the main pancreatic duct, and empties into the second part of the duodenum.

Spleen.   The **spleen** (Fig. 7-4) is about the size of a fist and is located in the left upper quadrant, completely above the subcostal margin where it is related to the posterolateral aspect of the diaphragm. Its outer convex surface corresponds to the contour of the diaphragm; its hilum is directed medially, and its visceral surface is indented by the stomach, left kidney, tail of the pancreas, and splenic flexure of the colon. This organ is completely peritonealized and attached to both the left kidney and the stomach by peritoneal ligaments.

Pancreas. The **pancreas** is a flattened and elongated organ that stretches across the posterior body wall from the right to the left upper quadrants. It is entirely retroperitoneal. Its rounded head occupies the curve formed by the duodenum, and its neck, body, and tail extend to the left and slightly superiorly. The tail is in contact with the spleen. The pancreas is related posteriorly to both kidneys as well as the inferior vena cava and aorta. Anteriorly, it is related to the stomach. The products of the pancreas are dispensed through the pancreatic ducts into the second part of the duodenum.

Kidneys, ureters, and suprarenal glands. The **kidneys** (Fig. 7-3) rest on the posterior body wall on either side of the vertebral column, are in contact with both the quadratus lumborum and psoas major muscles, and are encased in a generous amount of perirenal fat. Both kidneys extend superiorly above the subcostal margin, with the left slightly more superior than the right. The hilum of each kidney is directed anteromedially, and the convex lateral border, posterolaterally. These organs are retroperitoneal and related to a variety of organs anteriorly. The right is in contact with the liver, duodenum, and hepatic flexure of the colon. The left kidney is related to the stomach, spleen, pancreas, left colic flexure, and usually the small intestine.

The **ureters** conduct urine from the kidneys to the urinary bladder, which is in the pelvis. The urine formed within the kidney drains toward the hilum, where it empties into the dilated proximal end of the ureter, the **renal pelvis.** The pelvis projects medially and narrows to the very small diameter ureter. The ureter then descends along the anterior aspect of the psoas major muscle, crosses the pelvic inlet, and passes anteriorly and then medially to reach the bladder.

The **suprarenal (adrenal) glands** (Fig. 7-3) are small endocrine glands that sit on the superior poles of the kidneys. These organs are retroperitoneal and encased within the same adipose layers as the kidneys.

Blood and Nerve Supply, Lymphatic Drainage of the Abdominal Viscera

The distribution of the blood vessels, autonomic nerves, and lymphatic vessels to the abdominal viscera is similar. This pattern of distribution corresponds to the arteries that supply the viscera and are all branches of the abdominal aorta. The veins, lymphatic vessels, and nerves all accompany the arteries to the organs.

The **abdominal aorta** (Fig. 7-3) is the continuation of the thoracic aorta and enters the abdomen by passing between crura of the diaphragm at vertebral level T12. It descends along the anterior aspect of the vertebral column and ends at vertebral level L4 where it bifurcates into the **common iliac arteries.** Each common iliac artery branches into the **external iliac artery,** which enters the thigh as the **femoral artery,** and the

internal iliac artery, which branches to supply the pelvic viscera, gluteal region, and perineum.

The **branches of the abdominal aorta** can be separated into parietal and visceral branches. The parietal branches are the paired **phrenic arteries** to the diaphragm and the multiple pairs of **lumbar arteries** that arise segmentally and pass laterally into the body wall. The visceral branches are both paired and unpaired. The paired branches supply the paired organs: The **suprarenal arteries** supply the suprarenal glands, the **renal arteries** the kidneys, and the **testicular** or **ovarian arteries** the gonads. The unpaired branches supply the unpaired organs, which are either part of, or related developmentally to, the GI tract. The three unpaired arteries branch from the anterior aspect of the aorta and include the **celiac trunk, superior mesenteric artery,** and the **inferior mesenteric artery** (Fig. 7-3). The celiac trunk arises at vertebral level T12 and has three main branches: The **common hepatic artery** passes to the right and supplies the liver, gall bladder, stomach, duodenum, and pancreas; the **left gastric artery** passes along the lesser curvature of the stomach; and the **splenic artery** supplies both the pancreas and stomach as it passes to the spleen. The **superior mesenteric artery** arises just inferior to the celiac trunk and supplies the pancreas and the GI tract as far distally as the splenic flexure of the colon; that is, it supplies the jejunum, ileum, ascending colon, and transverse colon. The **inferior mesenteric artery** branches from the aorta at vertebral level L3 and supplies the descending and sigmoid portions of the colon as well as the upper portion of the rectum.

Although all venous blood from the abdominal cavity eventually empties into the inferior vena cava, the venous drainage initially involves two separate systems: the **systemic** and **portal systems.** The systemic blood drains into the **inferior vena cava,** and the portal blood, into the **portal vein.** In both systems the venous tributaries are similar to the branches of the aorta. The inferior vena cava (Fig. 7-3), the major systemic vein below the diaphragm, returns venous blood to the right atrium of the heart. This large vein is positioned to the right of the aorta and is formed by the union of the common iliac veins. (Each common iliac vein is formed by the union of the internal and external iliac veins.) The inferior vena cava receives blood from the gonads (testicular or ovarian veins), kidneys and suprarenal glands (renal veins), and body wall (lumbar and phrenic veins). Just before passing through the diaphragm into the thorax, the inferior vena cava also receives the hepatic veins. The portal vein conveys blood from the GI tract, spleen, pancreas, and gall bladder to the liver. As a result, its primary tributaries are the superior and inferior mesenteric, left gastric, and splenic veins. The portal vein is formed posterior to the pancreas and then passes into the liver through the porta hepatis. The portal blood, rich in nutrients absorbed in the intestine, passes through the hepatic sinusoids, where it is exposed to the cells of the liver. It then is collected by the tributaries of the hepatic veins, which convey it to the inferior vena cava.

The **nerve supply** to the abdominal organs is provided by the **aortic (preaortic) autonomic plexus,** which is located on the anterior aspect of the full length of the abdominal aorta. The subdivisions of this plexus, which are segments of a single continuous plexus, are named by the branches of the aorta—for example, celiac, superior mesenteric, renal. In addition to general visceral afferent fibers, this plexus contains parasympathetic fibers from the vagus nerve and sympathetic fibers from branches of the sympathetic trunk. Certain parts of plexus, such as the celiac and superior mesenteric, contain ganglia that are the ganglia of the sympathetic system. The distribution of the fibers from the plexus to the organs is via periarterial plexuses along the branches of the aorta.

The **lymphatic fluid** from the abdominal viscera empties into the **thoracic duct,** the lymphatic vessel that drains the entire body below the diaphragm. The beginning of this duct is the dilated **cisterna chyli,** which usually is positioned between the aorta and right crus of the diaphragm. Small lymphatic vessels from the viscera follow the branches of the aorta toward the cisterna chyli. The lymphatic fluid then enters the thoracic duct, ascends through both the abdomen and thorax, and in the neck empties into the junction of the left internal jugular and subclavian veins.

The pelvis and perineum are the most inferior regions of the trunk. Delimited primarily by the bones of the pelvis, these two regions are separated by only the pelvic diaphragm. Both regions contain the terminal portions of the gastrointestinal tract as well as most of the organs of the urogenital system.

Pelvis

The **pelvic bones** (Figs. 4-5 through 4-8) are described on page 169. The **pelvic canal,** the bony portion of the birth canal, is inferior to the pelvic inlet. Its dimensions dictate the movements of the fetus during the birthing process. The orientation of this canal corresponds to the ventral surface of the sacrum (Fig. 8-1). From the pelvic inlet the canal initially is directed posteriorly and inferiorly and then curves anteriorly and inferiorly. The boundaries of this canal are defined by three planes: (1) The **plane of the pelvic inlet** is formed by the sacral promontory, iliopectineal line, and the body of the pubis and its symphysis. In the female pelvis the length of the lateral diameter of this plane exceeds that of its anteroposterior diameter. (2) The **plane of the pelvic outlet** is not a single plane because its anterior portion faces anteriorly and inferiorly and its posterior portion, posteriorly and inferiorly. The borders of this plane are the inferior aspect of the symphysis pubis, the ischiopubic rami, ischial tuberosities, sacrotuberous ligament, and inferior aspect of the sacrum. (3) The **plane of the midpelvis** is of particular clinical importance because it is the pelvic plane of least dimension. This plane passes through the midpelvis, extending from the inferior aspect of the symphysis pubis to the sacrum, at the level of the ischial spines. The anteroposterior diameter, from the symphysis to the sacrum, is longer than the transverse diameter,

Pelvis and Perineum

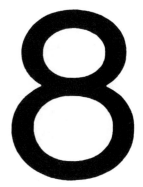

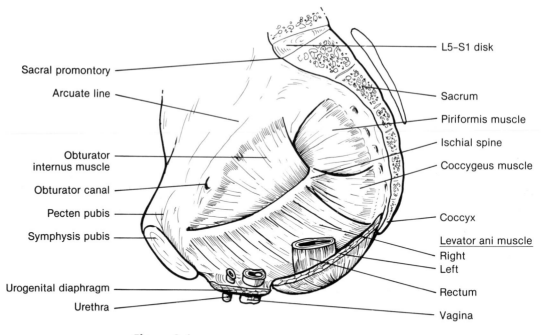

Sacral promontory

Arcuate line

Obturator
internus muscle

Obturator canal

Pecten pubis

Symphysis pubis

Urogenital diaphragm

Urethra

L5–S1 disk

Sacrum

Piriformis muscle

Ischial spine

Coccygeus muscle

Coccyx

Levator ani muscle
Right
Left

Rectum

Vagina

Figure 8-1
Sagittal section through the sacrum and pubis showing the muscles of the
lateral pelvic wall and the pelvic floor.

which is the distance between the ischial spines and the shortest dimension of the pelvis.

The **pelvic cavity** (Figs. 7-3, 8-1) is bounded superiorly by the pelvic inlet; anteriorly, laterally, and posteriorly by the bones of the pelvis and the obturator internus and piriformis muscles; and inferiorly by the pelvic diaphragm. The **pelvic diaphragm** (Figs. 7-3, 8-1) is the muscular floor of the pelvis and formed by the **levator ani** and **coccygeus muscles.** From attachments along the lateral walls of the pelvis, the muscles from the two sides slope medially and inferiorly and then unite in the midline. This arrangement results in a trough-shaped floor. In addition to sloping medially, the pelvic floor slopes inferiorly from posterior to anterior, which provides a soft tissue continuation of the slope of the sacrum and the birth canal. Contraction of the muscles that form the pelvic diaphragm elevate the pelvic floor and thus the pelvic organs. Since the skeletal muscle sphincter (external anal sphincter) of the anal canal is derived from the muscle of the pelvic floor, contraction of the pelvic diaphragm also tightens this sphincter.

The **sacral plexus** and the **internal iliac artery** and **vein** along with their branches are related to the walls of the pelvis. The sacral plexus is located on the posterolateral wall, on the ventral aspect of the piriformis muscle (Fig. 4-9). The components of this plexus converge toward the large terminal sciatic nerve, which exits from the pelvis by passing inferior to the piriformis muscle and through the greater sciatic foramen. The internal iliac artery and vein are located on the lateral pelvic wall. These vessels have branches to the gluteal region (superior and inferior gluteal), the perineum (internal pudendal), medial thigh (obturator), and pelvic viscera.

The **rectum** and **urinary bladder** are found in both the male and female pelves (Figs. 8-2 and 8-3). The rectum descends through the posterior aspect of the pelvis, on the pelvic surface of the sacrum, and passes through the posterior aspect of the pelvic diaphragm. The bladder is positioned anteriorly, immediately posterior to the symphysis pubis. When empty, the bladder is confined to the pelvic cavity. When full, it enlarges and usually extends above the pelvic inlet into the abdominal cavity. The ureters pass through the posterolateral walls of the bladder; the urethra begins at the bladder's most inferior aspect. Also found in varying amounts in the pelvis are portions of the small intestine and sigmoid colon.

The organs found only in the male pelvis are the **prostate, seminal vesicles,** and pelvic portion of the **ductus deferens** (Fig. 8-2). The prostate is a small, firm organ, about the size of a chestnut, that is positioned between the bladder and the anterior aspect of the pelvic diaphragm. It is immediately anterior to the most inferior portion of the rectum, so it is palpable upon rectal examination. The **prostatic portion of the urethra** descends through the center of the prostate. Both the seminal vesicles and dilated terminal portions (ampullae) of the ductus deferens are anchored to the posterior aspect of the bladder. The ducts of these two

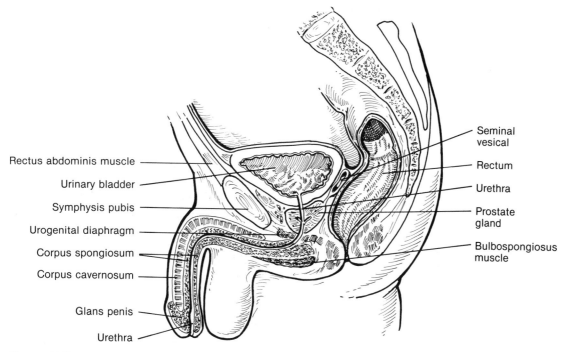

Rectus abdominis muscle
Urinary bladder
Symphysis pubis
Urogenital diaphragm
Corpus spongiosum
Corpus cavernosum
Glans penis
Urethra

Seminal vesical
Rectum
Urethra
Prostate gland
Bulbospongiosus muscle

Figure 8-2
Sagittal section through the male pelvis and perineum.

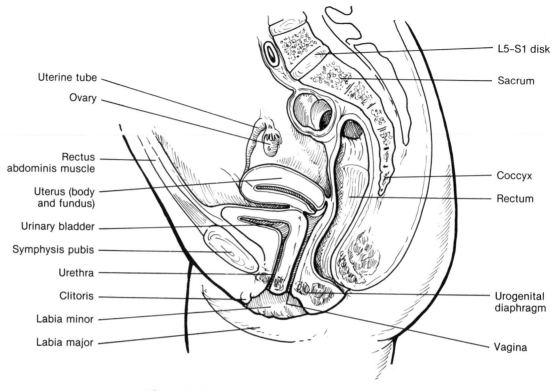

Figure 8-3
Sagittal section through the female pelvis and perineum.

structures join to form the **ejaculatory duct.** The ejaculatory duct then passes into the prostate, where it joins the urethra.

The organs specific to the female pelvis are the **vagina, uterus, uterine (fallopian) tubes,** and **ovaries** (Fig. 8-3). Viewed together, these organs are shaped like the letter **T** and, for the most part, are interposed between the bladder and rectum. The thin-walled vagina passes through the pelvic diaphragm anterior to the rectum and posterior to the urethra, then extends superiorly for approximately 7 to 10 cm. At that point it joins the thick-walled and muscular uterus. From its junction with the vagina, the uterus extends anteriorly on the superior surface of the bladder. The uterus is composed of a body, the fundus superiorly, and the cervix inferiorly. The cervix actually extends into the cavity of the vagina so a circular trough, which is part of the vaginal cavity and called the **fornices of the vagina,** surrounds the most inferior portion of the cervix. From the superolateral aspects of the uterus, the uterine tubes extend laterally toward the lateral pelvic walls, where they are related to the ovaries.

The **peritoneum** from the abdomen swoops down into the pelvis, where it is attached to the pelvic walls and related variably to the pelvic organs. In men (Fig. 8-2) the peritoneum passes from the anterior wall to the superior and posterior aspect of the bladder. It then passes from the bladder to the rectum, which it partially surrounds. In women (Fig. 8-3) the peritoneum also is related to the bladder and rectum. However, between the bladder and rectum, the peritoneum passes over the uterus, uterine tubes, and ovaries, forming a curtain (the broad ligament) that extends from side to side across the pelvic cavity. Posteriorly, where the peritoneum passes from the uterus to the rectum, it crosses the most superior part of the vagina (posterior fornix). This point is important clinically because infection from the vaginal cavity can be introduced into the peritoneal cavity through the thin wall of the posterior fornix, as in a "back-room" abortion.

The nerve supply to the pelvic viscera is provided by the inferior continuation of the aortic plexus. The plexus extends inferiorly into the pelvic cavity, where it is called the **inferior hypogastric** or **pelvic plexus.** It passes laterally on both sides of the viscera and provides branches to the viscera. The plexus receives input from the sacral parasympathetics and the sacral portion of the sympathetic trunk.

Perineum

The **perineum** is the region bounded by the pelvic outlet and located inferior to the pelvic diaphragm; the pelvic diaphragm, therefore, forms both the floor of the pelvis and the roof of the perineum (Fig. 8-1). The anterior, lateral, and posterior borders of the perineum are diamond shaped. The anterior triangle of the diamond is called the **urogenital triangle** because it contains components of the urogenital system. The posterior **anal triangle** contains the anal canal.

The urogenital triangle, bounded by the inferior aspect of the symphysis pubis and the ischiopubic rami, has a musculofascial shelf that stretches between the rami. This shelf, the **urogenital diaphragm,** transmits the urethra (membranous part) in men (Fig. 8-2) and both the urethra and vagina in women (Fig. 8-3). The portion of the urogenital triangle inferior to the urogenital diaphragm contains the testis in the man and the erectile bodies and related muscles in both sexes: the crura, bulb, and body of the penis in the man (Fig. 8-2), and the crura and body of the clitoris in the woman (Fig. 8-3).

The anal triangle is composed of the wedge-shaped **ischiorectal fossae** that are filled with fatty tissue. These fossae are bounded by the ischia laterally, the pelvic diaphragm medially and superomedially, and the skin inferiorly. These fossae extend posteriorly, deep to the gluteus maximus muscles and anteriorly, between the urogenital and pelvic diaphragms.

The blood supply to the perineum is provided by the **internal pudendal artery,** a branch of the internal iliac artery. The primary nerve supply is the **pudendal nerve** (S2–S4) from the sacral plexus. Both the internal pudendal artery and pudendal nerve exit from the pelvis through the greater sciatic foramen, curve around the ischial spine, and then enter the perineum by passing through the lesser sciatic foramen. A pudendal block, as sometimes used in childbirth, is accomplished by infiltrating the area around the ischial spine with anesthetic.

Bibliography

This bibliography is separated into topics so the interested reader can quickly identify sources of additional information. The information provided in each reference generally is more comprehensive than that included in this book, and the authors are authorities in their respective fields.

Musculoskeletal Anatomy

Brownstein B, Mangine RE, Noyes FR, Kryger S: Anatomy and biomechanics. In Mangine RE (ed): Clinics in Physical Therapy, vol 2, Physical Therapy of the Knee. New York, Churchill Livingstone, 1988

Hollinshead WH: Anatomy for Surgeons, ed 3, vol 1. Philadelphia, Harper & Row, 1982

Hollinshead WH: Anatomy for Surgeons, ed 2, vol 2. New York, Harper & Row, 1971

Hollinshead WH: Anatomy for Surgeons, ed 3, vol 3. Philadelphia, Harper & Row, 1982

Insall JN (ed): Surgery of the Knee. New York, Churchill Livingstone, 1984

Moore KL: Clinically Oriented Anatomy, ed 2. Baltimore, Williams & Wilkins, 1985

O'Rahilly R: Basic Human Anatomy—A Regional Study of Human Structure. Philadelphia, WB Saunders, 1983

Rockwood CA, Matsen FA (eds): The Shoulder. Philadelphia, WB Saunders, 1990

Sarrafian SK: Anatomy of the Foot and Ankle. Philadelphia, JB Lippincott, 1983

Snell, RS: Clinical Anatomy for Medical Students, ed 3. Boston, Little Brown, 1986

Spinner M (ed): Kaplan's Functional and Surgical Anatomy of the Hand, ed 3. Philadelphia, JB Lippincott, 1984

Tubiana R (ed): The Hand, vol 1. Philadelphia, WB Saunders, 1981

Nerve Injuries

Haymaker W, Woodhall B: Peripheral Nerve Injuries, ed 2. Philadelphia, WB Saunders, 1956

Omer GE, Spinner M: Management of Peripheral Nerve Injuries. Philadelphia, WB Saunders, 1980

Sunderland S: Nerves and Nerve Injuries, ed 2. Edinburgh, Churchill Livingstone, 1978

Muscle Functions

Basmajian JV, DeLuca CJ: Muscles Alive, ed 5. Baltimore, Williams & Wilkins, 1985

Kendall FP, McCreary EK: Muscles—Testing and Function, ed 3. Baltimore, Williams & Wilkins, 1983

Gross Anatomy Atlases

Anderson JE: Grant's Atlas of Anatomy, ed 8. Baltimore, Williams & Wilkins, 1983

Clemente CD: Anatomy—A Regional Atlas of the Human Body, ed 3. Baltimore, Urban & Schwarzenberg, 1987

Gosling JA, Harris PF, Humpherson JR, Whitmore I, Willan PTL: Atlas of Human Anatomy. Philadelphia, JB Lippincott, 1985

McMinn RMH, Hutchings RT: Color Atlas of Human Anatomy. Chicago, Year Book, 1977

Netter FH: The Ciba Collection of Medical Illustrations, vol 8, part 1. Summit, NJ, Ciba-Geigy Corporation, 1987

Netter FH: Atlas of Human Anatomy. Summit, NJ, Ciba-Geigy Corporation, 1989

Page numbers followed by an "f" indicate figures.

ISBN 0-397-54825-7

90000

CAYUGA COMMUNITY COLLEGE

3 2551 00117678 7

DATE DUE

DEC 1 8 2007

QM
100
.P73
1990

Pratt, Neal E.

Clinical musculoskeleta
anatomy

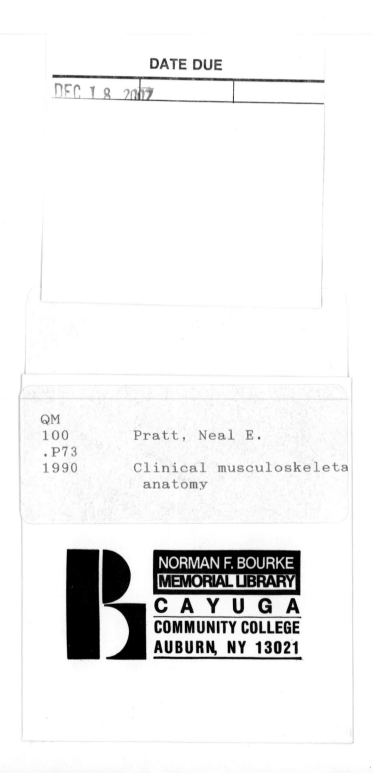

NORMAN F. BOURKE
MEMORIAL LIBRARY
CAYUGA
COMMUNITY COLLEGE
AUBURN, NY 13021